Innovative Strategies for Promoting Health and Mental Health Across the Life Span

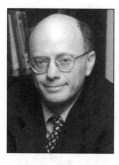

Leonard A. Jason is a professor of psychology and director of the Center for Community Research at DePaul University. He received his doctorate in clinical and community psychology from the University of Rochester. Dr. Jason is a past president of the Division of Community Psychology of the American Psychological Association and a former editor of *The Community Psychologist*. He has been the recipient of the Distinguished Contributions to Theory and Research Award from the Division of Community Psychology of APA and of the CSN ACTION Champion Award from the Chronic Fatigue Immune Dysfunction Syndrome Association of America. His extensive research and writing have focused on chronic fatigue syndrome; preventive school-based interventions; the prevention of alcohol, tobacco, and other drug use; media interventions; and program evaluation.

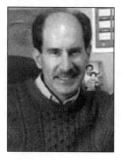

David S. Glenwick is a professor of psychology at Fordham University. He received his doctorate in clinical and community psychology from the University of Rochester. Dr. Glenwick is a past president of the American Association for Correctional Psychology and a former editor of *Criminal Justice and Behavior* and has been director of the graduate program in clinical psychology at Fordham University. He has published extensively in the areas of clinical child psychology, community-based interventions, and developmental disabilities.

Innovative Strategies for Promoting Health and Mental Health Across the Life Span

Leonard A. Jason, PhD
David S. Glenwick, PhD
Editors

 Springer Publishing Company

Springer Publishing Company, Inc.
536 Broadway
New York, NY 10012-3955

Acquisitions Editor: Sheri W. Sussman
Production Editor: Janice Stangel
Cover design by Susan Hauley

01 02 03 04 05 / 5 4 3 2 1

Library of Congress Cataloging-in-Publication Data

Innovative strategies for promoting health and mental health across
    the life span / Leonard A. Jason, David S. Glenwick, editors.
        p. cm.
    Includes bibliographical references.
    ISBN 0-8261-4491-8
    1. Medicine, Preventive.   2. Health promotion.   3. Mental
health promotion.   4. Health behavior.   I. Jason, Leonard.
II. Glenwick, David.

    RA427.8 .I56 2002
    613—dc21   2002022804

Printed in the United States of America by Sheridan Press.

In memory of Emory Cowen (1926–2000), who, as teacher,
researcher, and disseminator, set a standard of excellence and
commitment in the field of prevention that inspired all who knew him

Contents

Contributors   ix

Foreword by James G. Kelly   xv

Acknowledgments   xviii

Part I   Prevention Science

1. Introduction: An Overview of Preventive and
   Ecological Perspectives   3
   Leonard A. Jason and David S. Glenwick
2. Making Effective Use of Prevention Science   17
   Anthony Biglan and Lisa James
3. Teaching About Prevention to Mental Health Professionals   37
   Jacob Kraemer Tebes, Joy S. Kaufman,
   and Matthew J. Chinman

Part II   Problems of Parenting and Youth

4. Promoting Effective Parenting Practices   63
   Lisa Sheeber, Anthony Biglan, Carol W. Metzler,
   and Ted K. Taylor
5. Preventing Physical and Sexual Abuse   85
   John R. Lutzker and Cynthia L. Boyle
6. Preventing School Failure and Promoting Positive Outcomes   106
   Lisa Machoian, Jean E. Rhodes, Nancy Rappaport,
   and Ranjini Reddy
7. Preventing Delinquency and Antisocial Behavior   126
   Jennifer J. Treuting, Tamara M. Haegerich,
   and Patrick H. Tolan

8. Preventing Depression in Youth   153
   W. LaVome Robinson and Mary H. Case
9. Preventing Alcohol, Tobacco, and Other Substance Abuse   176
   Caryn C. Blitz, Michael W. Arthur, and J. David Hawkins

Part III   Problems in Adulthood

10. Preventing HIV and AIDS   205
    Eric G. Benotsch and Seth C. Kalichman
11. Preventing Chronic Health Problems   227
    Joel A. Minden and Leonard A. Jason
12. Preventing Marital Disorder   245
    Peter Fraenkel and Howard J. Markman
13. Promoting Mental Health in Later Life   272
    Margaret Gatz, Michael Crowe, Amy Fiske,
    Wendy Fung, Christopher Kelly, Boaz Levy,
    Michele Maines, Gia Robinson, Derek D. Satre,
    Juan Pedro Serrano Selva, Kristen Suthers,
    Kecia Watari, and Julie Loebach Wetherell

Part IV   Community and Societal Issues

14. Preventing Racist, Sexist, and Heterosexist Behavior   301
    Doreen D. Salina and Linda M. Lesondak
15. Promoting Healthy Communities Through Community
    Development   324
    Maury Nation, Abraham Wandersman,
    and Douglas D. Perkins

Afterword by Michael C. Roberts   345

Index   349

Contributors

Michael W. Arthur is a research associate professor and a member of the Social Development Research Group at the University of Washington. He received his Ph.D. in community psychology from the University of Virginia. His research focuses on community-level approaches to the prevention of adolescent drug use, violence, and delinquency and on prevention services research methods.

Eric G. Benotsch is an assistant professor of psychiatry and behavioral medicine at the Center for AIDS Intervention Research, affiliated with the Medical College of Wisconsin. He received his Ph.D. in clinical psychology from the University of Iowa. His research interests include HIV primary prevention, behavioral medicine, and adult psychopathology.

Anthony Biglan is a senior research scientist at the Oregon Research Institute. He received his Ph.D. in social psychology from the University of Illinois. His primary research interests include community interventions on childrearing.

Caryn C. Blitz is a research scientist at the University of Washington's Social Development Research Group. She received her Ph.D. in clinical and community psychology from DePaul University. Her main research interests are prevention services research methods and prevention policy at the local, state, and federal levels.

Cynthia L. Boyle is a doctoral student in human development and family life at the University of Kansas. Her research interests are in the area of child maltreatment.

Mary H. Case is a project director in the Department of Psychology at DePaul University. She received her Ph.D. in clinical psychology from DePaul University. Her principal research interests include the primary prevention of depression, risk and resiliency factors in inner-city youth, and the cultural adaptation of intervention/prevention programs.

Matthew J. Chinman is an associate behavioral scientist at the RAND Corporation and a health science specialist at the West Los Angeles Veterans Administration Medical Center. He received his Ph.D. in community psychology from the University of South Carolina. He has published in the area of program evaluation methodology in prevention, adolescent empowerment, and case management and mutual support for those with serious mental illnesses.

Peter Fraenkel is an associate professor of psychology at the City College of the City University of New York; director of the Center for Time, Work and the Family at the Ackerman Institute for the Family; and director of the Prevention and Relationship Enhancement Program (PREP) at the New York University Child Study Center. He received his Ph.D. in clinical psychology from Duke University. His research centers on community-based prevention and intervention programs for couples and for families moving from welfare to work.

Margaret Gatz is a professor of psychology at the University of Southern California. She received her Ph.D. in clinical psychology from Duke University. Her research interests include community-based interventions in geropsychology. All of the co-authors of her chapter were students in a doctoral seminar on mental health and aging. Crowe, Fiske, Fung, Levy, Robinson, Satre, Watari, and Wetherell are from the USC Department of Psychology; Kelly, Maines, and Suthers are from the USC School of Gerontology; and Serrano was a visiting student from the University of Castilla-La Mancha in Spain.

Tamara M. Haegerich is a doctoral student in social psychology at the University of Illinois at Chicago. Her primary research interests are in the perceptions and experiences of youth in the legal system.

J. David Hawkins is the director of the Social Development Research Group and a professor of social work at the University of Washington. He received his Ph.D. in sociology from Northwestern University. His research has focused on the prediction and prevention of child and adolescent health and behavior problems.

Lisa James is a project manager at the Oregon Research Institute. Her research interests center on school- and community-based tobacco prevention strategies.

Seth C. Kalichman is a professor of psychology at the University of Connecticut. He received his Ph.D. in clinical-community psychology from the University of South Carolina. He has published extensively on the psychological aspects of the HIV-AIDS epidemic and is the author of several books including, *Preventing AIDS: A Sourcebook for Behavioral Interventions*. His research focuses on identifying factors that determine HIV risk behavior, testing theoretically derived intervention models, and examining the psychological adjustment of people with HIV infection.

Joy S. Kaufman is an assistant professor of psychology at the Yale University School of Medicine and the director of service system evaluation at the Consultation Center of Yale University. She received her Ph.D. in clinical and community psychology from DePaul University. Her research emphasis is the evaluation of community-based systems of care.

Linda M. Lesondak is the director of evaluation for the Chicago Department of Public Health in its STD/HIV/AIDS Public Policy and Programs Division. She is completing her Ph.D. in community psychology at Georgia State University. Her research centers on the promotion of women's health behavior.

John R. Lutzker is chief of the Prevention Development and Evaluation Branch of the Division of Violence Prevention, National Center for Inquiry Prevention and Control, Center for Disease Control and Prevention. He received his Ph.D. in developmental psychology from the University of Kansas. He co-authored this chapter while he was at the University of Judaism, where he was a distinguished professor of psychology. His research interests are in the prevention of violence.

Lisa Machoian is a lecturer in human development and psychology at Harvard University. She received her Ed.D. in human development and psychology from Harvard University. Her research focuses on trauma, coping, and resilience in children and adolescents.

Howard J. Markman is a professor of psychology and director of the Center for Marital and Family Studies at the University of Denver. He is also the co-developer of the Prevention and Relationship Enhancement Program (PREP). Dr. Markman received his Ph.D. in clinical psychology from Indiana University. His research interests include the prediction and prevention of relationship discord and divorce, the effects of divorce and discord on children, and the dissemination of empirically based interventions.

Carol W. Metzler is a research scientist at the Oregon Research Institute. She received her Ph.D. in clinical psychology from the University of Oregon. Her primary research focus is the evaluation of the efficacy of interventions for improving child outcomes, including the prevention of substance use, aggression, and other youth problem behaviors.

Joel A. Minden is a doctoral student in clinical-community psychology at DePaul University. His research interests include health promotion, developmental psychopathology, and quantitative research methods.

Maury Nation is an assistant professor of Psychology and the director of the counseling psychology program at the University of North Florida. He received his Ph.D. in clinical/community psychology from the University of South Carolina. His main research interests are community assessment and development and the impact of racial and social characteristics on the perception of neighborhood quality and desirability.

Douglas D. Perkins is an associate professor of human and organizational development and the director of the graduate program in community research and action at Vanderbilt University. He received his Ph.D. in community psychology from New York University. His research interests include community development and empowerment and policy uses of research.

Nancy Rappaport is a clinical instructor of psychiatry at Harvard University School of Medicine. She received her M.D. from Tufts University School of Medicine. Her primary research interests are the interface of education and psychiatry and the creation of infrastructures to support at-risk children and adolescents.

Ranjini Reddy is a research associate in psychology at the University of Massachusetts, Boston. She received her Ph.D. in developmental psychology from St. Louis University. Her research interests lie in the influences of school climate on adolescent development and the role of nonparental adults in adolescents' lives.

Jean E. Rhodes is an associate professor of psychology at the University of Massachusetts, Boston. She received her Ph.D. in clinical psychology from DePaul University. Her research interests include mentoring, middle-school students' adjustment, social support, and intergenerational influences on youth development.

W. LaVome Robinson is a professor of psychology and the director of the graduate program in clinical psychology at DePaul University. She received her Ph.D. in clinical psychology from the University of Georgia. Her chief research interests are the development and evaluation of school-based prevention and treatment programs and mental health promotion for African American adolescents.

Doreen D. Salina is an assistant professor of psychiatry and behavioral sciences at Northwestern University School of Medicine. She received her Ph.D. in clinical psychology from DePaul University. Her research centers on community-based HIV/AIDS prevention, with a particular focus on programs for women.

Lisa Sheeber is a research scientist at the Oregon Research Institute. She received her Ph.D. in clinical psychology from the University of Florida. Her research focuses on family processes related to child development and adjustment.

Ted K. Taylor is a research scientist at the Oregon Research Institute. He received his Ph.D. in clinical psychology from York University. His principal research interests are the design, implementation, and evaluation of community-based prevention projects for children, families, and schools.

Jacob Kraemer Tebes is an associate professor of psychology at the Yale University School of Medicine and the deputy director of the Consultation Center of Yale University. He received his Ph.D. in clinical/community psychology from the State University of New York at Buffalo. His research interests are in the areas of prevention research methodology, resilience promotion among at-risk groups, and the prevention of adolescent substance abuse.

Patrick H. Tolan is the director of the Institute for Juvenile Research and a professor of psychology at the University of Illinois at Chicago School of Medicine. He received his Ph.D. in school/community psychology from the University of Tennessee. His major research interests include prevention research and policy related to urban children and families, with a particular focus on violence prevention.

Jennifer J. Treuting is a visiting research assistant professor of psychology at the University of Illinois at Chicago School of Medicine. She received her Ph.D. in clinical psychology from the University of California at Berkeley. Her research interests lie in the areas of developmental psychopathology and prevention among urban children and families.

Abraham Wandersman is a professor of psychology at the University of South Carolina. He received his Ph.D. in social psychology from Cornell University. His research has focused on citizen participation in community organizations, community coalitions and interagency collaboration, and program implementation and evaluation.

Doreen D. Salina, Ph.D.
Northwestern University Medical School
Assistant Professor of Psychiatry and Behavioral Sciences

333 North Michigan Avenue, Suite 1801
Chicago, Illinois 60601
(312) 346-1881
d-salina@northwestern.edu

Foreword

After World War II a new way of addressing personal and social problems began to develop among psychologists. Instead of viewing a solution as primarily to treat the already "sick" or "disabled" individual, the focus shifted to preventing a problem at the community level. A public health approach replaced a clinical emphasis.

This book is a portfolio of informative and challenging examples of how psychologists—most often community psychologists—carry out prevention research. The book represents broad coverage of approaches to individual and community problems that limit us as persons and as members of our communities.

The material presented in these 15 chapters brings the reader up to date on the knowledge now available about carrying out these preventive programs. The history of the evolution of doing preventive efforts in real-life circumstances is quite a story—and that story is discussed here with a self-critical sensitivity.

The authors have a shared point of view: Knowledge of how to prevent a difficult and challenging problem—such as physical or sexual abuse, school failure, depression among adolescents, chronic health problems, HIV-AIDS, mental health in later life, or racist or sexist behavior—can be most directly and persuasively addressed by carrying out randomized trials.

This method of doing research makes it possible to compare individuals or groups who have and who have not been the subject of a particular prevention program. There is an explicit value expressed in this volume that community psychologists who employ randomized designs are a major source of knowledge and understanding about preventing a specific condition. These community psychologists are credible because, according to the authors' view, the best knowledge comes from the application of rigorous research procedures adapted from the laboratory and conducted in the community. This usually translates to involving people or organizations, such as schools, or even school districts, in a fixed number of sessions or programs where the content is preset and the method already pretested. The participants learn specific skills to be evaluated in post-tests after the sessions have been completed. This does not always work out cleanly and neatly as in some idealized view of science. It is often an awkward, tentative, and inconclusive process. So, when there is evidence of salutary and solid results, it is an achievement. The book notes these achievements in a writing style which extracts from the scientific results the palpable and useful findings.

The writing is not abstract or technical. Each of the chapters has been prepared for both scholars and citizens who wish to try out prevention programs, or develop and evaluate a program for themselves. The editors and chapter authors have succeeded in making the findings and the significance of these findings clear and cogent. It is reassuring that there are a variety of tested and tried efforts that can be used as points of reference in the reader's own community.

The review of the current research literature on each chapter topic is followed by a case example which brings out in more detail the key elements of prevention programs for that particular topic. This is very helpful for those who desire to pursue a topic or problem further.

The frankness with which unresolved problems are addressed in each chapter gives a forthright view of the challenges that remain. This is the most important quality in the book. There are hints and references to the fact that prevention efforts, to be effective, emerge not from one isolated prevention program, but from a multifaceted array of efforts such as local ordinances, TV announcements, or movie clips, which take into account the ways of thinking about and doing everyday tasks in communities.

In some cases, such as preventing racist or sexist behaviors, using legal mechanisms to combat illegal discrimination is recommended. In the case of reducing tobacco use by teenagers, a state ballot was established to add 30 cents to the cost of a pack of cigarettes, with 10% of revenues dedicated for prevention activities. While knowledge gained from randomized trials is a significant start, prevention efficacy is also realized through public policies, which means community development, community organizing, and advocacy. This is true because, as many of the authors point out, a successful prevention program in one community may not be as effective in another locale because of differences in values, traditions, and customs surrounding community problem-solving.

This book lays the groundwork for continuing expeditions to create, design, and evaluate prevention programs that can reduce difficulties and promote competencies that, in turn, enable us to live healthier and more satisfying lives, and save resources that focus primarily on later casualties. This volume lays the foundation for the next adventure: to understand more fully how to implement and sustain community-based prevention efforts—prevention efforts which work for the poor and for people from different ethnic backgrounds and life circumstances, as well as for those who have varying political views and who are from diverse cultural contexts. It motivates us to renew our efforts to create dialogues between citizens and community psychologists about how to share in the creative acts of inventing preventive solutions at the local level that are systemic for their community.

James G. Kelly
Emeritus Professor of Psychology
University of Illinois at Chicago

Acknowledgments

We are deeply appreciative of our chapter authors, who worked on tight time schedules to produce stimulating, integrative, and readable contributions, and who graciously worked to comply with our length and style requests. We also are indebted to James Kelly and Michael Roberts for their thoughtful Foreword and Afterword commentaries. In addition, we thank our many colleagues who have helped us think through many of the issues in the book, including Brad Olson, Meg Davis, Josefina Alaverez, Steven Pokorny, Susan Torres-Harding, Peter Ji, and Renee Taylor.

Rosa Pugliese of Fordham University deserves many thanks for her skill, patience, and "grace under pressure" (to borrow Hemingway's phrase) in handling many of the "nitty gritty" tasks involved in producing this volume. Finally, we greatly appreciate the unflagging support and encouragement of Springer's editorial staff, particularly Sheri Sussman and William Tucker.

PART I

Prevention Science

CHAPTER 1

Introduction:
An Overview of Preventive and
Ecological Perspectives

Leonard A. Jason and
David S. Glenwick

Amerian society is faced with numerous, seemingly insurmountable problems, including homelessness, AIDS, gang activity, and domestic violence (Levine
& Perkins, 1997). More and more people face battles related to substance abuse,
physical and mental illness, and other challenging conditions (Glenwick & Jason,
1993). Seemingly safe and healthy communities are feeling the full force of these
problems (Dugger, 1995), with even sheltered or isolated citizens experiencing
their effects (Duffy & Wong, 2000). Although communities try to mobilize against
these problems, individuals often appear less connected, lacking direction and
certainty about how to proceed (Jason, 1997).

In addition to these community-wide problems, we also face many individual and family problems. For example, Etzioni (1993) claimed that, for
many people, marriage has become a disposable relationship, with divorce and
the preceding years of conflict often leading to heightened psychological and
physiological distress. According to a report by the National Advisory Mental
Health Council (NAMHC, 1993), mental disorders affect 22% of the population within a given one-year period; 2.8% have severe mental illness, but only
20% of all mental disorders and 62% of severe mental disorders are treated
within a given year. Nearly four million American students drop out of high
school each year (Rossi & Montgomery, 1994). In addition, our nation's
children spend more time watching television and surfing the Internet than

3

engaging in any other activity except sleep, and the images they see are filled with high levels of violence and sexuality (Jason & Hanaway, 1997). Thus, despite our country's comparative economic prosperity during the past decade, its report card with respect to its citizens' and communities' social, psychological, and physical well-being is considerably less sanguine.

Over the past 20 years, a number of edited volumes and special issues of scholarly journals (e.g., Felner, Jason, Moritsugu, & Farber, 1983; Glenwick & Jason, 1980, 1984, 1993) have advocated, and presented research grounded in, a preventively oriented approach to these types of problems. Mental health professionals have increasingly explored the possibilities of intervening before problems become evident in order to prevent their appearance in the first place and, ideally, to enhance the growth of competencies in both individuals and social systems. This represents a shift in emphasis from repairing and rehabilitating those who have acquired disability labels and diagnoses to building in strengths to ward off the development of dysfunction (Caplan, 1964). In the last decade, a new set of terms has gained currency for describing various types of preventive interventions (Mrazek & Haggerty, 1994). Specifically, *universal interventions* target the general population regardless of risk status, *selective interventions* target subgroups whose risk of developing a particular disorder is above average, and *indicated interventions* target high-risk individuals who have minimal but detectable signs indicating a predisposition for mental disorder. As noted by Tebes, Kaufman, and Chinman in their chapter on training, this taxonomy allows investigators to place preventive interventions along a continuum, although all three types are initiated prior to the onset of a psychiatric disorder.

Since our initial survey in 1980 of community interventions from a behavioral perspective (Glenwick & Jason, 1980), the field of prevention has continued to mature, with well-controlled investigations increasing in number. The present volume represents an attempt not only to provide an update of preventive and community-based research in those areas covered in our earlier reviews (Glenwick & Jason, 1980, 1984, 1993; Jason & Glenwick, 1984) but also to demonstrate how the field has branched out in innovative ways into new and exciting areas. Setting the stage for the chapters that follow, in this chapter we provide an overview of the principal contemporary perspectives on prevention and the current trends in the field.

FOUNDATIONS OF PREVENTION:
ACTION-ORIENTED AND THEORETICAL PERSPECTIVES

The beginning development of many of the core areas of prevention can be traced to the birth of community psychology in the 1960s (Bennett, Anderson, Cooper, Hassol, Klein, & Rosenblum, 1966). Albee (1967), for example, critiqued the status quo in human services, observing that the number of human service professionals trained by our institutions of higher education would be increasingly insufficient to meet the evergrowing population of those experiencing some form of suffering or being judged by society as in need of services. By devoting most of our mental health resources to those with longstanding disorders, we were giving ourselves the daunting challenge of attempting to cure refractory, entrenched problems—problems with which our track record of success had been less than glowing. Furthermore, not only were traditional services inadequate in amount and limited in efficacy, but they also were receiving a disproportionately smaller share of our society's resources (Heller et al., 1984).

The development of the field of community psychology represented an effort to become more active in addressing the social and community problems confronting our country during the 1960s and 1970s (Duffy & Wong, 2000; Tolan, Keys, Chertok, & Jason, 1990). This perspective, first explicitly formulated in 1965 at a conference in Swampscott, Massachusetts (Levine & Perkins, 1997), stressed the need to emphasize prevention and widen our scope of intervention to encompass supraindividual target levels. A core belief of this approach was that by either (a) modifying social systems to make them more responsive and health inducing or (b) teaching persons how to live behaviorally healthier lifestyles, the flow of human casualties could be reduced (Cowen, 1973). Thus, it was hoped that, through community-based prevention and promotion, services could be implemented that were cost-effective, with fewer resources ultimately having to be devoted to remediating hard-to-cure, entrenched problems.

Among professionals and scholars in this field, there is much diversity of views about how to actually effect prevention and community change (Dalton, Elias, & Wandersman, 2001). Cook and Shadish (1986) suggested three ways of implementing social change. The most successful model, they claimed, involves making incremental modifications in existing social problems. Advocates of this approach believe that few policies are approved if they call for more than marginal changes in the status quo. A bolder approach is the use of demonstration programs to test the efficacy of a planned innovation. On the other end of the spectrum, as a third approach, are interventions that alter basic social structures. Albee (1986) argued that, in the absence of fundamental change, we will always have excessive amounts of psychopathology as long as we have excessive concentrations of economic power, nationalism, and institutions that perpetuate powerlessness, poverty, discrimination, sexism, racism, and ageism.

From a more theoretical perspective, several models of prevention have been advanced, the principal ones being *social competence, empowerment, developmental,* and *ecological*. Some theorists focus on a social competence model, where the goal is to prevent disorders by enhancing individuals' competencies (Duffy & Wong, 2000). Examples of such approaches include drug abuse prevention programs that concentrate on teaching skills to youngsters to resist pressure to take drugs (Bogat & Jason, 2000). Favored by many behavior-oriented psychologists because of its emphasis on explicit skills, the social competence approach can assist persons in gaining more resources and increasing their competence and independence.

Those psychologists adopting the empowerment model attempt to enhance justice and people's sense of control over their own destinies (Rappaport, 1981). Some clinical-community psychologists feel more comfortable with this type of model, because it is action-oriented and above the individual level emphasized by the social competence model. One difficulty for practitioners of the empowerment model involves deciding which groups to help empower. In many communities there are opposing groups, each regarding its perspective as correct, as is illustrated by the ongoing conflict in the Middle East.

Many prevention-oriented mental health professionals have aligned themselves with a developmental model. In an early influential review paper, Sameroff and Chandler (1975) found that infants with pregnancy or perinatal complications had few, if any, negative long-term effects if they came from intact families of high socioeconomic status. The same complications often led to later retardation or personality problems if the parents were of low socioeconomic status in unstable environments. These findings point to inadequacies in a main-effects model (i.e., one which posits that a child's constitution and his/her environment exert independent influences) and an interactional model (i.e., one which considers the combination of constitution and environment, but does not include the possibility that the characteristics of each might change over time). Within what Sameroff and Chandler (1975) termed a transactional model, however, reciprocal changes are posited. For example, as a parent begins to modify a child's behavior, these changes in the child begin to bring about changes in the parent. The transactional model focuses on those breakdowns in continuous organism-environment transactions over time which prevent children from organizing their worlds adaptively. A transactional approach focuses not just on children or parents, but also on the transactions of both over time.

Sameroff (1987) proposed three preventive strategies—*remediation, redefinition*, and *reeducation*—that incorporate transactional concepts. Remediation involves changing the child to adhere to the normative codes of parents. Redefinition consists of helping parents use existing regulatory systems to guide the child toward normative developmental outcomes (e.g., identifying for parents the possibilities of normal child rearing within what appear to be deviant situations). Finally, reeducation entails teaching parents the cultural code that regulates a child's development from birth to maturity (e.g., how to raise their children). Although societal-level influences can be added to family regulatory systems, their influences are not as precisely indicated by the model. It is curious that in these types of interventions, efforts are targeted primarily at either the child or the parent, but not both child and parent. Lorion (1990), however, defined risk using the transactional model, as the simultaneous presence and reciprocal influence of individual and environmental characteristics which, if unaltered, can lead to dysfunction. In the current volume, the chapter by Treuting, Haegerich, and Tolan on the prevention of antisocial behavior provides further elaboration of a developmental and life-course framework that emphasizes a dynamic relationship between individuals and the social systems, settings, and contexts in which they live.

Another paradigm that has captured the attention of many prevention practitioners and clinical-community psychologists is the ecological model (Kelly, 1985, 1990). Kelly's aim has been to develop theories of how people become effective and adaptive in diverse social environments. The ecological paradigm is a guiding framework for understanding behavior in interaction with its social and cultural contexts. Kingry-Westergaard and Kelly (1990) suggested that a principle fundamental to ecological approaches is the need to use multiple methods to understand the complex qualities of relationships and systems.

One aspect of the ecological approach for increasing the validity of our understanding of social phenomena is its emphasis on the collaborative relationship between researcher and participants. In such a relationship, concepts and hypotheses are developed and tested jointly by the investigator and the participants. This feature of the ecological model also has been espoused by many feminists, among others, who recommend that we listen to and understand people first and foremost from their points of view (Spretnak, 1991). When people are involved in research projects, they should be included as participants, not as subjects, whereby the process of being understood and represented is considered to be empowering.

Ecological principles can be used by professionals who join in long-term collaborative relationships with persons and settings (Kelly, 1985). By being actively involved in the planning of intervention programs, the recipients receive support, learn to identify resources, and become better problem-solvers who are more likely to be able to manage future challenges and issues. Interventions that have been generated from collaboratively defined, produced, and implemented change efforts are more apt to endure. An ecological approach analyzes community traditions for responding to community problems, helps evaluate or create settings that provide individuals with opportunities to continue receiving support after the termination of formal programs, works closely with community leaders in all aspects of health care intervention, and assesses positive and negative second-order ripple effects of interventions (Burgoyne & Jason, 1991).

The interventions described in this book illustrate the application of the social competence, empowerment, developmental, and ecological paradigms for the amelioration of many of the social ills noted earlier in this chapter. Such research is especially exciting and promising on three counts: (a) its melding of theory and action, (b) its willingness to confront difficult social problems, and (c) its incorporation of innovative approaches (such as the media, community development, and social support promotion) as intervention mechanism (see the chapter, for example, by Rhodes, Reddy, & Rappaport on the prevention of academic failure).

CURRENT TRENDS IN PREVENTION

In the following chapters, several recurrent themes emerge that appear to be characteristic of the field as it enters its adolescence. The first is the importance of involving the target populations themselves (i.e., the consumers and recipients of programs) in all phases of the intervention process (Kelly, 1990). There is a growing willingness by psychologists involved in health and mental health promotion to turn to the target populations for input concerning such aspects as problem identification, information on the problem, intervention design, and intervention acceptability (see, for instance, the chapter by Nation, Wandersman, & Perkins on community development). The result is a collaborative process in which (a) consensus between the applied interventionist (i.e., the mental health professional) and the target population is sought at each step and (b) the intervention process is more sensitive to the local culture and environment.

The values that underlie such efforts emphasize a willingness to understand people from their own vantage points. By actively working with people as engaged participants rather than as subjects, researchers and interventionists can empower those whom they are trying to help. Such involvement of participants increases the possibility that (a) they will have the skills to continue solving their problems even after the outside interventionists have departed and (b) the research findings will be used to benefit the community.

A second feature is the increasing collaboration occurring between psychologists and other professions/disciplines concerned with prevention and promotion. Among these are educators, medical personnel, communications experts, and epidemiologists (see the chapter by Tebes, Kaufman, & Chinman). Psychologists are evidencing greater awareness that by themselves they possess only a limited perspective on a particular social problem and that collaboration with other professions and disciplines can have synergistic effects, producing a more potent intervention than would otherwise be possible (Jason, Hess, Felner, & Moritsugu, 1987).

The increased fostering of target groups' sense of personal control is a third hallmark of much recent research (see, for example, the chapter by Lutzker &

Boyle on preventing abuse). Current projects are placing conspicuous emphasis on encouraging internal control—that is, control by the participants—as part of the behavioral change process. Thus, target populations are given the skills to act on and mold, rather than be passively shaped by, their environment (see the chapters by Sheeber, Biglan, Metzler, & Taylor on parenting, and by Fraenkel & Markman on marriage). The process becomes a bidirectional, transactional one between individuals and their ecological contexts.

A fourth distinguishing characteristic of the present generation of preventive interventions is a greater emphasis on antecedent behavioral change procedures as opposed to consequence procedures (i.e., ones that employ rewards or penalties). Psychologists have developed an awareness of how changing setting factors (i.e., aspects of the contexts and environments in which behavior occurs) can increase the likelihood of desirable behavioral change. In a review of interventions aimed at preventing youth violence, Embry (2001) found that the most successful interventions employ structured systems, which can come from arranging antecedents or the differential reinforcement of other, nonviolent behaviors. Thus, many of the projects outlined in the following chapters incorporate into the environment such components as prompting, modeling, role-playing exercises, and problem-solving training as ways of fostering the development of health and mental health competencies (see for instance, the chapter on aging by Gatz et al.).

A fifth theme involves understanding that our preventive interventions frequently have to compete with high-density alternative messages that might overwhelm and nullify our interventions. That is, there are multiple ecological systems that impact health care systems and other human services, and their messages are often not consistent (see the chapter by Biglan & James on the dissemination of research findings). One example involves youth access to tobacco (Jason, Berk, Schnopp-Wyatt, & Talbot, 1999). For many years, smoking prevention interventions have been implemented in schools, and yet children report that they are almost always sold cigarettes by store vendors (Jason, 1991). By sending youngsters conflicting messages (i.e., vendors selling minors cigarettes when school-based programs indicate that youths should not be smoking), our society diminishes the effectiveness of school-based smoking prevention interventions. An ecological assessment evaluates the complex and sometimes conflicting streams of messages targeted at the recipients of our health care services.

Respect for diversity is an important sixth theme in the prevention field. Salina and Lesondak's chapter on the prevention of racism, sexism, and heterosexism points to the increasing interest in decreasing such behaviors. Preventive interventions in general are becoming more culturally sensitive and appropriate, as is evidenced in Robinson and Case's chapter on the prevention of depression. The validation of different styles of living, distinctive world views, and diverse social arrangements is an important goal for prevention professionals (Duffy & Wong, 2000), since prejudice and discrimination have many detrimental effects on individuals' and social groups' physical and mental well-being.

A seventh theme is the realization that many children who develop problems in one area of functioning seem to be at risk for other difficulties as well. Longitudinal and epidemiological studies indicate that substance abuse, school failure, juvenile delinquency, depression, and other problems share many developmental roots (Embry, 2001). Unfortunately, school personnel are increasingly being provided with programs that deal with each of these problems as separate entities, since many officials are concerned that children might be overwhelmed with multiple interventions, some of which might be incompatible with each other. There is a clear need to better coordinate and integrate the multiple initiatives that are being marketed for the prevention of problems in children and adolescents, particularly given that many of these problems might share similar causes.

In summary, the field today seems to be marked by greater awareness, heterogeneity, and flexibility with regard to such questions as (a) how interventions are developed, (b) with whom one develops them, (c) what behavioral change techniques are employed, (d) how much interventions should depend on external versus internal controls, and (e) what process and outcome variables are appropriate to measure when evaluating projects. In the following section we consider some of the principal challenges facing preventive psychology as it continues to mature.

FUTURE DIRECTIONS

Despite the progress that the prevention field has made in the past decade, noteworthy challenges remain for mental health professionals interested in facilitating health and mental health in communities. The first is the need to develop more multilevel interventions. Thus, for example, a substance abuse or AIDS prevention program could involve both the media (a community-level component) and participating schools (an organizational-level component) (see, for example, the chapters by Benotsch & Kalichman on HIV/AIDS prevention and Blitz, Arthur, & Hawkins on substance abuse prevention). Multilevel interventions potentially have the twin virtues of targeting many persons while influencing them with maximally effective behavioral change techniques.

A second challenge stems from the unfortunate, but not surprising, finding that many creative projects mounted by psychologists during the past 20 years have all too seldom been adopted by the host settings on an ongoing basis. The challenge is to devise cost-effective, user-friendly interventions and to work with the target populations involved to enhance their desire and ability to retain the program without, or with minimal, outside assistance. Such empowerment efforts increase stakeholders' sense of ownership of the program and the probability that the program will become incorporated into the setting's routine mode of functioning.

As important as program maintenance is the challenge of program dissemination, both within and outside of psychology, to relevant applied researchers, human service organizations, governmental bodies, and the like. Transmitting information about effective preventive programs and techniques to those who might profit by such knowledge is a vital initial step in the adoption process and requires psychologists to venture beyond conventional professional outlets such as journals and conventions (see the chapter by Biglan & James). Attempting to influence legislative or regulatory policies, for example, can be one way of initiating higher-level changes and expanding our programs' reach.

As we noted above, mental health professionals engaged in prevention have developed an increasing openness toward collaboration with professions and disciplines outside of psychology. However, there remains room for further incorporation of concepts and theories from other subdisciplines *within* psychology. The challenge is to draw creatively from those areas that would appear to have especially heuristic value. These include social psychology (e.g., the concepts of psychological reactance and intrinsic motivation), environmental/ecological psychology (e.g., the concept of the interdependence of systems), and developmental psychology (e.g., the notion of transactional influence processes between persons and their environmental contexts) (Jason, 1992). Embry and Flannery (1999) also suggested that we consider an evolutionary psychology perspective in our conceptualizations, as some human behavioral adaptations might have evolved over thousands of years, and our preventive interventions might work with or against these ancient evolutionary patterns.

Another challenge concerns the importance of appreciating the complexity of settings and the impact of such complexity on both researchers and participants. The term *contextualism* has received much currency in recent writings on the philosophy of psychology as a science. It refers to the idea that knowledge is relative to a given frame of reference (Kingry-Westergaard & Kelly, 1990). According to this view, rather than discovering knowledge of the objective world, investigators are gathering knowledge of their interactions with the world. This somewhat humbling perspective suggests that several of the traditional goals of scientific research—such as the external control of phenomena, the identification of universal principles, and the replicability of specific findings—may be elusive when mounting applied interventions. For example, the complexity of social environments may limit the robustness of general principles identified in laboratory settings and may alter or moderate their expression. Thus, the characteristics of the social settings in which we work, and the multiple contingencies that may simultaneously be in effect in any setting, need to be carefully analyzed to uncover the operative factors influencing behavior in that setting. An awareness of the complexity of settings can aid prevention-oriented behavioral researchers in better comprehending and considering those contextual issues (e.g., entry issues, the process of target problem selection, larger systemic forces influencing the selected problem) that frequently determine a project's outcome (Bogat & Jason, 2000).

The health promotion and preventive interventions described in this book represent only a few of the multitude of influences on community members' health behavior. For example, individuals successfully completing substance abuse treatment programs are subjected to high-risk environments that encourage engaging in substance abuse. Viewers of television are bombarded with messages to use products that are primarily processed, often having minimal nutritional value (Schlosser, 2001). We are all deluged with inaccurate information and unhealthy behavior messages from a variety of corporations trying to promote their products and services. These enterprises have considerably more resources available to them than do the collaborators of the described health promotion projects. Negative alternative ecological influences need to be recognized because they undoubtedly have a counterproductive impact on health promotion interventions. At a very minimum, interventions should allude to such forces and assist participants in dealing with them. Such conflicting adverse influences are legitimate targets of our health delivery interventions.

The potential impact of preventive principles and strategies on health and mental health promotion would appear to be considerable. Indeed, much current activity in health and education is already grounded in the application of these types of perspectives by intervention agents and service deliverers. The challenge is to develop more interventions in which preventive approaches are applied systematically and thoughtfully. Such interventions are exemplified by the projects highlighted in the following chapters. Increasing preventive psychology's influence in the promotion of health and mental health represents an exciting opportunity for contributing to social change in the coming decade.

PURPOSE AND ORGANIZATION OF THIS BOOK

This volume is intended to reach two critical audiences. The first includes scholars and students desiring a summary of the existing empirical literature on preventive interventions addressing a variety of health and mental health issues. Many of those comprising this audience may themselves be among those conducting such interventions. The second audience consists of those on the front lines, including program developers and evaluators, human service administrators, and community organizers, advocates, and educators. These groups seek innovative, practical approaches to preventing psychological problems.

Our aims in producing this work are to summarize the latest findings in the field and to provide recommendations for the assessment and prevention of problems. The topics included are ones in which substantial investigation has been carried out, and the chapters' authors are among the cutting-edge researchers in the field. We have added several chapters since our last edited volume (Glenwick & Jason, 1993), now with coverage of aging, chronic health problems, marital disorder, delinquency and antisocial behavior, depression, racism and sexism, community disintegration, research dissemination, and prevention training, in addition to updating of research on such topics as physical and sexual abuse, school failure, substance abuse, and AIDS. Although these topics typify current research in the field, they are meant to be illustrative rather than exhaustive of the totality of prevention-oriented applied behavioral research. For example, biopsychosocial-oriented interventions are not the explicit focus of any of the chapters, although Minden and Jason's chapter on chronic illness does include consideration of health-related issues. Clearly, the neuroscience revolution has not yet been well-captured in our prevention theories and interventions, and the next generation of studies might indicate how genes could be activated using environmental stimuli (Embry, 2001).

Many of the interventions and programs reviewed in this book adopt a perspective of social change that is wider than the more typical, person-centered health and clinical interventions. In the reviews and recommendations presented here, there is attention to the public policy implications of the interventions. A number of the chapters direct us toward thinking about instituting changes by means of legislative or regulatory policies, where our impact and reach might be greatest (Jason, 1991). There is a critical need to reconsider and expand how we conceptualize and implement our programs so that they can be maximally effective in bringing about needed change.

To provide consistency in format and presentation, all of the chapters include four sections: a description of the problem, a review and evaluation of the literature, a discussion of a case example, and suggestions for future directions. The initial section of each chapter defines the problem that is that chapter's focus, presenting its salient characteristics and current status and emphasizing why it merits attention. The second section presents a critical review of the empirical literature on the topic, highlighting accomplishments and central findings, on the one hand, but also the shortcomings of research to date, on the other. Each chapter then describes an applied intervention project in its area, considering the issues (e.g., ethical, logistical, political, and financial) involved in actually designing and implementing such a project in the "real world." The objective of this third section is to convey a sense of both (a) the potential pitfalls that can endanger a project's success and (b) concrete recommendations for preventing or surmounting such stumbling blocks. Finally, the chapters conclude with a fourth section discussing unresolved issues and future research directions, pointing the way to the next steps that empirical investigations and applied interventions might profitably take. Our hope is that the readers of this book will be among those involved in taking these steps.

We are extremely enthusiastic about this volume, since prevention appears to be on the forefront of current health care discussion. It is our hope that this book will stimulate even more academically based psychologists, mental health professionals, preventionists in other disciplines, and students to contribute to the field's further maturation by the development of strategies and applications that are theoretically sound and creative, empirically valid and innovative, and beneficial to the communities of which we are a part.

REFERENCES

Albee, G. W. (1967). The relation of conceptual models to manpower needs. In E. L. Cowen, E. A. Gardner, & M. Zax (Eds.), *Emergent approaches to mental health problems* (pp. 63–73). New York: Appleton-Century-Crofts.

Albee, G. W. (1986). Toward a just society. *American Psychologist, 41,* 891–898.

Bennett, C. C., Anderson, L. S., Cooper, S., Hassol, L., Klein, D. C., & Rosenblum, G. (Eds.) (1966). *Community psychology: A report of the Boston Conference on the Education of Psychologists for Community Mental Health.* Boston: Boston University Press.

Bogat, G. A., & Jason, L. A. (2000). Towards an integration of behaviorism and community psychology: Dogs bark at those they do not recognize. In J. Rappaport & E. Seidman (Eds.), *Handbook of community psychology* (pp. 101–114). New York: Plenum.

Burgoyne, N. S., & Jason, L. A. (1991). Incorporating the ecological paradigm into behavioral preventive interventions. In P. M. Martin (Ed.), *Handbook of behavior therapy and psychological science: An integrative approach* (pp. 457–472). New York: Pergamon.

Caplan, C. (1964). *Principles of preventive psychiatry.* New York: Basic Books.

Cook, T. D., & Shadish, W. R. (1986). Program evaluation: The worldly science. In M. R. Rosenzweig & L. W. Porter (Eds.), *Annual review of psychology* (Vol. 37, pp. 193–232). Palo Alto, CA: Annual Reviews.

Cowen, E. L. (1973). Social and community interventions. In P. Mussen & M. Rosenzweig (Eds.), *Annual review of psychology* (Vol. 24, pp. 423–472). Palo Alto, CA: Annual Reviews.

Dalton, J. H., Elias, M. J., & Wandersman, A. (2001). *Community psychology: Linking individuals and communities*. Belmont, CA: Wadsworth.

Dugger, R. (1995). Real populists please stand up. *The Nation, 261*, 159–164.

Duffy, K. G., & Wong, F. Y. (2000). *Community psychology* (2nd ed.). Boston: Allyn and Bacon.

Embry, D. D. (2001). *The next generation multi-problem prevention: A comprehensive science-based, practical approach*. Manuscript submitted for publication.

Embry, D. D., & Flannery, D. J. (1999). Two sides of the coin. Multi-level prevention and intervention to reduce youth violent behavior. In D. J. Flannery & C. R. Huff (Eds.), *Youth violence: Prevention, intervention and social policy* (pp. 47–72). Washington, DC: American Psychiatric Press.

Etzioni, A. (1993). *The spirit of community*. New York: Crown.

Felner, R. D., Jason, L. A., Moritsugu, J., & Farber, S. S. (Eds.) (1983). *Preventive psychology: Theory, research and practice*. New York: Pergamon.

Glenwick, D. S., & Jason, L. A. (Eds.) (1980). *Behavioral community psychology: Progress and prospects*. New York: Praeger.

Glenwick, D. S., & Jason, L. A. (1984). Behavioral community psychology: An introduction to the special issue. *Journal of Community Psychology, 12*, 103–112.

Glenwick, D. S., & Jason, L. A. (Eds.) (1993). *Promoting health and mental health in children, youth, and families*. New York: Springer Publishing.

Heller, K., Price, R. H., Reinharz, S., Riger, S., Wandersman, A., & D'Aunno, T. (1984). *Psychology and community change: Challenges of the future* (2nd ed.). Homewood, IL: Dorsey.

Jason, L. A. (1991). Participating in social change: A fundamental value for our discipline. *American Journal of Community Psychology, 19*, 1–16.

Jason, L. A. (1992). Eco-transactional behavioral research. *Journal of Primary Prevention, 13*, 37–72.

Jason, L. A. (1997). *Community building: Values for a sustainable future*. Westport, CT: Praeger.

Jason, L. A., Berk, M., Schnopp-Wyatt, D. L., & Talbot, B. (1999). Effects of enforcement of youth access laws on smoking prevalence. *American Journal of Community Psychology, 27*, 143–160.

Jason, L. A., & Glenwick, D. S. (1984). Behavioral community psychology: A review of recent research and applications. In M. Hersen, R. M. Eisler, & P. M. Miller (Eds.), *Progress in behavior modification* (Vol. 18, pp. 85–121). New York: Academic Press.

Jason, L. A., & Hanaway, E. K. (1997). *Remote control: A sensible approach to kids, TV, and the new electronic media*. Sarasota, FL: Professional Resource Press.

Jason, L. A., Hess, R., Felner, R. D., & Moritsugu, J. N. (Eds.) (1987). *Prevention: Toward a multidisciplinary approach*. New York: Haworth.

Kelly, J. G. (1985). The concept of primary prevention: Creating new paradigms. *Journal of Primary Prevention, 5,* 269–272.

Kelly, J. G. (1990). Changing contexts and the field of community psychology. *American Journal of Community Psychology, 18,* 769–792.

Kingry-Westergaard, C., & Kelly, J. G. (1990). A contextualist epistemiology for ecological research. In P. Tolan, C. Keys, F. Chertok, & L. Jason (Eds.), *Researching community psychology: Issues of theory and methods* (pp. 23–31). Washington, DC: American Psychological Association.

Levine, M., & Perkins, D. V. (1997). *Principles of community psychology: Perspectives and applications* (2nd ed.). New York: Oxford University Press.

Lorion, R. P. (1990). Developmental analyses of community phenomena. In P. H. Tolan, C. Keys, F. Chertok, & L. A. Jason (Eds.), *Researching community psychology: Integrating theories and methodologies* (pp. 32–41). Washington, DC: American Psychological Association.

Mrazek, P. J., & Haggerty, R. J. (1994). *Reducing the risks for mental disorder: Frontiers for preventive intervention research.* Washington, DC: Institute of Medicine, National Academy Press.

National Advisory Mental Health Council (1993). *Health care reform for Americans with severe mental ilnesses.* Bethesda, MD: National Institute of Mental Health.

Rappaport, J. (1981). In praise of paradox: A social policy of empowerment over prevention. *American Journal of Community Psychology, 9,* 1–25.

Rossi, R., & Montgomery, A. (1994). Educational reforms and students at risk: A review of the current state of the art. (Available at *http://www.ed.gov/pubs/EDReformStudies/EdReforsms/*)

Sameroff, A. J. (1987). Transactional risk factors and prevention. In J. A. Steinberg & M. M. Silverman (Eds.), *Preventing mental disorders: A research perspective* (pp. 74–89) (DHHS Publication No. 87–1492). Washington, DC: U.S. Government Printing Office.

Sameroff, A. J., & Chandler, M. J. (1975). Reproductive risk and the continuum of caretaking casualty. In F. D. Horowitz, M. Hetherington, S. Scarr-Salapatek, & G. Siegel (Eds.), *Review of child development research* (Vol. 4, pp. 187–244). Chicago: University of Chicago Press.

Schlosser, E. (2001). *Fast food nation.* Boston: Houghton Mifflin.

Spretnak, C. (1991). *States of grace.* New York: HarperCollins.

Tolan, P., Keys, C., Chertok, F., & Jason, L. (Eds.) (1990). *Researching community psychology: Issues of theories and methods.* Washington, DC: American Psychological Association.

CHAPTER 2

Making Effective Use of Prevention Science

Anthony Biglan

and

Lisa James

DESCRIPTION OF THE PROBLEM

The present volume describes numerous interventions that could help to reduce the prevalence of human behavior problems. If they were widely implemented, it might be possible to lower the incidence of divorce, reduce delinquency and substance abuse, ensure a more pleasant old age, prevent much anxiety and depression, and ensure greater health for most of the population. However, translation of current scientific knowledge into widespread benefits to society will require new initiatives on the part of the scientific community and some major transformations in the practices of the rest of society. Rather than simply exporting programs and policies from research to practice settings that remain otherwise unchanged, the practices of science will need to become an integral part of how society goes about ensuring people's well-being.

In this chapter, we describe cultural practices that would be involved in society making full use of prevention science. For each practice, we provide a brief description and discuss its value for reducing human behavior problems. Then we suggest ways to develop these practices, including research and coordinated efforts of scientific, governmental, and non-governmental organizations.

REVIEW AND CRITIQUE OF THE LITERATURE

Articulating What Works

As knowledge has accumulated, many organizations have begun to articulate what works. Perhaps the most fully developed system for organizing outcome research is the Cochrane Collaboration, a worldwide network of centers that are creating a database of randomized controlled trials in medicine (http://hiru.mcmaster.ca/cochrane/). Only about half of the existing randomized trials can be identified as such because many papers don't indicate in the title or abstract that they employed randomized trials. For this reason the Cochrane Collaboration has been systematically hand-searching every journal in medicine. The reports of the trials are then coded and put into the Cochrane database so that they are available to reviewers. As a result of this effort, it is increasingly possible for the medical community to accurately characterize the effects of tested treatments. It is hoped that such information will facilitate the spread of effective treatments.

In the behavioral sciences, there are numerous efforts to identify empirically supported treatment and preventive interventions. They include meta-analyses (e.g., Derzon, Wilson, & Cunningham 1999; Durlak & Wells, 1997; Lipsey & Wilson, 1993; Tobler & Stratton, 1997). In clinical psychology, the American Psychological Association, Division of Clinical Psychology, developed criteria for empirically supported interventions (Chambless & Hollon, 1998) and identified treatment procedures that have been shown in multiple randomized trials or interrupted time-series experiments to be efficacious. At the same time, the Practice Guidelines Coalition, a cooperative effort of managed care providers and clinical researchers, has begun creating practice guidelines for managed care organizations (Hayes, personal communication, November 15, 2000).

Numerous organizations have implemented formal processes to identify empirically supported practices. The Blueprints Project at the Center for the Study and Prevention of Violence identified 10 empirically supported prevention programs. It made information about them available on a Web site (*http://www.colorado.edu/cspv/blueprints/*) and through center publications. The Center for Substance Abuse Prevention has had the Program Enhancement Protocols, which summarize the evidence on preventing specific substance use problems. The U.S. Department of Education's Safe and Drug Free Schools program has identified programs that it believes are effective (http://www.ed.gov/offices/OESE/SDFS/). The National Institute on Drug Abuse has produced a redbook that summarize principles for effective prevention (National

Institute on Drug Abuse, 1997). The National Institute on Alcohol Abuse and Alcoholism is creating a similar summary of principles for the prevention of alcohol problems (J. Howard, personal communication, November 8, 2001).

Thus, the practice of summarizing and disseminating information about treatment and prevention is growing. The growth of this practice appears to be due to several factors. First, there is a critical mass of empirical evidence about efficacious prevention practices. Recognition of this fact by the scientific community has prompted efforts to articulate what is known and to advocate the adoption of empirically based practices. Second, there is increasing demand for accountability for social programs.

Necessary Further Developments

The further development of a system for identifying empirically supported preventive interventions is vital to realizing their benefits. Three things are needed. First, we need a registry of preventive trials similar to that of the Cochrane Collaboration in medicine. Several efforts are underway. The Cochrane Collaboration has assisted in the creation of such a registry—the Campbell Collaboration. The Centers for Disease Control and Prevention is maintaining a database of studies relevant to AIDS prevention and treatment, and is building one on preventive trials. Under the auspices of the Society for Prevention Research, Brown and Mrazek have been attempting to obtain funding for the creation of a registry of prevention trials (Biglan, Brown, Maibach, & Mrazek, 1999). However, it has been difficult to obtain adequate funding for these efforts. Perhaps a more concerted effort by the prevention science community can convince federal agencies and foundations of the value of such a registry.

Second, articulation of what works would be facilitated by consensus standards for identifying programs or policies worthy of dissemination. There is considerable variability in the standards used to identify interventions. Many summaries include programs that have only been shown to produce pre-post changes for a single sample. This encourages organizations to continue the use of inadequately evaluated programs. If prevention scientists spoke with one voice about standards for selecting programs and policies, it would promote their adoption.

Elsewhere, we have suggested a set of standards that derive from discussions in clinical psychology (Biglan, Mrazek, Carnine, & Flay, in press; Chambless & Hollon, 1998) and the Institute of Medicine report on prevention (Mrazek & Haggerty, 1994). Briefly, we have suggested that in order for scientific organizations to advocate widespread adoption of a program or policy, there should be evidence from multiple well-designed randomized controlled trials or multiple well-designed interrupted time-series experiments that were conducted by two or more independent research teams.

Third, it will do little good to articulate what works if the scientific community remains mute in public discussion. Organizations of scientists such as the American Psychological Association, the Society for Community Research and Action, and the Society for Prevention Research, are becoming increasingly sophisticated in advocating the use of science in human affairs. Information about effective preventive practices needs to be presented in effective ways in the media and in regular presentations to decision makers. Policy makers and journalists need to be informed, through briefings and workshops, about the value of choosing programs and policies that have been experimentally evaluated, as well as about the most appropriate techniques for evaluating programs. Ultimately, we will want the policy makers who have responsibility for people's psychological and behavioral well-being to be behavioral scientists themselves, just as those who are responsible for public health are trained in public health, medicine, and biology.

The Dissemination of Empirically Supported Prevention Practices

As we advocate for the use of empirically based practices we must build an infrastructure that ensures that they are effectively implemented. The beginnings of that infrastructure can be discerned, but considerable research and much more funding will be needed if the best science is to be effectively translated into practice.

One of the best organized efforts to disseminate empirically supported interventions is being conducted by the Center for the Study and Prevention of Violence at the University of Colorado, which was described above. It is providing training and technical assistance for a total of 50 implementations of eight of the empirically supported programs they identified. Other organizations that are actively providing assistance to communities and organizations in the implementation of research-based practices include the Collaborative to Advance Social and Emotional Learning (CASEL), the Center for Substance Abuse Prevention, the Community Tool Box at the University of Kansas (*http://ctb.lsi.ukans.edu/*), the National Center for Improving the Tools of Educators at the University of Oregon, the Social Development Research Group at the University of Washington, and the Society for Prevention Research.

The Need for Research on the Effectiveness of Interventions

Research evaluating preventive interventions is usually done in such well-controlled and well-funded implementations that we cannot be sure that the interventions will be effective when implemented under more typical conditions. Regular classroom teachers or clinic-based therapists may not have as much experience, training, supervision, or preparation time as interventionists in research evaluations, and some decrement in effectiveness may result. The recognition of this problem has prompted calls for effectiveness trials in which apparently efficacious interventions are evaluated when they are implemented by service providers (Flay, 1986; Holder et al., 1999).

Traditionally, such studies have been seen as intermediary between efficacy studies and dissemination. However, we believe that they should be conceptualized as part of the process of dissemination. We can never be sure that an implemented intervention is achieving its desired outcomes unless we continue to collect outcome data. Thus, rather than assuming that one or more successful tests of an intervention's effectiveness in a field setting will guarantee its continued success, we should assume that no practice will maintain its effectiveness. For example, elementary schools that adopt programs to reduce aggressive behavior will have to regularly assess the incidence of aggressive behaviors and the prevalence of overly aggressive children. Such a stance is in keeping with continuous quality improvement systems that have come to be widely used to ensure the quality of most manufactured goods (e.g., Halberstam, 1987). Why should we not have the same systematic concern with quality for practices, which are designed to affect people's physical and psychological well-being?

Below we describe the development of systems for assessing human well-being and the growing use of experimental techniques to evaluate programs and policies. As these practices grow, continuous assessment of the effectiveness of preventive practices will grow too.

The Need for Implementation Specialists

Effective dissemination will require a new specialty in prevention science and community psychology. One might call them "implementation specialists." They would need to be skilled both in implementing empirically supported interventions and in training and consulting with others who are going to implement them. Moreover, if we are correct that continuous evaluation of implemented programs will become more common, specialists of this sort will have to be skilled in helping organizations set up systematic evaluations.

The reinforcing contingencies that would foster the development of such a cadre of people do not yet exist. Researchers are not particularly motivated to train people to disseminate their programs or policies because there is little economic incentive and little likelihood that their efforts will result in highly valued outcomes such as publication and recognition from one's peers. Universities have little current incentive to set up training programs because the demand for such professionals does not yet exist. We suggest that a set of pilot programs in which people are trained and highly paid to disseminate empirically supported programs might get the process started.

The Need for Experimental Research on Dissemination Strategies

Experimental evaluations of the effects of dissemination strategies are exceedingly rare (E. Rogers, personal communication, October 3, 2000). About the only area of dissemination research where experimental evaluations of dissemination strategies seem to be taking place is medicine. To give some flavor of the work in this area, here are two examples: Randomized controlled trials have been used to evaluate the impact of computerized feedback and newsletters on physician prescribing behavior (Hershey, Goldberg, & Cohen, 1988) and personal educational visits by clinical pharmacists were shown in a randomized trial to reduce excessive use of three drugs (Avorn & Soumerai, 1983).

Not all experimental evaluations of dissemination strategies have targeted medical practices, however. In an innovative study, Jason and Rose (1984) evaluated a strategy for influencing state legislatures to adopt laws requiring the use of child passenger restraints. They randomly assigned 59 senators in the Illinois legislature to receive or not to receive information about the value of child restraint. Those who received it were significantly more likely than those who did not to vote in favor of a bill requiring child safety restraints.

Despite these few experimental studies, the stark fact is that there has been very little progress in understanding how to bring about the effective implementation of empirically-supported interventions in practice settings. The paucity of experimental evaluations of dissemination strategies may be because they are not encouraged by the National Institutes of Health schema for phases of research (Greenwald & Cullen, 1985; Hoagwood & Koretz, 1996; Holder et al., 1999). According to the schema, research on a topic begins with hypothesis and method development. It then proceeds to testing interventions for efficacy and effectiveness (Flay, 1986). In theory, once an intervention has been shown to be effective, it becomes widely implemented, possibly through demonstration projects. This schema has been valuable for moving the field toward tests of interventions. However, it implies that implementation is not in itself a topic for research (Biglan & Glasgow, 1991; Flay, 1986; Holder et al., 1999). As a result, few experimental evaluations of dissemination strategies are undertaken, and knowledge of how to influence effective implementations remains limited.

Progress requires use of the same scientific tools that helped us identify effective programs and policies in the first place, namely, valid experimental evaluations. To foster such research, we need to specify the organizations that are expected to adopt the empirically supported intervention, a theory of the variables that would influence effective implementation, and valid measures of implementation. Once we have these conceptual and methodological tasks accomplished, we should be able to experimentally evaluate the effects of well-defined procedures for fostering effective implementation (Biglan & Taylor, 2000).

Another reason for the lack of experimental evaluations may be the perceived cost and difficulty of conducting such experimental evaluations. Many of the targeted practices involve whole organizations, rather than individuals, and therefore seem to require randomization of entire organizations (Murray & Wolfinger, 1994). For example, one might test a strategy for influencing clinics to adopt empirically supported parenting practices (e.g., Taylor & Biglan, 1998). Obtaining the cooperation of organizations for such studies could be difficult. Even where the focus is on influencing the practices of individuals (e.g., therapists or teachers), it is important to determine whether the practices are effective when implemented by those individuals. This requires assessing not only the practices being disseminated but also their effects on the recipients of the services. For example, a study to test a strategy for influencing teachers' use of empirically supported reading instruction practices would need to assess both teacher behavior and student learning. This type of assessment can be costly.

We cannot, however, repeal the principles of experimental design simply because they are costly or inconvenient. If we want to know the factors that influence the adoption of specific programs or policies, experimental studies are essential (Cook & Campbell, 1979).

There are other research problems for which experimental designs were once considered unfeasible. For example, only during the past 20 years have randomized controlled trials have been used to evaluate community interventions (e.g., Biglan, Ary, Smolkowski, Duncon, & Blach, 2000; COMMIT, 1991; Forster, Murray, Wolfson, Blaine, & Wagenaar, 1998; Perry, Williams, Veblen-Mortenson, & Toomey, 1996; Wagenaar, Murray, Wolfson, & Forster, 1994).

Moreover, randomized controlled trials are not the only option for experimentally evaluating dissemination strategies. Interrupted time-series experimental designs provide useful methods for identifying influential variables, especially when we are trying to identify variables that influence a practice (Biglan, Ary, & Wagenaar, 2000). In these designs, the behavior of an individual or the practice of an organization is monitored regularly over time. Once a baseline has been obtained, the presumed influence on the practice is introduced and its effect on the practice is assessed. (The time series is "interrupted" by the intervention.) For example, one might explore whether giving bonuses to health care providers for advising smokers to quit increases the practice. Following a baseline, one might offer incentives for a period of time, withdraw the offer, and then reimplement it. Evidence that the incentives made a difference would be provided by changes in the rate of advice-giving that coincided with the instatement and withdrawal of the incentive.

Ongoing Monitoring of Human Well-Being

The systematic dissemination of empirically supported programs and policies may not be the only, or even the primary, means by which prevention science will improve human well-being. We believe that much of the improvement will result from systems of monitoring human well-being that motivate and guide communities, states, and the nation to adopt practices that have measurable benefits.

The development of such monitoring systems is well under way. According to O'Malley, Bachman, Johnston, and Schulenberg (in press), systematic population-based assessments of populations began in the 1960s with three projects that assessed national samples. Now such systems for monitoring population well-being are proliferating. At the national level, there is Monitoring the Future, which obtains data on most youth problem behaviors from representative samples of 8th-, 10th-, and 12th-grade students. The Youth Risk Behavior Survey (*http://www.cdc.gov/nccdphp/dash/yrbs/*) attempts to obtain data on most youth problem behaviors from a representative sample of schools in each state every other year. In Oregon, that effort has been integrated with a longstanding state initiated effort to assess schools in the alternate years. The integrated assessment will provide annual data on a representative sample of 8th- and 10th-grade students in Oregon. A proposal is being made to the state legislature to conduct such surveys in every school in the state.

The monitoring of adult well-being is less developed, perhaps because obtaining data on adults is more expensive. We are aware of two surveys of psychological disorders that employed representative samples of adults. The Epidemiological Catchment Area study obtained data from samples in five metropolitan areas, and the National Comorbidity Survey obtained data from a sample of 8,000 respondents age 15 to 54 years. Although these efforts are providing important information about the prevalence of most problems of adults, state and local systems for the ongoing monitoring of such functioning do not appear to have been developed. As the cost of such systems is reduced and their value for the well-being of human populations becomes more widely understood, it is conceivable that most communities will establish such systems.

In our view, such assessment systems are a fundamental first step in reducing the incidence and prevalence of psychological and behavioral problems. Only through ongoing monitoring can we know whether efforts to address human problems are bringing about the improvements we desire. Moreover, the release of the data can increase public awareness of the need to prevent or remediate problems.

Thus, we foresee a society in which the incidence and prevalence of human behavior problems are monitored in every community. This will be no different from what is already the case in the management of our economy. Key indicators of economic health are collected at the state and local levels and aggregated up to the national level. Economic policies are modified in light of minute changes in these indicators. As a result, the frequency and depth of economic downturn has been reduced over the last 50 years (Monyihan, 1996).

Similarly, annual information about the extent of drug abuse, crime, depression, and so on could influence private and public organizations toward coordinated prevention efforts. In the absence of such information, communities will be unable to know whether they are having any impact on the problems they are charged with preventing or ameliorating.

Thus, it is essential that the scientific community organize to further validate, standardize, and refine methods for monitoring important aspects of human psychological and behavioral functioning so that data can be obtained, analyzed, and publicized inexpensively. The creation of a set of standard indicators of human well-being would appear to be a critical step. The indicators would need to reflect key aspects of human behavior that have been empirically demonstrated to be (a) costly to society and (b) judged as important by representative samples of the public. The measures would have to be validated. Also, the indicators would have to be readily understood by policy makers and political leaders not trained in the behavioral sciences. A task force of scientists and policy makers established through an act of Congress would be helpful in moving such efforts forward.

Toward the Experimenting Society

We could evolve improved social conditions more rapidly if the practice of experimentally evaluating programs and policies were widespread. Imagine that every new program or policy intended to affect important human behavior were experimentally evaluated. Programs and policies that had a detectable impact would tend to receive continued support and would be more likely to be adopted by others. Those that had no impact or deleterious effects would wither. Experimental evaluation of programs and policies is no less than what is required of every prescription drug. Why should we not demand of our educational, mental health, and criminal justice systems that they too use the tools that are available to select more effective policies and programs?

Our evolution toward an experimenting society already can be discerned. The other chapters in this volume describe the numerous policies and programs that have been shown through experimental evaluation to be of value for prevention. Above we described the growing number of experimental evaluations of community interventions and the increasing use of experimental evidence to guide the selection of programs and policies. As the value of experimental evidence becomes more widely understood and accepted, it will further increase demand and support for experimental evaluations.

Earlier, in our discussion of the need for research evaluating dissemination strategies, we described two types of experimental designs that are particularly important to encourage. The first, and better known, is the randomized controlled trial, in which cases are randomly assigned to different programs (or to no program) and the effects of each condition are compared. It is most easily used to evaluate the effects of programs for individuals or small groups, such as families, although it also has been used to evaluate the effects of community interventions (Biglan, Ary, Smolkowski et al., 2000). The other experimental design is the interrupted time-series experiment, in which measures of the target process are obtained repeatedly over an extended time and the effect of the introduction of the policy or program on the slope or level of the time-series is observed (Biglan, Ary, & Wagenaar, 2000b). This form of experimental design has made important contributions to our understanding of the effects of policies such as laws involving alcohol (e.g., Holder, 1998) and can be of considerable value for assessing the effects of interventions in communities (e.g., Biglan, 1995; Biglan et al., 1996).

The increased use of experimental evaluations involves a breakdown of the traditional distinction between research and practice. Increasingly, practice will be conducted in the context of organized efforts to evaluate its effects. Thus, science will inform practice, not simply through the export of knowledge from research to practice settings but through the integration of scientific methods into the management of practice settings.

In sum, we need to promote the practice of continuous quality improvement among all organizations that affect human health or behavior. The well-functioning society of the future will be one in which organizations that affect human well-being routinely and experimentally evaluate the effects of their programs and policies, and modify them in light of what they learn. This will require that those who manage such organizations are trained in measurement and experimental evaluation.

We can move toward such a society if prevention scientists organize to promote the use of experimental designs. They need to inform legislators and foundations about the value of experimental design and the rudiments of appropriate designs. They need to increase journalists' understanding of experimental evaluations. Ultimately, they need to push for making funding contingent on organizations experimentally evaluating their policies and programs.

A Framework for Choosing Programs and Policies

Our vision of a society, which is increasingly managed by behavioral scientists raises the specter of behavior control, as well it should. Legions of behavioral scientists, teachers, therapists, and policy makers are working hard to ensure that certain types of behavior occur less often and others occur more often. There is no guarantee that the behaviors they target and the practices that they implement to achieve those goals will be in the best interests of the people whose behavior they try to influence (Biglan, 1995). For example, recent movements toward mandatory minimum sentences and treating juvenile offenders as adults are predicated on the notion that such policies will reduce crime. The harm that these policies do to society and individual young people is seldom considered. Along with the development of practices such as monitoring of problem behavior, dissemination of empirically supported practices, and increased experimental evaluation of policies and programs, we need to specify how decisions will be made about behavioral objectives and strategies for achieving those objectives.

Elsewhere, Biglan (1995) has described a set of principles for intentional efforts to bring about changes in cultural practices. Those of us who are seeking to bring about beneficial outcomes for populations should adhere to a set of procedures that prevent the exploitation of the populations that we set out to assist. We would do well to (a) eschew the use of coercive means to bring about change, (b) provide informed consent to those who would be affected by a change effort, (c) obtain review of proposed cultural change efforts by disinterested parties, (d) involve representatives of the target population in decisions about the goals of any effort and the strategies to be used in pursuing those goals, (e) empower disadvantaged populations to effectively pursue their own well-being, and (f) provide decision makers with empirical evidence relevant to the choice of goals for change and strategies for achieving change.

These principles define a set of cultural practices that should accompany organized efforts to bring about changes in the physical or psychological well-being of populations in communities. To the extent that they are adopted, they will prevent exploitation of disadvantaged groups and individuals and will foster greater support over time for organized efforts to bring about changes in our communities. Indeed, they may contribute to the success of change efforts by ensuring understanding of and commitment to the effort by key members of the community.

CASE EXAMPLE

In this section, we describe efforts in the state of Oregon to reduce illegal sales of tobacco to young people as one example of an effort to translate research into practice. Our experience exemplifies many, but not all, of the points made above about how science might be better used in prevention.

Cigarette smoking is the number one preventable cause of disease and death, and is firmly established as a cause of numerous cancers, heart disease, emphysema, and pulmonary disease (Centers for Disease Control and Prevention, 1989, 1990). Most smokers become addicted during adolescence (U.S. Department of Health and Human Services, 1994). Thus, it is likely that many of the deaths due to tobacco product use could be prevented if we could prevent young people from becoming addicted.

One avenue to preventing teenage addiction involves decreasing adolescents' access to tobacco products. All 50 states have laws prohibiting the sale of tobacco to those under 18. However, studies of teen access to tobacco have shown that from 57% to 100% of outlets in communities are willing to make these sales (Forster & Wolfson, 1998). As evidence has become available that decreasing such sales can contribute to lowering the prevalence of youthful tobacco use (Jason, Salina, Hedecker, & Kimball, 1991), the importance of reducing illegal sales has been increasingly recognized.

For these reasons, we included a program to reduce illegal sales of tobacco to young people as one component of a community intervention to prevent adolescent tobacco use that we experimentally evaluated (Biglan, Ary, Smolkowski, Duncan et al., 2000). When we began the project in 1991, laws prohibiting such sales were seldom enforced. Law enforcement officials argued that the time and effort required to patrol stores and cite offenders had to be devoted to more serious crimes. Moreover, they did not believe that there was sufficient community support to justify enforcement. We therefore developed an approach to reducing illegal sales that did not involve law enforcement. Instead, it involved mobilizing reinforcement for clerks not making illegal sales.

The program had five components: (a) mobilization of community support, (b) education of merchants, (c) changing consequences to clerks for selling and not selling to those under 18 years, (d) publicity about clerks refusals to sell, and (e) feedback to store owners or managers about the extent of clerks' sales to adolescents. The program was evaluated in eight small Oregon communities using multiple baseline designs (Biglan, Ary, & Wagenaar, 2000). In four of the communities, the average baseline sales rate of 62% was reduced to 24% during the intervention (Biglan et al., 1995). These effects were replicated in the second set of four communities (Biglan et al., 1996). Across all eight communities the percentage of outlets willing to sell tobacco to young people was reduced from a baseline level of 57% to 22%.

Disseminating the Program in Oregon

Having established some confidence that the approach could reduce illegal tobacco sales, we tried to make it available to other communities in Oregon. At the time that we developed it, some argued that it would not be very useful for other communities because it required paid staff that would not be available in most communities. We could say little in rejoinder; the analysis was accurate. However, a number of developments have made it more likely that communities could mount such efforts. First, the passage of the Synar Amendment to the federal Health and Human Services appropriation required each state to assess and reduce illegal sales of tobacco to young people or lose some of its federal subsidy for drug abuse treatment (Federal Register, 1993). This led to a substantial increase in the efforts of the State of Oregon and local communities to reduce illegal sales. Second, in 1996 Oregonians approved a ballot measure that added 30 cents a pack to the price of cigarettes and dedicated 10% of that revenue to tobacco reduction activities. These funds made it possible to hire staff in every county and in most larger communities to work on tobacco control. Thus, an infrastructure had become available for implementing our access reduction program.

These developments suggest a general principle about translating prevention science into practice. Many communities lack resources to pay, train, and supervise the skilled people who are needed to successfully implement research-based interventions. Although these barriers have typically been taken to imply that researchers should develop cheaper, more foolproof interventions, it is also possible to develop the infrastructure that is needed to implement the interventions. The identification of an effective, yet expensive social intervention need not imply that its dissemination is impossible. It might rather be taken to define the community infrastructure which further research must figure out how to achieve.

Initial Dissemination Efforts

In 1996 and 1997, we implemented the access reduction intervention in three communities under a contract from the Oregon Office of Alcohol and Drug Abuse Programs. In Salem a paid staff person implemented the program with the assistance of numerous adolescent and adult volunteers. Sales were reduced approximately 66% by implementation of the program, and, by follow-up, sales were only 14.5% of what they had been at the outset. In Bend, where our Salem staff person worked with local community members, sales decreased from 73% of stores to 0% after reward and reminder visits, and sales remained at 11% at follow-up. In Tillamook, sales were reduced by about 89% by the program, although 17% of stores remained willing to sell at follow-up.

Subsequent Efforts

In 1998 and 1999, tobacco prevention funds were available to counties thanks to the increased tobacco tax. Four Oregon counties chose to use some of the money to contract directly with our organization to conduct the entire access intervention. As contractors, we were given responsibility either to carry out or to be involved in all five components of the intervention. Thus, we were able to ensure maximum adherence to the empirically evaluated model and to use our own methods of data collection, allowing us to evaluate the results based on the same criteria used in our research.

There was, however, wide variation in the level of implementation desired by each contracting county. The local coalitions directing the contracts varied in composition, in the priority they gave to reducing youth access to tobacco within their grant work plan, and in the level of available funding for the project. In addition, there was variation in county demographic composition.

Unfortunately, in three of these counties, we were not asked to collect baseline data prior to implementing the program. However, in all but one county, the proportion of stores willing to sell tobacco after the program was implemented was below 17%. In the fourth county it was 30.3% and 27.3% in the two post-intervention assessments.

We provided training to personnel in seven other counties that chose to implement the program on their own. Data are available from the state assessments of sales that were done in each of these counties in each of 4 years, but data from the results of the actual reward and reminder visits were not available. The state's assessments were only conducted in a random sample of stores in the county, and thus provided only an estimate of the sales rate. In three of the seven counties which received training in the program, the proportion of outlets willing to sell was clearly lower after the intervention than before. In the remaining counties, the sales rates across years were quite variable and not clearly related to the provision of training.

The Generic Features of This Effort

Oregon's effort to reduce illegal sales of tobacco exemplifies many of the practices we believe are needed to translate science into effective practice. The decision to reduce illegal sales of tobacco was dictated by the Synar Amendment. However, the decision was based on epidemiological and etiological evidence about the extent of illegal sales of tobacco and their role in the addiction of young people to tobacco. A state-level task force was created that allowed for representatives of all sectors of the state to give input, and local tobacco control coalitions made the decisions about the strategies to be used in reducing sales in individual communities. Thanks to tax-generated funds, an infrastructure of staff was created to work on tobacco control. Prompted by the Synar Amendment, the state set up a scientifically valid system for monitoring the level of illegal sales in the state—although its accuracy at the community level was limited due to sample size in communities. Because the first author was on the state's task force implementing the Synar Amendment, information about our reward and reminder intervention was communicated to state and community leaders. Although this falls short of scientists providing a meta-analysis of all available evidence, it put practitioners in closer contact with empirical evidence than often has been the case. Finally, the access reduction intervention was evaluated through the collection of data on outlets' willingness to sell.

FUTURE DIRECTIONS

This chapter has described a set of practices which would make it more likely that our society will make effective use of prevention science. These practices can be established through further research and through government and private sector funding. The practice of clearly articulating what programs and policies are likely to be effective will be facilitated by: (a) the creation of a registry of prevention trials, (b) the development of consensus about standards for identifying disseminable programs and policies, and (c) increased advocacy by scientific organizations for the adoption of empirically supported interventions.

The dissemination and effective implementation of empirically supported interventions will be enhanced by: (a) effectiveness studies in which further evaluations of programs are conducted in and by the organizations that will ultimately be providing the intervention, (b) the development of specialists in dissemination within the prevention science community, and (c) experimental evaluations of strategies for dissemination.

If states and communities increase their monitoring of human well-being, it will focus public attention on the prevention of human behavior problems and favor the selection of effective methods of preventing those problems. These developments will be facilitated by research that identifies systems for quickly and efficiently gathering assessment data and making such systems effectively available to all decision makers and by the appropriation of funds to help states and communities create such monitoring systems.

Improvements in our ability to prevent human behavior problems will accelerate if experimental evaluations of policies and programs become commonplace. A concerted effort on the part of scientific organizations to advocate the value of experimental evaluations is needed.

Finally, we must recognize that scientists' ability to assist society in solving its problems requires a high degree of public trust. Thus, prevention scientists must adhere to ethical principles that ensure respect for the privacy and autonomy of individuals and meaningful participation of all stakeholders in decisions about the programs, policies, and evaluation procedures that states or communities adopt.

ACKNOWLEDGMENT

This chapter was prepared while the first author was a Fellow at the Center for Advanced Study in the Behavioral Sciences. Financial support was provided by the Robert Wood Johnson Foundation (Grant # 034 248) and the National Institutes of Health (Grant # BCS 960 1236). It also was supported, in part, by the National Cancer Institute (Grant # CA38273).

REFERENCES

Avorn, J., & Soumerai, S.B. (1983). Improving drug-therapy decisions through educational outreach: A randomized controlled trial of academically based "detailing." *New England Journal of Medicine, 308,* 1457–1463.

Biglan, A. (1995). *Changing cultural practices: A contextualist framework for intervention research*. Reno, NV: Context Press.

Biglan, A., Henderson, J., Humphreys, D., Yasui, M., Whisman, R., Black, C., & James, L. E. (1995). Mobilising positive reinforcement to reduce youth access to tobacco. *Tobacco Control, 4*, 42–48.

Biglan, A., Ary, D. V., Koehn, V., Levings, D., Smith, S., Wright, Z., James, L., & Henderson, J. (1996). Mobilizing positive reinforcement in communities to reduce youth access to tobacco. *American Journal of Community Psychology, 24*, 625–638.

Biglan, A., Brown, H., Maibach, E., & Mrazek, P. (1999). *Translating prevention science into effective prevention practices: A proposal from the society for prevention research*. Unpublished grant proposal.

Biglan, A., Ary, D. V., Smolkowski, K., Duncan, T. E., & Black, C. (2000). A randomized control trial of a community intervention to prevent adolescent tobacco use. *Tobacco Control, 9*, 24–32.

Biglan, A., Ary, D. V., & Wagenaar, A. C. (2000). The value of interrupted time-series experiments for community intervention research. *Prevention Research, 1*, 31–49.

Biglan, A., & Glasgow, R. E. (1991). The social unit: An important facet in the design of cancer control research. *Preventive Medicine, 20*, 292–305.

Biglan, A., Mrazek, P., Carnine, D. W., & Flay, B. R. (in press). The integration of research and practice in the prevention of youth problem behaviors. *American Psychologist*.

Biglan, A., & Taylor, T. (2000). Increasing the use of science to improve child rearing. *Journal of Primary Prevention, 21*, 207–226.

Centers for Disease Control and Prevention (1989). *Reducing the health consequences of smoking: 25 years of progress. A report of the Surgeon General* (DHSS Publication No. CDC 89–8411). Washington, DC: U.S. Department of Health and Human Services.

Centers for Disease Control and Prevention (1990). Cigarette smoking-attributable mortality and years of potential life cost–United States, 1990. *Morbidity and Mortality Weekly Report, 42*, 645–649.

Chambless, D. L., & Hollon, S. D. (1998). Defining empirically supported therapies. *Journal of Consulting and Clinical Psychology, 66*, 7–18.

COMMIT (1991). Community Intervention Trial for smoking cessation (COMMIT): Summary of design and intervention. *Journal of the National Cancer Institute, 83*, 1620–1628.

Cook, T. D., & Campbell, D. T. (1979). *Quasi-experimentation: Design and analysis issues for field settings*. Chicago: Rand McNally.

Derzon, J. H., Wilson, S., & Cunningham, C. A. (1999). *The effectiveness of school-based interventions for preventing and reducing violence*. Nashville,

TN: Vanderbilt University, Center for Evaluation Research and Methodology, Vanderbilt Institute for Public Policy Studies.

Durlak, J. A., & Wells, A. M. (1997). Primary prevention mental health programs for children and adolescents: A meta-analytic review. *American Journal of Community Psychology, 25,* 115–152.

Federal Register (1993). Substance abuse prevention and treatment block grants: Sale or distribution of tobacco products to individuals under 18 years of age. *Federal Register, 45, 58, 156.*

Flay, B. R. (1986). Efficacy and effectiveness trials (and other phases of research) in the development of health promotion programs. *Preventive Medicine, 15,* 451–474.

Forster, J. L., Murray, D. M., Wolfson, M., Blaine, T. M., Wagenaar, A. C., & Hennrikus, D. J. (1998). The effects of community policies to reduce youth access to tobacco. *American Journal of Public Health, 88,* 1193–1198.

Forster, J. L., & Wolfson, M. (1998). Youth access to tobacco: Policies and politics. *Annual Review of Public Health, 19,* 203–235.

Greenwald, P., & Cullen, J. W. (1985). The new emphasis in cancer control. *Journal of National Cancer Institute, 74,* 543–551.

Halberstam, D. (1987). *The reckoning.* New York: Morrow Avon.

Hershey, C. O., Goldberg, H. I., & Cohen, D. I. (1988). The effect of computerized feedback coupled with a newsletter upon outpatient prescribing charges: A randomized controlled trial. *Medical Care, 26,* 88–94.

Hoagwood, K., & Koretz, D. (1996). Embedding prevention services within systems of care: Strengthening the nexus for children. *Applied and Preventive Psychology, 5,* 225–234.

Holder, H. D. (1998). *Alcohol and the community: A systems approach to prevention.* Cambridge: Cambridge University Press.

Holder, H., Flay, B., Howard, J., Boyd, G., Voas, R., & Grossman, M. (1999). Phases of alcohol problem prevention research. *Alcoholism: Clinical & Experimental Research, 23,* 183–194.

Jason, L., Salina, D., Hedecker, D., & Kimball, P. (1991). Designing an effective worksite smoking cessation program using self-help manuals, incentives, groups and media. *Journal of Business & Psychology, 6,* 155–166.

Jason, L. A., & Rose, T. (1984). Influencing the passage of child passenger restraint legislation. *American Journal of Community Psychology, 12,* 485–495.

Lipsey, M. W., & Wilson, D. B. (1993). The efficacy of psychological, educational, and behavioral treatment: Confirmation from meta-analysis. *American Psychologist, 48,* 1181–1209.

Monyihan, D. P. (1996). *Miles to go: A personal history of social policy.* Cambridge, MA: Harvard University Press.

Mrazek, P. J., & Haggerty, R. J. (1994). *Reducing risks for mental disorders: Frontiers for preventive intervention research.* Washington, DC: National Academy Press.

Murray, D. M., & Wolfinger, R. D. (1994). Analysis issues in the evaluation of community trials: Progress toward solutions in SAS/STAT MIXED. *Journal of Community Psychology, 22,* 140–154.

National Institute on Drug Abuse (1997). *Drug abuse prevention package* (NTIS Publication No. 97–209605). Rockville, MD: U.S. Department of Health and Human Services, National Institutes of Health.

O'Malley, P. M., Bachman, J. G., Johnston, L. D., & Schulenberg, J. (in press). Studying the transition from youth to adulthood: Impacts on substance use and abuse. In J. F. House, T. Juster, H. Schuman, E. Singer, & R. Kahn (Eds.), *A telescope on society: Survey research and social science in the 20th & 21st centuries.*

Perry, C. L., Williams, C. L., Veblen-Mortenson, S., & Toomey, T. L. (1996). Project Northland: Outcomes of a communitywide alcohol use prevention program during early adolescence. *American Journal of Public Health, 86,* 956–965.

Taylor, T. K., & Biglan, A. (1998). Behavioral family interventions: A review for clinicians and policymakers. *Clinical Child and Family Psychology Review, 1,* 41–60.

Tobler, N. S., & Stratton, H. H. (1997). Effectiveness of school-based drug prevention programs: A meta-analysis of the research. *Journal of Primary Prevention, 18,* 71–128.

U.S. Department of Health and Human Services (1994). *Preventing tobacco use among young people: A report of the Surgeon General.* Atlanta, GA: U.S. Department of Health and Human Services, Public Health Service, Centers for Disease Control and Prevention, National Center for Chronic Disease Prevention and Health Promotion, Office of Smoking and Health.

Wagenaar, A. C., Murray, D. M., Wolfson, M., & Forster, J. L. (1994). Communities mobilizing for change on alcohol: Design of a randomized community trial. *Journal of Community Psychology, 22,* 79–101.

CHAPTER 3

Teaching About Prevention to Mental Health Professionals

Jacob Kraemer Tebes,

Joy S. Kaufman, and

Matthew J. Chinman

DESCRIPTION OF THE PROBLEM

For the past four decades, there has been tremendous growth in prevention research and practice (Albee, 1996; Glenwick & Jason, 1993; National Institute of Mental Health [NIMH], 1998). Prevention has emerged as an important professional activity in a variety of disciplines, including psychology, public health, medicine, nursing, social work, and education. Prevention and health promotion also are widely accepted as integral components of American mental health policy and are viewed as critical to the nation's health and welfare in the 21st century (U.S. Surgeon General, 1999).

However, during this same period, teaching about prevention has not progressed in a manner commensurate with its growth in research and practice. There are two primary reasons for this: (a) there is currently no consensus on what the essential knowledge in prevention is (NIMH, 1998; Price, 1986), and (b) because prevention training today occurs across so many different disciplines, there is no consensus on how teaching should occur, what its components should be, and what the key professional roles and competencies for prevention professionals should be.

In this chapter, these issues are addressed by summarizing core concepts in prevention and by describing how they are conceptualized and taught across several disciplines and in various professional contexts. The chapter is timely for several reasons. First, the field continues to grow at a pace so rapid that its successful integration across disciplines and professional endeavors remains in doubt. Our attempt at integration is intended to form the basis for integrating teaching about prevention to mental health professionals. Second, recent efforts that have emphasized theoretical and methodological pluralism within the social sciences in general, and prevention and health promotion in particular (Hays, 1994; Humphreys, 1993; MacLachlan, 2001; Rosnow, 1993; Royce, 1987; Sechrest & Sidani, 1995; Tebes, 1997; Tebes & Kraemer, 1991), provide a conceptual framework consistent with the adoption of an integrative approach to teaching about prevention.

The term "teaching about prevention" is used (as opposed to training in prevention or teaching prevention skills) to underline the broader educative purpose in this endeavor. The domain of "mental health professional" is defined more expansively than is typically the case, in order to include professionals from a range of disciplines who, in the course of their research or practice, concern themselves with issues in mental health.

To provide a context for understanding the current state of education in prevention, we begin by briefly tracing its history in America.

A Synopsis of 20th Century Prevention in America

Prevention in mental health had its roots in the mental hygiene, child guidance, and settlement house movements in the early part of the last century (Levine & Levine, 1970; Long, 1989; Mrazek & Haggerty, 1994; NIMH, 1998). These "first generation" efforts (NIMH, 1998) were essentially humanitarian. Citizens and some professionals intervened to relieve human suffering among the poor and most vulnerable in the general population in order to promote "positive mental health" and well-being (Levine & Levine, 1970; NIMH, 1998). Virtually none of this work was based on scientific research, very little was professionalized, and most of it did not involve government intervention.

Prevention emerged as a major scientific and professional activity in its own right when it was included prominently in the report of the President's Joint Commission on Mental Illness and Health (1961). The report maintained that the mental health needs of the public were too great in number, too diverse in kind, and too rooted in the social context to be addressed only with individual treatment delivered by highly trained professionals. As a result, it recommended the development of larger-scale, community-based interventions aimed at preventing problems before treatment was necessary (Joint Commission on Mental Health & Illness, 1961; Levine & Perkins, 1987).

The report also stimulated a variety of innovative approaches to meet the mental health needs of the general population. Congressional approval of the Community Mental Health Centers Act in 1963 was an outgrowth of these developments and established an active federal role for prevention. This act divided population centers into roughly equal catchment areas to be served by a community mental health center. Each qualifying center received federal funds for a range of direct clinical services and for mandated indirect services in consultation and education. These latter services usually were initiated before the onset of specific problems or disorders and, thus, were preventive interventions. However, most federal funding for consultation and education terminated after eight years, causing many mental health centers to eliminate prevention services (Snow & Newton, 1976; Zolik, 1983). Nevertheless, prevention had become a formal part of U.S. policy.

Prevention also had taken hold among the public, practitioners, and scientists. It was championed by advocacy groups, such as the National Mental Health Association (Long, 1989), and was the focus of a variety of scientific and professional meetings in the 1970s and 1980s, such as the Vermont Conference on the Primary Prevention of Psychopathology (Albee, 1996). Prevention also featured prominently in the report of the President's Commission on Mental Health (1978). The commission report recommended an expanded federal role for prevention efforts, including increased federal support for the training of prevention researchers and establishment of an Office of Prevention Research at the National Institute of Mental Health, which came to pass in 1982. Beginning in the 1980s and continuing to the present, this office and its various institutional successors established a strong track record for promoting prevention research, training, and practice (NIMH, 1998). The federal role in prevention and health promotion was further strengthened after the reorganization of NIMH as a research institute within the National Institutes of Health (NIH) in 1992 and the subsequent establishment of the Substance Abuse and Mental Health Services Administration (SAMHSA) as a separate agency that supported prevention services as one of its activities (through its Center for Mental Health Services [CMHS] and Center for Substance Abuse Prevention [CSAP]). Federal leadership in prevention and health promotion also was fostered through dramatic increases in funding for prevention services or research by such agencies as NIMH, CMHS, CSAP, the former Alcohol, Drug Abuse, and Mental Health Administration (ADAMHA), the National Institute on Drug Abuse (NIDA), the National Institute on Alcohol Abuse and Alcoholism (NIAAA), the Department of Justice (DOJ), and the Department of Education (DOE). During the 1980s and continuing to the present, many of these federal agencies also provided funding for prevention training at the pre- and postdoctoral levels, and sponsored conferences to promote prevention research and practice. These federal initiatives have stimulated and, in some cases, paralleled state initiatives to increase the availability of prevention and health promotion services.

The Emergence of Prevention Science

Governmental and advocacy efforts to enhance prevention services and research during this "second generation" of prevention (NIMH, 1998) have mirrored an explosive growth in prevention research over the past quarter century. Among the most important developments in this growth over the past 15 years has been the emergence of prevention science (Heller, 1996; Reiss & Price, 1996). Recent reports issued by two independent panels on prevention research—one convened by the Institute of Medicine (Mrazek & Haggerty, 1994), the other by NIMH (1996)—have further elaborated the basis for the new prevention science. Both reports were subsequently consolidated into a Report to the National Advisory Mental Health Council entitled *A Plan for Prevention Research for the National Institute of Mental Health* (NIMH, 1996), and were summarized in the scholarly literature (Munoz, Mrazek, & Haggerty, 1996; Reiss & Price, 1996). A more recent report by the Council entitled *Priorities for Prevention Research at NIMH* (NIMH, 1998), provides the most comprehensive statement to date of the new prevention science.

Prevention science represents a shift in the field's conceptualization of preventive research and practice. Priority is now given to individual change as opposed to social change and, specifically, to individual change as it pertains to psychiatric disorder (NIMH, 1996). Preventive interventions are no longer classified as primary, secondary, or tertiary, but rather are divided into three types: *universal, selective*, and *indicated* (Gordon, 1987; NIMH, 1996). Universal interventions target the general public or entire population groups regardless of risk status; selective interventions target individuals or population subgroups whose risk of developing the disorder may be higher than average; and indicated interventions target high-risk individuals who have "minimal, but detectable signs, or biological markers, indicating predisposition for the mental disorder, but who do not meet diagnostic criteria" (NIMH, 1996, p. 6). This taxonomy represents a conceptual shift, which makes it possible to regard preventive intervention as part of a continuum, which includes individual mental health treatment and maintenance services, including rehabilitation (Munoz, Mrazek, & Haggerty, 1996). All three types of preventive interventions involve varying levels of primary prevention; that is, they are initiated prior to the onset of a psychiatric disorder. Individual treatment includes case findings and standard approaches to intervention, all of which usually take place during an acute episode of disorder (NIMH, 1996). Maintenance interventions are delivered after an acute episode has passed, with the goal of reducing relapses or recurrences of the disorder, and also may include rehabilitative services (NIMH, 1996).

The primary focus of intervention in prevention science is risk reduction. Risk is defined as "those characteristics, variables, or hazards that, if present for a given individual, make it more likely that this individual, rather than someone selected from the general population, will develop a disorder" (NIMH, 1996, p. 6). Whenever possible, risk and protective factors should be considered in their interaction, even though the primary aim of research and intervention is the reduction of risk (Mrazek & Haggerty, 1994; Reiss & Price, 1996). For risk reduction to be most effective, it should be implemented in developmentally appropriate contexts which address the transactional nature of both risk and protection (Mrazek & Haggerty, 1994). It also should be informed by epidemiological data about the distribution of mental disorders and patterns of risk in a given population (Kellam, Koretz, & Moscicki, 1999; Mrazek & Haggerty, 1994; NIMH, 1996).

Finally, prevention science advances knowledge through adherence to the "preventive intervention research cycle" (Mrazek & Haggerty, 1994; NIMH, 1996). The first phase of this cycle is the identification of a problem or disorder that is to be the target of intervention. This is followed by a review of risk and protective factors that are associated with the onset of the disorder or the problem being considered. In the cycle's third phase, pilot, confirmatory, and replication studies of the preventive intervention are conducted to determine its efficacy. During this phase, a theoretical model is specified to guide the research, and, if possible, randomized controlled efficacy trials are completed and then followed by a replication study. In the fourth phase, large-scale field trials of efficacious preventive interventions are implemented and evaluated for their effectiveness in a real-world setting. Whenever possible, effectiveness trials should be implemented under controlled conditions, particularly in the case of indicated or selective interventions. In the final phase of the cycle, effective preventive interventions are implemented in the community. Large-scale, community-based interventions should be initiated only after partnerships have been developed between researchers and community members to ensure that the interventions that are implemented are attuned to local conditions, and that appropriate measures of program monitoring and evaluation are included (Fawcett, Paine, Francisco, Richter, & Lewis, 1994; Reiss & Price, 1996).

The most recent report by the National Advisory Mental Health Council which established NIMH priorities for prevention research has proposed an expanded definition of prevention research that goes beyond what historically was known as "primary prevention" (NIMH, 1998). This definition includes: (a) studies of basic biological and clinical processes that may inform subsequent efficacy and effectiveness trials and (b) studies of already diagnosed populations who may be at risk for comorbid disorders or treated through service systems. The former expands the conceptual framework for pre-intervention research, while the latter divides intervention studies into preventive intervention research and preventive services research. The resulting continuum of pre-intervention, preventive intervention, and preventive services research with both asymptomatic and diagnosed individuals offers new opportunities for improving mental health and preventing mental disorders.

This conceptual continuum also contains new possibilities and perils for the training of prevention professionals. Prevention can now more easily be integrated into university training programs and post-degree professional offerings that emphasize treatment and rehabilitation services and research. This also may foster integration of the prevention knowledge base across disciplines and training programs, particularly among those in medicine and psychology. However, there are at least two risks associated with this development as well. First, integration of prevention training into more clinical- and rehabilitation-based programs of study and post-degree offerings may disperse even further the types of roles and competencies expected from prevention professionals. This may make it virtually impossible to develop a consensus about what the knowledge base for prevention is and how prevention professionals should be trained.

A second risk associated with adopting the conceptual continuum described above is that the field will eschew prevention efforts aimed at changing "problems in living" (Heller & Monahan, 1977)—such as poverty, unemployment, social isolation, and racism—that may not involve diagnosable mental disorders but that do have an impact on the public's mental health and general welfare. This original framework for prevention has directed efforts beyond intra-individual and interpersonal processes to social processes and structures (Albee, 1996; Heller & Monahan, 1977). Within this latter perspective, mental disorders share something in common with other problems in living; both were caused, exacerbated, or maintained by social factors such as social institutions, community settings, the peer group, the school, and the family (Albee, 1982; Cowen, 1980; Levine & Perkins, 1987; Price, 1974). This emphasis on the prevention of problems in living as rooted in individual responses to social structures and processes also made explicit the view that such problems were intrinsic to political systems and to the maldistribution of power within those systems (Albee, 1982; Dohrenwend, 1978; Rappaport, 1977). A prevention science focused on the prevention of individual mental disorders—defined within a classification system in which illnesses are diagnosed essentially in isolation from their sociopolitical context, for example, the *DSM-IV* (American Psychiatric Association, 1994)—is likely to devalue or dismiss claims about the social causes of problems in living and attempts to address them through social action. It is also not likely to foster the training of prevention professionals in these approaches.

REVIEW AND CRITIQUE OF THE LITERATURE

We will review teaching about prevention in two areas: (a) graduate training within universities and (b) post-degree professional training. The former includes educational experiences within graduate and professional schools and affiliated institutions, while the latter refers to selected training offerings for individuals who have obtained a professional degree or have worked in a professional capacity in a given field. When possible, we summarize this literature by discipline and identify key roles and competencies for each. This is intended to provide an initial basis for a subsequent interdisciplinary, integrative understanding of prevention education for professionals.

Graduate Training Within Universities

Graduate training in prevention takes place at the master's and doctoral levels in several disciplines, including psychology, public health, preventive medicine, public health nursing, social work, and education. Training experiences also occur at the postdoctoral or post-residency level, but these are too varied and specialized to be reviewed here.

Community psychology

In graduate psychology programs, the greatest emphasis on prevention training comes from the field of community psychology. When community psychology was established at the 1965 Swampscott Conference as a separate field of study, a commitment to prevention was a major impetus in its formation (Bennett et al., 1966). The new Community Mental Health Centers Act, calling for community-based treatment, consultation, and education services, recently had been passed by Congress. Conference participants, many of whom were trained in clinical psychology, recognized an urgent need not only to develop innovative community-based programs to meet the needs of persons already in treatment, but also to prevent or reduce the incidence of problems in living (Bennett et al., 1966). Community psychology's commitment to prevention as a central focus in graduate training was restated at a subsequent national conference on training in 1975 (Iscoe, Bloom, & Spielberger, 1977). Within a decade, the new field of community psychology had become the leading institutional voice within psychology for prevention (Cowen, 1984; Price, 1983; Zolik, 1983).

Price (1983, 1986) articulated perhaps the most comprehensive framework for graduate psychology training in prevention. He proposed four major domains of activity for prevention research and practice: (a) problem analysis, (b) intervention design, (c) field trials, and (d) diffusion of preventive interventions. Each domain corresponds to specific roles that may be carried out by prevention professionals and overlaps, partially, in theory and practice with a subsequent domain. The problem analyst identifies and assesses risks that may lead to negative psychological outcomes. The analyst's primary tools are survey and epidemiological research concerning risk factors for a given problem or disorder. In contrast, the interventionist spans two roles, that of innovation designer and implementer of field trials. Price (1986) argued that these two roles may overlap because innovations are often developed to be implemented as a field trial. What distinguishes these roles is that designing an intervention involves implementation planning and attention to program theory that is relatively independent of a subsequent evaluation, whereas conducting a field trial is explicitly focused on evaluating the intervention. A final role for the prevention professional involves the diffusion of an innovation. This role requires the preventionist to be able to understand and negotiate larger systems in which interventions will be disseminated.

Although Price's (1986) framework is useful in the graduate training of prevention scientists, it does not adequately address domains of prevention practice in which both applied and academic psychologists are likely to find themselves. At The Consultation Center at Yale, we have built on Price's (1986) framework to develop a model for predoctoral training in prevention that balances more effectively scientist and practioner roles and expected competencies. Details about this training program are provided in the Case Example section below.

Finally, prevention is also a focus within other fields of psychology, such as developmental psychology, school psychology, health psychology, and clinical psychology, as well as various subfields such as developmental psychopathology, the study of addictive disorders, and the psychological study of social issues. In contrast to community psychology, in which prevention has a central focus, in these other fields this is usually not the case.

Public Health

Public health is the profession dedicated to the promotion of health and the prevention of disease. Although most professional activities in public health involve physical health and illness, an increasing focus within public health is mental health (Perry, Albee, Bloom, & Gullotta, 1996). Graduate training in public health takes place in a university school of public health or a medical school, which awards a master's (MPH, MHS, or MS) or doctoral degree (PhD, ScD, or DrPH). In addition, advanced professional training is also available through various public and private health service agencies and institutions, such as the Centers for Disease Control and Prevention.

Several fields of study within public health have particular relevance to mental health prevention. Mental health epidemiology is concerned with: (a) the distribution of mental disorders within population groups and (b) the variation in risk and protective factors associated with specific disorders and groups. The former is characteristic of descriptive epidemiology, whereas the latter is emblematic of analytical epidemiology, in that it provides a basis for the identification of causal relationships among risk, protective factors, and health outcomes (Kellam, Koretz, & Moscicki, 1999). Health care policy and administration is concerned with training professionals in skills essential to management in health care settings and effective policy development and analysis. Applied prevention and preventive services research provides graduate training in the design, implementation, and evaluation of preventive interventions and preventive services in community settings. An underlying principle in public health practice is the commitment to social justice. As a result, public health professionals are trained to be able to move conceptually and pragmatically from epidemiological research and problem analysis to policy change and social action (Cwikel, 1994).

Competencies in public health have much in common with those obtained through graduate training in community psychology. For example, training in applied prevention and preventive services research prepares one for competency in the implementation of field trials of preventive interventions and services. Similarly, aspects of health care policy and administration involve competencies in organizational and systems consultation and advocacy.

Preventive Medicine

In this section we describe "postgraduate" (internship and residency) medical training, which takes place after the completion of medical school. "Undergraduate" training in medicine refers to the completion of 4 years of medical school after obtaining a baccalaureate degree and is not discussed here.

Preventive medicine is the specialty within medicine that is committed to disease prevention and health promotion. It includes specialties in general medicine/public health, occupational medicine, and aerospace medicine. According to the American College of Preventive Medicine (Lane, Ross, Chen, & O'Neill, 1999), specialists in preventive medicine have competencies and knowledge in one or more of the following areas: biostatistics; epidemiology; environmental and occupational health; planning, administration, and evaluation of health services; the social and behavioral aspects of health and disease; and the practice of prevention in clinical medicine. Several of these competencies overlap with roles and competencies described above for graduate training in community psychology and public health. For example, one core competency for residents emphasizes that preventive medicine specialists should be able to identify "the processes by which decisions are made within an organization or agency and their points of influence" (Lane, Ross, Chen, & O'Neill, 1999, p. 369). This competency is comparable to community psychology training in organizational and systems consultation or public health training in health policy administration. Another core competency is the ability to communicate effectively with target groups, such as health professionals, the public, and the media, about matters of public health and the rationale for selected interventions. This corresponds to training in community psychology and public health which emphasizes one's role as an advocate. Furthermore, competencies in clinical preventive medicine are comparable to those required in community psychology training in prevention that focus on developing effective intervention designs. Finally, competencies in biostatistics/epidemiology resemble those essential for a problem analyst and also overlap significantly with competencies established through graduate training in public health.

Public Health Nursing

In the nursing profession, public health (or community health) nursing emphasizes health promotion and disease or injury prevention. A specialization in public health nursing prepares the nurse to apply population-based interventions for the promotion of physical health and the prevention of disease, such as cancer screening, immunizations, and the prevention of lead poisoning (Gerrity & Kinsey, 1999). Increasingly, however, public health nurses are involved in mental health-related interventions, such as the promotion of positive parenting and the prevention of family violence, and have developed practice guidelines resembling competencies found in community psychology, public health, and preventive medicine (Lia-Hoagberg, Schaffer, & Strohschein, 1999). For example, effective public communication and media advocacy is increasingly considered to be an important competency for public health nurses (Flynn, 1998).

Social Work

Dating back to the settlement house movement, social workers have a long tradition of community-based services to promote the public welfare (Levine & Levine, 1970). Social workers' involvement in community outreach, advocacy, and community organizing with vulnerable populations are exemplars of macro-level approaches to prevention. More recent developments have established a more explicit focus on prevention and health promotion in graduate programs of social work (Bowker, 1983). In 1985, the Division of Maternal and Child Health of the U.S. Public Health Service sponsored a conference to develop a plan for public health social work practice, which resulted in recommendations for the training of social workers in prevention and public health approaches (Gitterman, Black, & Stein, 1985), a plan that accelerated the development of graduate-level public health social work training programs (Siefert, Jayarante, & Martin, 1992). Many of these programs offer a joint MSW/MPH degree to train public health social workers in the development, implementation, management, and evaluation of prevention and health promotion programs in social service organizations (Hooyman, Schwanke, & Yesner, 1980; Siefert, Jayarante, & Martin, 1992). Expected competencies for graduate training in public health social work are established by individual degree programs.

Education

Educational settings, such as schools and early childhood centers, represent the most common institutional basis for preventive and health-promotive interventions. Perhaps the most widely implemented and successful early childhood preventive intervention is Project Head Start (Zigler & Styfco, 1998). This intervention provides a range of educational, health, and social services to young children and their families living in poverty and has been shown to promote social competence in millions of children and parents (Zigler & Styfco, 1998). More recent preventive interventions that are being implemented in schools include "full-service schools," which provide a variety of integrated health, supportive, and preventive services to children, families, and especially youth (Dryfoos, 1994), and "21st century community learning centers," which provide supervised and structured after-school care and family support to school-aged children (U.S. Department of Education, 2000).

The development and implementation of these types of interventions in educational settings involve collaboration across several disciplines. Programs of study in graduate schools of education increasingly are training educators to design, implement, and manage preventive interventions. Doctoral and master's programs which train educators in these skills include programs of study in administration, planning, and public policy; early childhood education; human development; and community education. Competencies in these areas are established by individual degree programs.

Post-Degree Professional Training

Once professionals have received their degree, they often need to obtain more focused training in specific prevention skills. For example, addiction counselors who work with chemically dependent families have been trained to identify and intervene with at-risk family members (Schiff, Cavaiola, & Harrison, 1989). Clergy have been trained in advocacy skills so that they can assist individuals who require pastoral counseling (Weaver & Koenig, 1996). Teachers have been trained to deliver various school-based programs in substance abuse prevention (e.g., Tobler et al., 2000), and parent educators have been trained to implement complementary school-based prevention programs (Tebes, Grady, & Snow, 1989). Finally, a variety of prevention professionals increasingly are being trained in cultural competence skills in order to deliver prevention and health promotion programs more effectively to diverse groups (Johnson, 1997).

Two of the current most common types of prevention training for mental health professionals, namely, training for certification as a prevention professional and training in science-based or evidence-based approaches to prevention.

Certification as a Prevention Professional

A recent development in the training of mental health professionals in prevention is the establishment of standards for certifying individuals as "prevention professionals." The largest accrediting body in this area is the International Certification and Reciprocity Consortium for Alcohol and Other Drug Abuse (IC&RC; *www.icrcaoda.org*). The IC&RC serves as a member association for prevention certification boards from 41 states and territories, seven international countries, all branches of the U.S. Military, the Indian

Health Service, the World Federation of Therapeutic Communities, and the United States Administrative Office of the Courts. This body establishes minimal standards for achieving the status of a Certified Prevention Professional, which include: (a) 1 year (2,000 hours) of general prevention training in alcohol, tobacco, and other drug (ATOD) relevant experiences; 100 contact hours of prevention-specific training (of which 50 hours must include ATOD training); a 120-hour practicum in six performance domains (i.e., program coordination, education and training, community organization, public policy, professional growth and responsibility, and planning and evaluation) and (b) passing the ICRC written prevention exam. Didactic and practicum experiences for certification are provided through institutions and sites who have been pre-approved as qualifying toward certification. Training that is not pre-approved must be demonstrated as relevant by the certification candidate. The uniform aspect of this certification across sites is the ICRC written exam, which covers content in the six performance domains relevant to certification. Other specific criteria for certification, as well as those for recertification, are left up to the individual certification boards.

Completion of the certification exam provides some assurance that prevention professionals have a basic understanding of prevention in different geographic localities. However, because there is currently no consensus as to the body of knowledge essential to prevention practice, the appropriateness of the content chosen for certification is open to debate. Some of the six content domains specified by the IC&RC stress professional competencies that have some relation to those covered in graduate training programs in community psychology, public health, and social work. However, certification does not emphasize knowledge of prevention program theory or preventive science, areas that are increasingly essential to effective prevention practice. We also do not know the professional value or prestige attached to one's certification as a prevention professional. Most mental health professionals who practice in prevention are unfamiliar with the term "certified prevention professional," and many do not list the initials of certification (CPP), along with any graduate degree they may have obtained. This may change if certification becomes more widely known and accepted.

Training in Science-Based Prevention

A growing emphasis in post-degree prevention training is on teaching mental health professionals about science-based or evidence-based approaches to prevention. These approaches involve interventions that have been shown to be effective using systematic research methods (Morrissey et al., 1997). With the current emphasis on accountability in public policy, prevention professionals are being called upon to identify, implement, and monitor—through continu-ous quality assessments—science-based or evidence-based approaches to pre-vention (Fraser & Richman, 1999). The interest in these approaches derives from the continuing gap in effectiveness found between prevention science tri-als and prevention practice (Mrazek & Haggerty, 1994). This gap refers to the observation that positive results from well-evaluated demonstration programs often are not found when these same programs are adopted by local commu-nities (Morrissey et al., 1997). Teaching mental health professionals about sci-ence-based approaches is believed to increase the chance that a program shown to be effective will be implemented in a manner that approximates the condi-tions under which it was successful.

Training in science-based approaches usually addresses one or more of the following skill areas: needs and resources assessment, selection of the most suitable science-based program, the assessment of organizational capacity to implement the program, program implementation, and program evaluation. These areas are discussed here in relation to science-based training in the pre-vention of adolescent substance abuse.

A comprehensive needs and resources assessment identifies the scope and nature of a given community problem or asset, assesses the relationship of related problems or assets to various risk and protective factors, and consid-ers the feasibility of potential solutions to address the problem (Wandersman, Imm, Chinman, & Kaftarian, 2000). This information then is used to inform program development so that an intervention targets the most appropriate risk and protective factors for the population of interest. Conducting and inter-preting a quality needs and resources assessment requires competencies in research design and problem analysis, particularly in understanding phenom-ena at multiple levels of analysis (e.g., from the individual to the policy level). Numerous resources are available to guide trainers to teach about needs and resources assessment, including written manuals (e.g., Office of Substance Abuse Prevention, 1989) and internet resources (e.g., the Community Tool Box, *www.ctb.lsi.ukans.edu* and the Aspen Institute, *www.aspenroundtable.org*).

Many mental health professionals charged with selecting a best practices program after having completed a needs and resources assessment, often are ill-equipped to do so. In part, this is because prevention practitioners may not have had much training in social science or health policy research and, there-fore, have trouble critically examining different programs. Another reason is that federal agencies do not always agree on what constitutes a science- or evi-dence-based program. In the field of substance abuse prevention, for exam-ple, the following six agencies have their own list: (a) the Office of National Drug Control Policy (*www.whitehousedrugpolicy.gov/policy/ndcs/html*), (b) the National Institute of Drug Abuse (*www.health.org/pubs/prev/prevopen.html*), (c) the National Institute of Alcohol Abuse and Alcoholism (*jhoward@willco.*

niaaa.nih.gov), (d) the Center for Substance Abuse Prevention (*www.white-housedrugpolicy.gov/prevent/progeval.html*), (e) the Department of Education (*www.ed.gov/legislation/fedregister/announcements/1998-2/060198c.pdf*), and (f) the Office of Juvenile Justice and Delinquency Prevention (*www.colorado.edu/cspv/ blueprints/index.html*).

In addition to having a sufficient understanding of what is meant by "science-based" when choosing programs to implement, prevention professionals often must determine how well a given science-based program meets the needs of the target population in their local community. A program that has been shown to be effective in one community may not be appropriate for implementation in another community because it may not target local risk or protective factors or be sensitive to specific ethnic, gender, or other local diversity issues. Although the former issue may be readily apparent based on a comprehensive needs and resources assessment, the latter may be unknown because research that takes diversity markers into account in examining program effectiveness is sparse (Tebes, 2000).

As different science-based models are being considered, prevention professionals at agencies or within communities need to assess their capacity to implement the model in question. Do they have the staff, the resources, and/or the knowledge of how to adapt it? The Northeast Center for the Application of Prevention Technology, funded by the Center for Substance Abuse Prevention, has developed a "feasibility tool" that can help mental health professionals answer some of these capacity questions (Goddard & McLean, 2000). The tool prompts program staff to consider the degree to which they meet the program of interest's requirements in terms of resources (financial, human, technical), target population, favorable community and organizational climate, evaluation capacity, and future sustainability. Although these various scale scores can be used to assess readiness, their relationship to program outcomes has not been established. Also, use of this tool requires training and some prerequisite knowledge of, and experience with, prevention programs.

Mental health professionals are often most familiar with how to implement a prevention program effectively, a factor that has been shown to be essential for a program's success (Gottfredson, Fink, Skroban, & Gottfredson, 1997). A number of issues that are amenable to training may influence a program's implementation. Prevention professionals may not attend to essential details of implementation or may adapt their program in such a way that it no longer retains critical elements of the original science-based model. Implementation staff also may not be fully conversant with the program theory underlying the program. As a result, they may fail to implement certain key aspects of the program because they do not believe them to be important for achieving positive outcomes. Various tools are available to help address these issues (e.g., Wandersman et al., 2000).

Finally, prevention professionals who implement programs are often least familiar with the essentials of program evaluation. Evaluation skills may be critical in a program's success, especially when data are used for ongoing program improvement. There are numerous barriers to successful staff participation in evaluating a prevention program. Staff may have insufficient time or resources to evaluate a program, they may lack an objective perspective to examine their own program critically and systematically, and they may have difficulty accessing a vast scholarly literature (Wandersman et al., 1998). Program evaluation requires an array of skills, some similar to those required for needs and resources assessments, such as knowledge of research design and measurement, understanding of quantitative and qualitative data collection and analysis methods, and the ability to collaborate and communicate effectively with stakeholders and constituent groups. A few evaluation guides for lay audiences have been published (e.g., Bond, Boyd, Raphael, & Sizemore, 1997; Linney & Wandersman, 1991), which, if accompanied by training, provide essential information for prevention professionals.

CASE EXAMPLE

A setting, which illustrates one successful approach to the training of mental health professionals in prevention, is The Consultation Center's training program for predoctoral psychology fellows. The Consultation Center is a multidisciplinary service, research, and training site that is a cooperative endeavor of a university (the Department of Psychiatry, Yale University School of Medicine), a state-funded community mental health center (the Connecticut Mental Health Center), and a private, nonprofit corporation (the Community Consultation Board, Inc.). The mission of the center, which was established in 1978, is to design and implement services and research in order to promote the psychosocial development of individuals and families, to prevent mental disorders and problem behaviors, and to enhance the effectiveness of mental health and other human service organizations and service systems (Snow, 2000). Center services and research involve individuals across the life span, as well as the organizations or systems that serve them.

The center is a multidisciplinary training site for pre- and postdoctoral psychology fellows and psychiatry residents, as well as master's level students from social work, nursing, education, divinity, and public health. The training program for predoctoral psychology fellows emphasizes the teaching of competencies in five areas related to prevention practice and research: professional training and community education, program development, organizational and systems consultation, advocacy and community organizing, and research and evaluation. Each of these competencies is reinforced through: (a) attendance at weekly staff or area meetings in which programs are presented for feedback and review, and guest speakers are invited to address relevant topics; (b) participation in a weekly, year-long seminar which covers each of the areas of competency above, as well as additional topics in human diversity and professional development; and (c) completion of supervised practicum experiences on specific projects.

Prior to the beginning of the training year, the Center's leadership identifies several dozen projects that provide excellent training opportunities for predoctoral psychology fellows. Each project is designed to require a commitment of about 6 hours per week, with primary placement fellows at the center required to complete four projects each and secondary placement fellows two projects each during the year. (Primary placement fellows spend approximately 3 days per week at the center and secondary placement fellows about 1 1/2 days per week at the center. Fellows accepted to the Yale Department of Psychiatry internship at the Connecticut Mental Health Center complete concurrent primary and a secondary placements in two sites during the year.) Within the first few weeks of the internship training year, fellows are introduced to the projects available for selection and meet with their primary advisors to clarify their goals for the year. During those meetings, they are encouraged to select about half of their projects to refine skills or knowledge they already have (e.g., professional training or program development) and to choose the other half of their projects to expand their training into new areas. After submitting their preferences to faculty, every effort is made to match fellows to projects so as to maximize the fellow's training goals.

Below are examples of prevention projects, listed by competency area, that are usually available for selection by fellows: (a) professional training (e.g., teacher training in such areas as peer mediation, crisis resource team development, or substance abuse prevention; training of youth service workers in positive youth development and skills essential in working with youth); (b) community education (e.g., providing workshops to parents, children, and youth on a variety of health promotion topics; conducting one or more workshop series in anger management for adult or juvenile offenders arrested under Connecticut's domestic violence law); (c) program development (e.g., implementation of family support services to at-risk children living with parents with serious mental disorders; development of school- and community-based programs for urban youth to promote academic achievement or prevent school failure); (d) consultation (e.g., program consultation to schools to implement school- or district-wide prevention programs; organizational consultation and technical assistance to human service agencies to restructure community-based services for youth; systems consultation to local and state governments or regional citizen coalitions to implement community-based and preventive services; policy development at the state and local level); (e) advocacy and community organizing (e.g., participation on foundation and nonprofit agency boards to promote a prevention perspective; lobbying in the state legislature to support prevention initiatives; assisting at-risk youth and adult program participants to obtain services and entitlements); (f) evaluation (e.g., completion of needs and resources assessments to develop town, regional, or state-wide prevention services in such areas as school readiness, housing, problem gambling, youth development, after-school programs, child abuse, substance abuse, and elderly services; program evaluations of community-based preventive services in areas such as substance abuse prevention, the promotion of academic achievement among urban youth, delinquency prevention, the prevention of child abuse and neglect, competence promotion among at-risk youth; service system evaluations of state and local community-based and preventive services for children, youth, and families); and (g) research (e.g., pre-intervention, preventive intervention, and preventive services research in adolescent and adult substance abuse prevention; the prevention of HIV/AIDS; the prevention of family violence; the promotion of resilience in at-risk groups, such as children of parents with serious mental disorders, and family caregivers and their children; cost-effectiveness studies).

FUTURE DIRECTIONS

The scope and diversity of research, practice, and training in prevention works against the development of a coherent knowledge base or framework for training prevention professionals. We agree with Price (1986) regarding the need for "boundary spanning" across disciplines and areas of expertise in prevention in order to move the field toward a consensual future. The recent emphasis on mental health epidemiology training for prevention researchers in psychology, the efforts to bring prevention science into the post-degree training of mental health professionals, and an increased focus on incorporating public health concepts into the training of social workers, nurses, and educators are all steps in this direction. A renewed commitment also must be made to strengthen prevention training for primary care physicians and other primary care professionals because these groups are often an individual's first contact with the health care system and, thus, a natural point for early identification and prevention of mental health concerns (e.g., Yager et al., 1989). Despite some of its drawbacks, the recent adoption by NIMH (1998) of an expanded continuum of preventive services that includes a focus on preventive interventions with individuals who have concurrent disorders may rekindle an earlier call (Adams, Chency, Tristan, Friese, & Schweitzer, 1978) to provide prevention training for primary care professionals.

Other examples of innovative boundary spanning and collaboration that have brought diverse perspectives together include use of the mass media and interventions to affect public policy. Jason (1998) has described in some detail how collaborative interventions involving the media can be effective in preventing substance use and HIV/AIDS and promoting health. Others have described how policy changes or the actions of community coalitions can have a substantial impact on the prevention of problems in living (Albee, 1996) or on the quality of life within communities (Dalton, Elias, & Wandersman, 2001). These examples illustrate the value of training the next generation of prevention professionals in the skills necessary to implement multidisciplinary, collaborative, and larger-scale innovations.

As the field enters the "third generation" of prevention in America (NIMH, 1998), we also must consider approaches in which new technologies can facilitate innovative formats for training and professional development. A variety of distance-learning technologies such as Web-based training and video teleconferencing may be particularly promising ways to expand post-degree prevention training. Increasingly, these approaches also are being considered by major research universities as a way to expand their educational offerings for established programs of study. Prevention professionals have long been at the cutting edge and, thus, may be open to newer educational formats.

New technologies also may be instrumental in bringing together prevention professionals across disciplines to establish "effective practice networks" or "prevention study groups" in which professionals with a common interest in prevention join together to share information, ideas, and expertise. These networks can be established on a regional, statewide, or global basis, and sustained through use of Web-based technologies, such as e-mail listservs, chat rooms, and distance-learning approaches. Such structures will enhance future education and training in prevention because of greater shared understanding of the domains of prevention research and practice.

Prevention carries within it the vision of a brighter future. Its proliferation across so many disciplines and professional endeavors signifies its promise. The fulfillment of that promise, however, depends on our commitment to educating the next generation of mental health professionals in its core principles and practices, its methods of knowledge generation and scientific understanding, and its utility for enhancing the public welfare.

REFERENCES

Adams, G. L., Cheney, C. C., Tristan, M. P., Friese, J., & Schweitzer, L. R. (1978). Mental health in primary care training and practice: An innovative approach. *International Journal of Psychiatry in Medicine, 9*, 49–60.

Albee, G. W. (1982). Preventing psychopathology and promoting human potential. *American Psychologist, 37*, 1043–1050.

Albee, G. W. (1996). Revolutions and counterrevolutions in prevention. *American Psychologist, 51*, 1130–1133.

American Psychiatric Association (1994). *Diagnostic and statistical manual of mental health disorders* (4th ed.). Washington, DC: Author.

Bennett, C. C., Anderson, L. S., Cooper, S., Hassol, L., Klein, D. C., & Rosenblum, G. (1966). *Community psychology: A report of the Boston conference on the education of psychologists for community mental health.* Boston: Boston University.

Bond, S. L., Boyd, S. E., Raphael, J. B., & Sizemore, B. A. (1997). *Taking stock: A practical guide to evaluating your own programs.* Chapel Hill, NC: Horizon Research.

Bowker, J. P. (Ed.) (1983). *Education for primary prevention in social work.* New York: Council for Social Work Education.

Cowen, E. L. (1980). The wooing of primary prevention. *American Journal of Community Psychology, 8*, 258–284.

Cowen, E. L. (1984). Training for primary prevention in mental health. *American Journal of Community Psychology, 12*, 253–259.

Cwikel, J. G. (1994). After epidemiological research: What next? Community action for health promotion. *Public Health Reports, 22*, 375–394.

Dalton, J. H., Elias, M. J., & Wandersman, A. (2001). *Community psychology: Linking individuals and communities.* Belmont, CA: Wadsworth/Thompson Learning.

Dohrenwend, B. S. (1978). Social stress and community psychology. *American Journal of Community Psychology, 6*, 1–14.

Dryfoos, J. G. (1994). *Full-service schools: A revolution in health and social services for children, youth, and families.* San Francisco: Jossey Bass.

Fawcett, S. B., Paine, A., Francisco, V., Richter, K., & Lewis, R. (1994). In P. J. Mrazek & R. J. Haggerty (Eds.), *Background materials for reducing risks for mental disorders: Frontiers for preventive intervention research* (pp. 39–68). Washington, DC: National Academy Press.

Flynn, B. C. (1998). Communicating with the public: Community-based nursing research and practice. *Public Health Nursing, 15*, 165–170.

Fraser, M. W., & Richman, J. M. (1999). Risk, protection, and resilience: Toward a conceptual framework for social work practice. *Social Work Research, 23*, 131–143.

Gerrity, P., & Kinsey, K. K. (1999). An urban nurse-managed primary health care center: Health promotion in action. *Family & Community Health, 21,* 29–40.

Gitterman, A., Black, R. B., & Stein, F. (Eds.) (1985). *Public health social work in maternal and child health.* Rockville, MD: Bureau of Health Care Delivery and Assistance, U.S. Department of Health and Human Services.

Glenwick, D. S., & Jason, L. A. (Eds.) (1993). *Promoting health and mental health in children, youth, and families.* New York: Springer Publishing.

Goddard, C. E., & McLean, D. (2000). *Science-based program implementation and adaptation.* New Britain, CT: Northeast Center for the Application of Prevention Technology.

Gordon, R. (1987). An operational classification of disease prevention. In J. Steinberg & M. Silverman (Eds.), *Preventing mental disorders: A research perspective* (DHHS Publication No. ADM 87–1492, pp. 20–26). Rockville, MD: Alcohol, Drug Abuse, and Mental Health Adminstration.

Gottfredson, D. C., Fink, C. M., Skroban, S., & Gottfredson, G. D. (1997). Making prevention work. In R. P. Weissberg, & T. P. Gullotta (Eds.), *Healthy children 2010: Establishing preventive services* (pp. 219–252). Thousand Oaks, CA: Sage.

Hays, B. J. (1994). The new paradigm: Concepts and application in community health nursing. *Public Health Nursing, 11,* 150–154.

Heller, K. (1996). Coming of age of prevention science. *American Psychologist, 51,* 1123–1127.

Heller, K., & Monahan, J. (1977). *Psychology and community change.* Homewood, IL: Dorsey Press.

Hooyman, G., Schwanke, R. W., & Yesner, H. (1980). Public health social work: A training model. *Social Work in Health Care, 6,* 87–99.

Humphreys, K. (1993). Expanding the pluralist revolution: A comment on Omer and Strenger (1992). *Psychotherapy, 30,* 176–177.

Iscoe, I., Bloom, B. L., & Spielberger, C. D. (Eds.) (1977). *Community psychology in transition.* Washington, DC: Hemisphere.

Jason, L. A. (1998). Tobacco, drug, and HIV preventive media interventions. *American Journal of Community Psychology, 26,* 151–173.

Johnson, R. L. (1997). Health perspectives on urban children and youth. In H. J. Wahlberg & O. Reyes (Eds.), *Children and youth: Interdisciplinary perspectives.* Thousand Oaks, CA: Sage.

Joint Commission on Mental Health & Illness. (1961). *Action for mental health.* New York: Basic Books.

Kellam, S. G., Koretz, D., & Moscicki, E. K. (1999). Core elements of developmental epidemiologically-based prevention research. *American Journal of Community Psychology, 27,* 463–482.

Lane, D. S., Ross, V., Chen, D. W., & O'Neill, C. (1999). Core competencies for preventive medicine residents: Version 2.0. *American Journal of Preventive Medicine, 16*, 367–372.

Levine, M., & Levine, A. (1970). *A social history of helping services*. New York: Appleton-Century-Crofts.

Levine, M., & Perkins, D. V. (1987). *Principles of community psychology*. New York: Oxford University Press.

Lia-Hoagberg, B., Schaffer, M., & Strohschein, S. (1999). Public health nursing practice guidelines: An evaluation of dissemination and use. *Public Health Nursing, 16*, 397–404.

Linney, J. A., & Wandersman, A. (1991). *Prevention plus III: Assessing alcohol and other drug prevention programs at the school and community level*. Washington, DC: U.S. Department of Health & Human Services.

Long, B. B. (1989). The Mental Health Association and prevention. *Prevention in Human Services, 6*, 5–44.

MacLachlan, M. (Ed.) (2001). *Cultivating health: Cultural perspectives on promoting health*. Chichester, England: John Wiley & Sons.

Morrissey, E., Wandersman, A., Seybolt, D., Nation, M., Crusto, C., & Davino, K. (1997). Toward a framework for bridging the gap between science and practice in prevention: A focus on evaluator and practitioner perspectives. *Evaluation and Program Planning, 20*, 3, 367–377.

Mrazek, P. J. & Haggerty, R. J. (Eds.) (1994). *Reducing risks for mental disorder: Frontiers for preventative intervention research*. Washington, DC: Institute of Medicine, National Academy Press.

Muñoz, R. F., Mrazek, P. J., & Haggery, R. J. (1996). Institute of Medicine report on prevention of mental disorders. *American Psychologist, 51*, 1116–1122.

National Institute of Mental Health (1996). *A plan for prevention research at the National Institute of Mental Health: A report by the National Advisory Mental Health Council* (NIH Publication No. 96-4093). Bethesda, MD: National Institutes of Health.

National Institute of Mental Health (1998). *Priorities for prevention research at NIMH: A report by the National Advisory Mental Health Council* (NIH Publication No. 98-2079). Bethesda, MD: National Institutes of Health.

Office of Substance Abuse Prevention (1989). *Prevention plus II: Tools for creating and sustaining drug-free communities* (DHHS Pub. No. ADM 89-1649). Rockville, MD: Author.

Perry, M. J., Albee, G. W., Bloom, M., & Gullotta, T. P. (1996). Training and career paths in primary prevention. *Journal of Primary Prevention, 16*, 357–371.

President's Commission on Mental Health (1978). *Report to the President*. Washington, DC: U.S. Government Printing Office.

Price, R. H. (1974). Etiology, the social environment, and the prevention of psychological dysfunction. In P. Insel & R. Moos (Eds.), *Health and the social environment* (pp. 74–89). Lexington, MA: Heath.

Price, R. H. (1983). The education of a prevention psychologist. In R. D. Felner, L.A. Jason, J. N. Moritsugu & S. S. Farber (Eds.), *Preventive psychology: Theory, research, and practice* (pp. 290–296). New York: Pergamon.

Price, R. H. (1986). Education for prevention. In M. Kessler & S. Goldston (Eds.), *A decade of progress in primary prevention* (pp. 289–306). Hanover, NH: University Press of New England.

Rappaport, J. (1977). *Community psychology.* New York: Holt, Rinehart & Winston.

Reiss, D., & Price, R. H. (1996). National research agenda for prevention research. The National Institute of Mental Health report. *American Psychologist, 51,* 1109–1115.

Rosnow, R. L. (1993). Toward methodological pluralism and theoretical ecumenism: A response to Leaf. *New Ideas in Psychology, 11,* 35–37.

Royce, J. R. (1987). A strategy for developing a unifying theory in psychology. In A. W. Staats & P. Leendert Mos (Eds.), *Annals of theoretical psychology* (Vol. 5, pp. 275–285). New York: Plenum.

Sechrest, L., & Sidani, S. (1995). Quantitative and qualitative methods: Is there an alternative? *Evaluation & Program Planning, 18,* 77–87.

Schiff, M., Cavaiola, A. A., & Harrison, L. (1989). Teaching prevention to professionals who work with chemically dependent families. *Alcoholism Treatment Quarterly, 6,* 41–52.

Siefert, K., Jayarante, S., & Martin, L. D. (1992). Implementing the Public Health Social Work Forward Plan: A research-based prevention curriculum for schools of social work. *Health & Social Work, 17,* 17–27.

Snow, D. L. (2000). The development of a community psychology setting: Integration of service, research, and training. In J. Rappaport & E. Seidman (Eds.), *Handbook of community psychology* (pp. 748–753). New York: Kluwer Academic/Plenum.

Snow, D. L., & Newton, P. M. (1976). Task, social structure, and social process in the community mental health center movement. *American Psychologist, 31,* 582–594.

Tebes, J. K. (1997, May). *Self-help, prevention, and scientific knowledge.* Paper presented at the Self-Help Pre-Conference of the 5th Biennial Conference of the Society for Community Research and Action, Columbia, SC.

Tebes, J. K. (2000). External validity and scientific psychology. *American Psychologist, 55,* 1508–1509.

Tebes, J. K., Grady, K., & Snow, D. L. (1989). Parents training in decision-making facilitation: Skill acquisition and relationship to gender. *Family Relations, 38,* 243–247.

Tebes, J. K., & Kraemer, D. T. (1991). Quantitative and qualitative knowing in mutual support research: Some lessons from the recent history of scientific psychology. *American Journal of Community Psychology, 19*, 739–756.

Tobler, N. S., Roona, M. R., Ochschorn, P., Marshall, D. G., Streke, A. V., & Strackpole, K. M. (2000). School-based adolescent drug prevention programs: 1998 meta-analysis. *Journal of Primary Prevention, 20*, 275–336.

U.S. Department of Education (2000) *21st century community learning centers: Providing quality afterschool learning opportunities for America's families*. Washington, DC: Author.

U.S. Surgeon General (1999). *Mental health: A report of the Surgeon General*. Washington, DC: U.S. Department of Health and Human Services.

Wandersman, A., Imm, P., Chinman, M., & Kaftarian, S. (2000). Getting to outcomes: A results-based approach to accountability. *Evaluation and Program Planning, 23*, 389–395.

Wandersman, A., Morrissey, E., Davino, K., Seybolt, D., Crusto, C., Nation, M., Goodman, R., & Imm, P. (1998). Comprehensive quality programming and accountability: Eight essential strategies for implementing successful prevention programs. *Journal of Primary Prevention, 19*, 3–30.

Weaver, A. J., & Koenig, H. G. (1996). Elderly suicide, mental health professionals and the clergy: A need for clinical collaboration, training, and research. *Death Studies, 20*, 495–508.

Yager, J., Linn, L. S., Leake, B., Goldston, S., Heinicke, C., & Pynoos, R. (1989). Attitudes toward mental illness prevention in routine pediatric practice. *American Journal of Diseases of Children, 143*, 1087–90.

Zigler, E., & Styfco, S. J. (1998). Applying the findings of developmental psychology to improve early childhood intervention. In S. G. Paris & H. M. Wellman (Eds.), *Global prospects for education: Development, culture, and schooling* (pp. 345–365). Washington, DC: American Psychological Association.

Zolik, E. S. (1983). Training for preventive psychology in community and academic settings. In R. D. Felner, L. A. Jason, J. N. Moritsugu & S. S. Farber (Eds.), *Preventive psychology: Theory, research, and practice* (pp. 273–289). New York: Pergamon.

PART II

Problems of Parenting and Youth

CHAPTER 4

Promoting Effective Parenting Practices

Lisa Sheeber,

Anthony Biglan,

Carol W. Metzler, and

Ted K. Taylor

DESCRIPTION OF THE PROBLEM

Nurturing and socializing children so that they develop the social, emotional, and academic competencies to function successfully is a goal for parents and society alike. There is substantial evidence (Collins, Maccoby, Steinberg, Hetherington, & Bornstein, 2000) that parenting behavior constitutes a considerable influence on child outcomes. The importance of parenting behavior has been demonstrated most clearly with regard to the development of antisocial and related behaviors. A large body of evidence has demonstrated that inadequate parental monitoring and high levels of harsh and inconsistent discipline predict association with deviant peers (e.g., Aryet al., 1999), substance abuse (e.g., Dishion, Patterson, & Reid, 1988), and antisocial behavior (e.g., Dishion, Patterson, & Kavanagh, 1992). More recently, evidence has been accumulating that childhood anxiety and depressive disorders are related to the nature of parent-child relationships and interactional patterns as well (Dadds & Barett,1996; Kaslow, Deering, & Racusin, 1994). For example, parent-child relationships characterized by low levels of warmth, high rates of conflictual behavior, and inadvertent reinforcement of depressive behavior appear to be associated with depressive symptomatology (Sheeber, Hops, & Davis, 2001). Additionally, effective parenting is critical in promoting children's competencies. Warm, structured child-rearing practices and high expectations for competence are associated with children's social and academic success (Masten & Coatsworth, 1998).

The relations between parenting behavior and child outcomes clearly indicate the need to direct societal resources to promoting and supporting effective parenting practices. It is time for behavioral scientists and policy makers to recognize how much is known about effective parenting and to work toward applying this information to supporting parents and improving child outcomes. This chapter addresses the question of how to go about doing so, examining both what *has* been done and, more important, what *could* be done. The question will be examined from both a clinical and a public health perspective.

The clinical perspective focuses on ensuring that families who seek treatment benefit from the services they receive. The public health perspective focuses on increasing the proportion of families that are raising academically and socially competent children. The public health perspective builds on the clinical perspective in that research on clinical interventions has clarified what families need to do in order to nurture their children to become competent, healthy, and productive adults. However, public health interventions seek to alter the prevalence of behavior by influencing a greater number of families than can be achieved through clinical means. It is characterized also by a preventive orientation, addressing difficulties before they necessitate clinical-level interventions.

Historically, the clinical perspective has predominated in efforts to promote effective parenting. This is largely because society was confronted with persons in need of treatment long before we understood how problems might be prevented or ameliorated more efficiently through nonclinical means (Biglan & Metzler, 1998). Therefore, many more of our organizational resources are committed to clinical interventions than might be the case if we made a fresh start and began with the question of how we could most efficiently promote effective parenting. Once we begin to think in terms of increasing the prevalence of effective families, it is apparent that intensive clinical interventions must coincide with more wide-reaching public health interventions.

REVIEW AND CRITIQUE OF THE LITERATURE

Clinical Approaches to Improving Parenting

If we are to use clinical interventions to improve parenting, then surely the first step is to ensure that effective parenting programs are available. As has been summarized in a number of recent reviews (e.g., Kazdin & Weisz, 1998; Taylor & Biglan, 1998), the research base offers strong empirical support for the efficacy of behavioral family interventions. This is most clearly the case for disruptive behavior problems, but successful outcomes also have been demonstrated for children with developmental disabilities, feeding and sleeping problems, and chronic physical illnesses (Taylor & Biglan, 1998). Moreover, it is apparent that the interventions are effective because they improve parenting behavior. Parents participating in behavioral family therapy have been shown to provide clearer limits and more praise for their children as well as to criticize and spank less often (Kazdin, Esveldt-Dawson, French, & Unis, 1987; Patterson, Chamberlain, & Reid, 1982; Sanders, Markie-Dadds, Tully, & Bor, 2000; Webster-Stratton, Kolpacoff, & Hollinsworth, 1988). Additional benefits, including reduced parental stress (Webster-Stratton, Kolpacoff, & Hollinsworth, 1988) and improved communication and conflict resolution between partners (Webster-Stratton, 1994), also have been noted.

A significant problem with clinical interventions, however, is that particularly troubled families are less likely both to participate in treatment and to benefit from their participation (Spoth & Redmond, 1995; Taylor & Biglan, 1998). Families who are experiencing the stressors of poverty, marital discord, maternal depression, or single parenthood are at particular risk in this regard. It is notable, therefore, that strides are being made in recruiting, retaining, and facilitating the success of such families (Taylor & Biglan, 1998). The structure and process of treatment appears to be relevant to this success. For example, group-based services seem to be more appealing to many families than is individual family therapy (Cunningham, Bremner, & Boyle, 1995). Strategies such as holding pre-treatment meetings with group leaders, making childcare and transportation available, and maintaining flexible scheduling options likewise facilitate families' engagement (Prinz et al., 2001; Reid, 1991; Webster-Stratton, 1995). Additionally, the opportunity to discuss concerns not directly related to parenting appears to be an effective means to prevent premature termination (Prinz et al., 2001). Similarly, augmenting behavioral parent-training with interventions that focus on nonparenting issues such as marital and personal adjustment improves the efficacy of parenting programs for multi-problem families (e.g., Dadds, Schwartz, & Sanders, 1987; Webster-Stratton, 1994).

Finally, with regard to providing clinical resources to families who for reasons of geography, culture, or stress are less likely to access community resources, it is notable that a developing research base (Sanders, 1999; Taylor & Biglan, 1998) suggests the potential of self-directed administrations of parent training programs. In particular, the provision of written and videotaped materials, especially in conjunction with brief therapist consultations, has been shown to be effective in improving parenting practices and reducing clinical-level behavioral problems. Additionally, it is likely that increasing access to materials and consultation will be provided to parents using interactive computer technologies (Gordon, 2000).

In contrast to the positive results obtained in controlled clinical trials, there is relatively little evidence for the efficacy of treatment as it is provided to families in "real-world" clinical settings (Weisz, Donenberg, Han, & Weiss, 1995; Weisz, Weiss, & Donenberg, 1992). There are very few studies evaluating treatment as it is typically administered, that is, the treatment of referred children, in clinical settings, by practicing clinicians. Significantly, the results of the available studies suggest that the large positive effects demonstrated in research settings are *not* being obtained in community settings. As noted by Weisz et al. (1992), the results cannot be accepted uncritically, since they are derived from a small, methodologically weak, and largely dated series of studies. Nonetheless, we curently lack convincing evidence that effective treatments are available to families in the community.

It is likely that the discrepancy between outcomes in experimental and clinical settings derives, in part, from the nature of treatments offered in clinical settings. Applied settings generally have not adopted behavioral family interventions as standard practice (Weisz et al., 1992). Instead, interventions available in applied settings typically have little, if any, empirical evidence to support their effectiveness (Taylor & Biglan, 1998; Weisz, 2000). In this regard, it is notable that in a recent effectiveness study (Taylor, Schmidt, Pepler, & Hodgins, 1998) an empirically supported behavioral family therapy program was more effective in reducing child behavior problems than the standard treatments offered by the children's mental health center. Obviously, to the extent that differences in outcome are a function of the nature of treatments provided, the implication for the improvement of clinical practice and outcome is clear.

To date, however, the limited number of effectiveness trials means that we know relatively little about how empirically supported programs operate in real-world settings. Given the number of differences between laboratory and clinical settings, it is unlikely that we can assume generalization (Weisz et al., 1992). Although some of the features (e.g., structure and monitoring to facilitate adherence) that characterize what Weisz et al. (1992) have termed "research therapy" may inform efforts to transfer empirically supported treatments to the clinic, others may represent constraints placed in laboratory-based studies that allow treatments to perform better than they could in the real world. One key concern in this regard is the restricted sample composition common in laboratory-based studies, by which, for example, participants experiencing comorbid disorders are excluded even though they represent the norm in community treatment settings (Burns, Hoagwood, & Mrazek, 1999). Additionally, participants in controlled trials tend to have less severe disorders and to come from homes characterized by less parental psychopathology, less family dysfunction, and less economic disadvantage than do participants seeking services in clinical settings (Kazdin, 2000). Thus, controlled clinical trials may overestimate our ability to provide effective interventions for the families who typically present for treatment, suggesting the need for treatment research that more accurately reflects the populations to be served.

Additional limitations, and hence directions for ongoing work, have to do with the range of populations who have access to effective interventions. For example, despite strong evidence of the role of family processes in depression, there has been limited headway made regarding the development of effective family interventions for youth with depressive disorders (Burns et al., 1999; Gillham, Shatte, & Freres, 2000). Furthermore, there are many groups of families that are difficult to reach and, however, are less likely to be included in clinical trials or to participate in treatment in applied settings. In addition to the multiproblem families discussed above, rural populations and members of minority ethnic and cultural groups are of particular concern in this regard (Biglan & Metzler, 1998; Sanders, 1997).

Public Health Approaches to Improving Parenting

There are at least two reasons for broadening our efforts beyond clinical services to include public health approaches to facilitating effective parenting. First, clinical interventions are likely to be more than is needed for many families who could still use support and guidance to promote competent academic, social, and emotional behavior in their children. As described by Sanders (1999) in providing the rationale for a multitiered set of interventions, determining the minimally sufficient intervention that parents require to deflect children away from trajectories of increasing difficulties is a means of maximizing efficiency—avoiding overservicing and ensuring wide reach. Second, even if we were to become extraordinarily skilled in disseminating effective clinical interventions, it is unlikely that this development, by itself, could provide sufficient reach to increase the prevalence of effective parenting practices to the extent needed. Resources are not available to pay for clinical interventions for the large number of youth who evidence significant behavioral or emotional problems, and, even if they were, many families would remain unwilling or unable to access services (Offord, Kraemer, Kazdin, Jensen, & Harrington, 1998; Sanders, 1997). As suggested by Offord et al., (1998), success will necessitate a multipronged approach in which effective clinical services are available for those in need, targeted programs are provided for those at risk, and universal programs are instituted to promote mental health across the community. Offord et al. (1998) noted, moreover, that providing interventions at multiple levels may have synergistic effects. As applied to the promotion of effective parenting, one could envision, for example, that a targeted intervention aimed at increasing the use of effective, noncorporal means of discipline in families at risk for child abuse might be more potent in a community in which a broad-based media campaign had sensitized parents to the deleterious effects of physical punishment and alerted them to alternatives.

Below we highlight some of the mechanisms being investigated to promote effective parenting behavior. The mediums in which these mechanisms operate share some important characteristics relating to their potential value as components of a public health campaign. In particular, they (a) are characterized by their wide reach, (b) use points of contact that are normative and non-stigmatizing, (c) rely on sources of information that have credibility to parents, and (d) are sufficiently flexible to be useful for both universal and targeted interventions. We would note here, however, that we consider this field to be in its infancy with regard to both application and science such that the work described represents but a sampling of what could be done.

Media

There is persuasive evidence that mass media can influence important health and social behaviors (Biglan & Metzler, 1998). For example, both the 1964 Surgeon General's Report and the introduction of television ads recommending smoking cessation were associated with reductions in the prevalence of smoking (Warner, 1977, 1989). Media effects also have been reported in studies of crime prevention (O'Keefe & Reid, 1990), alcohol consumption (Barber, Bradshaw, & Walsh, 1989), and drunk driving (Niensted, 1990).

To date, the professional community has made very little use of mass media to improve parenting behavior. This gap is noteworthy, not only because of the media's potentially powerful influence, but also because the enormous expansion in the marketing of child development and parenting guidance materials to parents in the form of print and, increasingly, electronic media suggests that there is a significant demand for parenting information (Simpson, 1997). There is, however, very little scientific information regarding either the quality of media messages parents are receiving or their impact on parental behavior. The quality question is aggravated, moreover, by the often contradictory nature of information conveyed by the media, a problem that may be due in part to the fact that parenting information is developed and disseminated by hundreds of organizations across dozens of disciplines (Simpson, 1997).

Though preliminary, efforts by the professional community to develop and evaluate media-based parenting programs are promising. For example, Pentz, Bonnie, and Shopland (1996) reported that a school and community intervention that included a media component had a significant impact on substance use; the design of the study, however, did not enable the researchers to isolate the unique effects of the media strategy. Initial investigations of age-paced newsletters and Web-based support programs similarly have demonstrated the potential of these media for providing education and support to at-risk families (Bogenschneider & Stone, 1997; Dunham et al., 1998; Riley & Meinhardt, 1991). For example, Bogenschneider and Stone (1997) found that parents of 9th- through 12th-graders who were randomized to receive a series of newsletters advocating parental monitoring, limit-setting on children's alcohol use, and networking with other parents reported increased monitoring compared with parents in a control group. In an unusually extensive use of the media, Sanders (1999) developed an "infotainment"-style television program that was aired as a prime-time series on commercial television. The program provided practical information and advice on handling a wide variety of common behavioral and developmental problems. Although the effects of the television show on viewers under natural conditions were not evaluated, a controlled follow-up examination in which parents observed the program on a series of videotapes indicated that parents who viewed the program reported a significant reduction in disruptive behaviors and an increase in parenting confidence (Sanders, Montgomery, & Brechman-Toussaint, 2000).

Media resources also could be used to convey information that might indirectly affect parenting behavior. For example, media campaigns could be an important means of motivating parents to participate in formal parenting programs by both normalizing the process of seeking help and increasing the visibility and acceptability of programs (Sanders, 1999). The media also could help parents by educating them about the availability of empirically supported programs. Such an education campaign, by increasing consumer demand, could be an important component in promoting the dissemination of effective interventions.

Schools and Community Organizations

Schools are increasingly becoming a hub for the delivery of a range of services to children and their families (Biglan & Metzler, 1998). Their credibility to parents as sources of information about child development, as well as the knowledge school personnel have regarding their students' well-being, places them in an excellent position to facilitate the provision of parenting guidance. One option is that schools could provide empirically supported parenting programs both universally and in the form of more intensive targeted interventions. Additionally, when schools are not in the position to provide the intervention themselves, they still could play an important role in identifying and referring children whose families could benefit from parenting interventions (Metzler et al., 1998).

Secondly, schools could provide a steady flow of information to parents about effective parenting through newsletters, handouts, and workshops. This approach may be particularly useful as children enter adolescence, in that the mass media provides less coverage directed to parents of this age group (Simpson, 1997). Likewise, it also may be possible to influence parenting practices through activities that are assigned in school (e.g., Holder, Perry, & Pirie, 1988; Perry, Finnegan, Forster, Wagenaar, & Wolfson, 1996). For example, Biglan et al. (1996) tested the effects of a school-prompted quiz about tobacco that middle-school students gave to their parents. The activity significantly increased the proportion of parents who were exposed to anti-tobacco messages, improved parents' knowledge about tobacco, increased their support for community efforts to prevent youth tobacco use, and increased parent-child communication about tobacco use.

Finally, schools are particularly well-situated to help parents become more involved in their children's education and to maintain this involvement through middle and high school, where parental involvement tends to decline (Eccles & Harold, 1996; Epstein & Dauber, 1991). As described by Metzler et al., (1998), schools can provide: (a) frequent progress reports; (b) varied schedules for school activities so more families can participate; (c) systematic information for parents on how to monitor, discuss, and help their children with homework; and (d) information on ways that parents can help students make informed decisions about school programs and activities.

It should be noted here that schools are not alone among community institutions in having the potential to reach and influence parents. For example, many churches already provide parenting skills and support programs, although little is known about the nature of existing programs or who they are serving (Biglan et al., 1997). Additionally, in much the same way that schools provide an access point for reaching families, work settings have the potential to facilitate access to parents for provision of universal parent education and support programs as well as referral services.

Medical Practitioners

Pediatric, obstetric, and family practice professionals provide another channel for promoting effective parenting (Biglan et al., 1997). For example, nurse visitation programs have demonstrated efficacy in the long-term prevention of developmental and behavioral problems (Reese, Vera, Simon, & Ikeda, 2000). These programs, in which nurses make home visits during pregnancy and early childhood, provide broad-based parent education and support to families at risk for adverse child outcomes.

As parents frequently turn to their children's physicians for assistance in dealing with children's behavioral difficulties (Sanders & Markie-Dadds, 1997), consultation regarding child behavior can be considered a vital component of well-child care. Assisting physicians and nurses both in the provision of brief counseling to parents regarding ways of handling normative behavioral and emotional problems, and in the identification of families who are in need of clinical interventions, represents an important component of work aimed at improving childrearing practices. As in school-based interventions, face-to-face meetings can be supplemented with newsletters, tip sheets, and video-based information that enable parents to review the information at home as well as share it with their children's other caregiver(s). Sanders (1999) is in the process of evaluating programs for training medical professionals to provide brief behavioral consultations for normative and subclinical behavior problems.

CASE EXAMPLE

The second and third authors recently implemented and evaluated the Community Action for Successful Youth (CASY) Project, which combined public health and clinical approaches to improve parenting practices in two entire communities.

Public Health Approach: Direct Mail and Parent-Child Homework Activities

We developed a series of integrated mailings and parent-child activities designed to build parents' skill in key practices for preventing aggressive behavior, deviant peer associations, and substance use. Consistent with the research on effective media communications (Flay & Burton, 1990; McGuire, 1985), these materials were designed to: (a) provide influential messages from credible sources (i.e., the school and community organizations), (b) be repeated frequently and consistently but with some novelty, (c) be sustained for a long period of time, (d) advocate a core set of specific behaviors, (e) be simple and attractive, (f) link advocated parenting skills to desired child outcomes, and (g) encourage positive discussions about the issue.

For each of five parenting topics, the materials consisted of a letter to parents, a fact sheet, a parent-child homework activity, and a postcard. Thus, parents received four "hits" on each topic, with the entire series paced across the school year. Each parenting topic was initiated by a letter to the parent from the school, advocating the targeted parenting practice, and promoting participation in the upcoming "homework" activity. One week later, the fact sheet was mailed to parents from the school. The fact sheets (a) included research-based information about the importance of the targeted parenting practice, (b) amplified existing community norms about the parenting practice by presenting data on the prevalence in that community of that practice and relevant parent beliefs, (c) gave concrete tips for implementing each skill, and (d) provided information that assisted parents in the upcoming parent-child homework activity.

Approximately 1 week later, teachers assigned the parent-child activities as homework. In these assignments, students and parents worked together on activities designed to encourage effective parenting (e.g., games to clarify rules; a parent quiz on substance use facts). Procedures also were established for parents to share their ideas about the advocated parenting skill with other parents. Students were provided a variety of incentives for returning the homework sheet (with parents' ideas) to the teacher. Parents' ideas then were summarized on a postcard which was mailed out to all families. This sharing of ideas was intended to amplify the norms among parents and to advocate further the targeted parenting practice.

In the first community in which these activities were implemented, participation rates among families were lower than desired and varied across activities and grades (from a low of 9% to a high of 73%). In order to increase participation in the second community, the authors (a) elicited a greater commitment from the teachers' to promote the parent-child homework activities, (b) obtained more teacher input in refining the content, format, and process of distributing the materials, (c) gave greater attention to integrating the series of materials, targeting them to parents' identified concerns, and making them more appealing, and (d) had focus groups of parents test the activities' appeal and clarity. Participation rates across all grades and activities were dramatically higher in the second community, ranging from 54% to 81%.

Analysis of the effects of these activities on parenting behavior and attitudes are underway. Initial results indicate that parents' reports of exposure to information about parenting increased during the intervention period, suggesting that efforts were successful in increasing the density of media about effective parenting. Preliminary analyses also suggest that parents' reports of their exposure to media on parenting were related to changes in parenting practices.

Clinical Intervention for an Indicated Population:
Behavioral Parent Training

Simultaneously with the implementation of the above activities, we also conducted community organizing to assist the communities in providing behavioral parent training to families whose children were exhibiting elevated levels of problem behavior. The Adolescent Transitions Program (ATP; Dishion & Kavanagh, in press) helps parents to develop consistent, nonharsh methods of setting limits on their children's behavior while increasing their reinforcement of appropriate social behavior. In two separate randomized controlled trials, ATP has been shown to improve parent-child problem solving and parents' positive feelings toward their children, to reduce parents' overreactivity and laxness toward their children's behavior, and to reduce parent- and teacher-reported child antisocial behavior (Dishion & Andrews, 1995; Irvine, Biglan, Smolkowski, Metzler, & Ary, 1999). Furthermore, Irvine et al. (1999) showed that nonprofessionals can be successfully trained to deliver the program effectively.

We worked with schools and community agencies to develop a community-wide referral system for identifying and engaging families most in need of parenting interventions. School staff and social service providers were asked to identify youth exhibiting behavioral difficulties such as substance use, aggression, and school failure. This step was critical because middle schools seldom have a systematic process for identifying students who would benefit from interventions for problem behaviors or for providing assistance to parents in improving these students' behavior.

Once the families were identified, we then used targeted outreach to encourage parents to participate in the program. Because simply issuing an invitation to parents to attend a parenting program and doing nothing further to facilitate their attendance typically results in poor attendance by those who would benefit most (Spoth & Redmond, 1995), the CASY project used a number of recruitment strategies that have been shown to be effective in previous research (Reid, 1991; Taylor & Biglan, 1998; Webster-Stratton, 1995). In particular, recruitment was facilitated by in-person contact with identified families to explain the program and invite participation, as well as by the provision of dinner, child care, and transportation assistance. Incentives for participation also were given in the form of drawings for inexpensive items and payments to families based on number of sessions attended. Despite these efforts, attrition was still notable; although approximately 85% of families agreed to participate in the program and approximately 75% of these came to the first session, only about 60% of those who began the program completed it. Average attrition was substantially higher in one community than another (66% vs. 30%), suggesting possible differences between communities regarding barriers to participation, competing demands on families, and/or the acceptability of the program and its leaders. Although progress has been made in identifying methods for increasing the engagement of families in parenting classes, more work in this area clearly is needed.

CASY Project staff also conducted community organizing to create partnerships to fund and deliver the ATP program free of charge to parents. The ATP classes were sponsored by mental health agencies and led by mental health professionals, with training and consultation from CASY staff. The classes themselves were held at the middle schools. Funding for the program and for the child care was a collaborative effort among the mental health agency, the schools, nonprofit family support agencies, and county and state governmental agencies. Business support helped to defray the costs of providing dinners to families. CASY staff took steps to strengthen these referral and funding partnerships to ensure that the ATP program remained when the research grant ended. In fact, foundation and governmental grants were obtained by collaboration among the school districts, local mental health providers, and family services organizations that allowed them to continue to provide the program.

FUTURE DIRECTIONS

As empirically supported parenting programs become more widely adopted and the skills that they promote become better understood by influential people in communities, it is likely that the programs will become more widely available and communities will develop additional practices to support effective parenting. The scientific community can take steps to increase the likelihood that communities put into place a set of practices that maximize the proportion of children who develop successfully.

Organizing Communities Around an Explicit Set of Goals

Prevention scientists are developing methods of assisting communities in articulating goals for preventing youth problems. These methods include (a) helping to organize community partnerships that identify important goals for community improvement and (b) informing that process with information about the prevalence and cost of specific youth problems, the risk and protective factors influencing those problems, and the programs and policies that could prevent or ameliorate them (Fawcett, Francisco, Paine-Andrews, & Schultz, in press; Hawkins, Catalano, & Associates, 1992). Inevitably, the importance of promoting nurturing families becomes clear in this process.

To the extent that a community articulates an explicit goal to ensure as many nurturing families as possible, it will organize efforts to achieve that goal. To be effective, however, this cannot be a one-time affair that simply leads to a "campaign." Rather, the goal of nurturing families needs to be built into the fabric of community life. As actions are taken that affect community life, the relevance of those actions to families' well-being must routinely be examined. In order to maintain attention to this goal, these should be an infrastructure of organizations and personnel who are formally vested with responsibility for examining how changes in the community affect families. We will need a growing cadre of prevention scientists and community psychologists to help communities establish and maintain goals in this way.

Research on the Dissemination of Empirically Based Parenting Programs

Given that there are empirically supported interventions worthy of dissemination, the scientific community must commit considerably more of its resources to facilitating the effective implementation of these programs in clinical settings. Several types of research studies are needed in this regard, and a number of pragmatic considerations must be addressed if programs are to be implemented with requisite fidelity.

First, research is needed on the organizations that are providing parenting programs (Biglan & Taylor, 2000; Burns et al., 1999). What types of organizations tend to do this (e.g., schools, churches, child protection agencies, clinics)? What proportion of the parents who would benefit from these programs are being reached in the typical community? How can we estimate the penetration or reach of these programs? To what extent are the organizations that are offering parenting programs providing ones that have been validated empirically?

A particularly important goal for research on organizational practices is the identification of the contingencies that influence organizations' adoption and maintenance of empirically supported programs (Biglan, 1995; Biglan & Taylor, 2000). For example, to what extent do funding sources influence the types of programs organizations provide to families? Could the availability of empirically supported programs be increased if those who funded mental health care, such as insurance companies and federal health programs, required that they be offered? Could a consumer population, better informed about empirically supported practices by the mass media, put pressure on clinical service providers and funders to provide access to such programs?

Increasing attention (e.g., Taylor & Biglan, 1998; Weisz, Donenberg, Han, & Weiss, 1995) also has been given to identifying practical barriers to the adoption of empirically-supported interventions, each of which provides an important avenue for research and advocacy. One set of issues relates to funding policies, such as those that restrict the spending of treatment monies on such expenses as child care or transportation necessary to engage parents in treatment, or that require the "identified patient" to be present although many effective treatments for children involve working primarily with the parents (Taylor & Biglan, 1998). A second set of issues relates to the training of clinicians in empirically supported interventions and the availability of materials to facilitate their use of these programs (Taylor & Biglan, 1998; Weisz, Donenberg, Han, & Weiss, 1995). As clinicians typically are not well-versed in the use of empirically supported methods (Weisz et al., 1995), attention must be directed in the short run toward developing and evaluating mechanisms for supporting training and supervision of clinicians (Taylor & Biglan, 1998). In the long run, this is an issue that should be addressed in the graduate training of future clinicians. It is likely that many of the same variables that need to be examined with regard to service organizations' program adoption will be relevant to influencing the behavior of graduate training programs.

Second, *experimental* research is needed that systematically tests strategies for influencing organizations to adopt and effectively implement parenting programs. Despite much research on factors associated with the adoption of practices (Rogers, 1995), experimental manipulations of variables that are thought to influence adoption are seldom done. We are not aware of any experimental studies testing strategies for fostering the adoption of empirically supported parenting programs by provider organizations. We need a series of studies in which well-defined strategies for influencing organizations to adopt such programs are experimentally evaluated, either in randomized trials or interrupted time-series analyses (Biglan, Ary, & Wagenaar, 2000). Variables that must be addressed include characteristics of both the program (e.g., ease of implementation) and the adopting agents (e.g., skill in providing administrative support), as well as the economic consequences of adoption (Biglan & Taylor, 2000). The proximal dependent variable in such studies would be the organizations' implementation of the program with fidelity.

This consideration points to a third facet of research that is needed, namely, demonstration that results similar to those achieved in laboratory-based trials can be obtained under real-world circumstances. To this end, an increase in effectiveness trials is called for in which interventions with demonstrated efficacy are conducted in clinical settings by practicing clinicians serving referred families (Weisz & Hawley, 1998). Such research is necessary to identify the structures necessary to maintain adequate fidelity of implementation (see Dumas, Lynch, Laughlin, Smith, & Prinz, 2001), as well as to determine whether currently available treatments will require modification to be effective under these conditions. Additionally, ongoing development and assessment of parenting interventions that can be self-administered via workbooks, videos, or internet technology are necessary to broaden our reach. Efforts to make laboratory-based treatment research more relevant for practice, for example by including samples of youth with comorbid disorders, are similarly necessary (Burns et al., 1999). Finally, research on parenting interventions for the prevention and amelioration of internalizing disorders also is warranted.

A fourth and final line of dissemination research involves the development of ongoing quality assurance systems for the provision of parenting programs. Even if the just-described studies show that empirically based programs can be disseminated in ways that maintain their effectiveness, it is unlikely that their effectiveness will be maintained over time in the absence of ongoing monitoring. Research is needed to develop and validate systems for assessing the outcomes of parenting programs and using the information from these assessments to maintain their quality.

Research on Mass Media

Research is needed on the extent to which mass media could be used to promote effective parenting. We are unaware of any experimental evaluations of the use of mass media to promote effective parenting, although there are now excellent examples available of the evaluation of media campaigns using either randomization of communities to conditions (Flynn et al., 1992) or time-series experiments (Palmgreen, Donohew, Lorch, Hoyle, & Stephenson, in press) in other public health areas.

Research also should be directed at evaluating the parenting information currently available through the mass media (e.g., parenting magazines, books, newsletters, news segments). For example, who is accessing these resources? What effect does access have on parenting behavior and child outcome? Similarly, mechanisms need to be developed to disseminate emerging scientific findings to media sources (Simpson, 1997), so that the media are provided with ongoing access to empirically derived information about child development, effective parenting behavior, and parent-training interventions.

Research on Community Organizations

Despite the fact that every community has numerous organizations whose actions affect families' well-being, there has been little systematic research on which organizations affect families and how they might be influenced to adopt practices that benefit families. Schools, social service agencies, medical practices, churches, and worksites are all potential contact points for the provision of parental education and support programs, as well as referral services. Research is needed to develop methods of identifying such organizations, measuring the services they provide to families, and estimating their success in assisting families. Research of this sort would then guide further research on how to influence the practices of these organizations and would be a basis for communities to assess how well they are meeting families' needs.

Ongoing Monitoring of Family Well-Being

If communities are going to work to ensure the largest possible proportion of nurturing families, they will need to develop better systems for monitoring families' well-being and nurturance. Ongoing surveillance is a vital feature of public health approaches to controlling disease. We track the incidence of disease in order to be able to prevent or ameliorate emerging patterns of disease. The monitoring of youth well-being is well-developed, with an increasing number of nationally representative surveys of youth substance use, antisocial behavior, and high-risk sexual behavior. Systems for accurate monitoring of the prevalence of youth problems are available at the state level for most states, and local systems are coming into use. These systems are an important guide to national, state, and community efforts to ensure optimal child and adolescent development. Systems for monitoring family well-being, however, are less developed. We need methods of estimating the proportion of families in each community that have problems that put them at risk to raise children unsuccessfully. These problems would include poverty, depression, divorce, spouse abuse, marital discord, and parental alcohol or drug abuse. At the same time, we need methods for estimating the prevalence of families that engage in problematic parenting practices, such as harsh and inconsistent discipline and inadequate monitoring.

In closing, we would reiterate the need for behavioral scientists and policy makers to recognize how much is known about both competent parenting and clinical approaches to promoting it. It is thus time to work toward ensuring that effective clinical approaches become widely available in community settings, and that public health approaches to promoting positive parenting be developed, implemented, and evaluated.

ACKNOWLEDGMENT

This research was supported by Grants Nos. MH4311 and MH57166 from the National Institute of Mental Health, Grants Nos. DA09306 and DA09678 from the National Institute on Drug Abuse, and Grant No. CA38273 from the National Cancer Institute. The authors wish to thank Elizabeth Mondulick for her contribution to the preparation of this manuscript.

REFERENCES

Ary, D. V., Duncan, T. E., Biglan, A., Metzler, C. W., Noell, J. W., & Smol-kowski, K. (1999). Development of adolescent problem behavior. *Journal of Abnormal Child Psychology, 27*, 141–150.

Barber, J. G., Bradshaw, R., & Walsh, C. (1989). Reducing alcohol consumption through television advertising. *Journal of Consulting and Clinical Psychology, 57*, 613–618.

Biglan, A. (1995). *Changing cultural practices: A contextualist framework for intervention research.* Reno, NV: Context Press.

Biglan, A., Ary, D. V., & Wagenaar, A. C. (2000). The value of interrupted time-series experiments for community intervention research. *Prevention Research, 1*, 31–49.

Biglan, A., Ary, D. V., Yudelson, H., Duncan, T. E., Hood, D., James, L., Koehn, V., Wright, Z., Black, C., Levings, D., Smith, S., & Gaiser, E. (1996). Experimental evaluation of a modular approach to mobilizing anti-tobacco influences of peers and parents. *American Journal of Community Psychology, 24*, 311–339.

Biglan, A., & Metzler, C. W. (1998). A public health perspective for research on family-focused interventions. In R. S. Ashery, E. B. Robertson & K. L. Kumpfer (Eds.), *Drug abuse prevention through family interventions. NIDA Research Monograph 177, NIH Publication NO. 994135* (pp. 430–458). Washington, DC: National Institute on Drug Abuse.

Biglan, A., Metzler, C. W., Fowler, R. C., Gunn, B., Taylor, T. K., Rusby, J., & Irvine, B. (1997). Improving childrearing in America's communities. In P. A. Lamal (Ed.), *Cultural contingencies: Behavior analytic perspectives on cultural practices* (pp. 185–213). Westport, CT: Praeger.

Biglan, A., & Taylor, T. K. (2000). Increasing the use of science to improve child-rearing. *The Journal of Primary Prevention, 21*, 207–226.

Bogenschneider, K., & Stone, M. (1997). Delivering parent education to low and high risk parents of adolescents via age-paced newsletters. *Family Relations, 46*, 123–134.

Burns, B. J., Hoagwood, K., & Mrazek, P. J. (1999). Effective treatment for mental disorders in children and adolescents. *Clinical Child and Family Psychology Review, 2,* 199–254.

Collins, W. A., Maccoby, E. E., Steinberg, L., Hetherington, E. M., & Bornstein, M. H. (2000). Contemporary research on parenting: The case for nature and nurture. *American Psychologist, 55,* 218–232.

Cunningham, C. E., Bremner, R., & Boyle, M. H. (1995). Large group community-based parenting programs for families of preschoolers at risk for disruptive behaviour disorders: Utilization, cost effectiveness, and outcome. *Journal of Child Psychology and Psychiatry and Allied Disciplines, 36,* 1141–1159.

Dadds, M. R., & Barrett, P. M. (1996). Family processes in child and adolescent anxiety and depression. *Behaviour Change, 13,* 231–239.

Dadds, M. R., Schwartz, S., & Sanders, M. R. (1987). Marital discord and treatment outcome in behavioral treatment of child conduct disorders. *Journal of Consulting and Clinical Psychology, 55,* 396–403.

Dishion, T. J., & Andrews, D. W. (1995). Preventing escalation in problem behaviors with high risk young adolescents: Immediate and 1-year outcomes. *Journal of Consulting and Clinical Psychology, 63,* 538–548.

Dishion, T. J., & Kavanagh, K. A. (in press). *Adolescent problem behavior: A family-centered intervention and assessment sourcebook.* New York: Guilford.

Dishion, T. J., Patterson, G. R., & Kavanagh, K. A. (1992). An experimental test of the coercion model: Linking theory, measurement, and intervention. In J. McCord & R. E. Tremblay (Eds.), *Preventing antisocial behavior: Interventions from birth through adolescence* (pp. 253–282). New York: Guilford.

Dishion, T. J., Patterson, G. R., & Reid, J. R. (1988). Parent and peer factors associated with drug sampling in early adolescence: Implications for treatment. *National Institute on Drug Abuse: Research Monograph Series, 77,* 69–93.

Dumas, J. E., Lynch, A. M., Laughlin, J. E., Smith, E. P., & Prinz, R. J. (2001). Promoting intervention fidelity: Conceptual issues, methods, and preliminary results from the Early Alliance Prevention Trial. *American Journal of Preventive Medicine, 20 (1S),* 38–47.

Dunham, P. J., Hurshman, A., Litwin, E., Gusella, J., Ellsworth, C., & Dodd, P. W. D. (1998). Computer-mediated social support: Single young mothers as a model system. *American Journal of Community Psychology, 26,* 281–306.

Eccles, J. S., & Harold, R. D. (1996). Family involvement in children's and adolescents' schooling. In A. Booth (Ed.), *Family school links: How do they affect educational outcomes?* (pp. 3–34). Mahwah, NJ: Erlbaum.

Epstein, J. L., & Dauber, S. L. (1991). School programs and teacher practices of parent involvement in inner-city elementary and middle schools. *Elementary School Journal, 91*, 289–305.

Fawcett, S. B., Francisco, V. T., Paine-Andrews, A., & Schultz, J. A. (2000). A model memorandum of collaboration: A proposal. *Public Health Reports, 115*, 174–179.

Flay, B. R., & Burton, D. (1990). Effective mass communication strategies for health campaigns. In C. W. Atkin & L. Wallack (Eds.), *Mass communication and public health: Complexities and conflicts* (pp. 129–146). Newbury Park, CA: Sage Publications.

Flynn, B. S., Worden, J. K., Secker-Walker, R. H., Badger, G. J., Geller, B. M., & Costanza, M. C. (1992). Prevention of cigarette smoking through mass media intervention and school programs. *American Journal of Public Health, 82*, 827–834.

Gillham, J. E., Shatte, A. J., & Freres, D. R. (2000). Preventing depression: A review of cognitive-behavioral and family interventions. *Applied and Preventive Psychology, 9*, 63–88.

Gordon, D. A. (2000). Parent training via CD-ROM: Using technology to disseminate effective prevention practices. *Journal of Primary Prevention, 21*, 227–251.

Hawkins, J. D., Catalano, R. F., & Associates (1992). *Communities that care: Action for drug abuse prevention.* San Francisco: Jossey-Bass.

Holder, W., Perry, C. L., & Pirie, P. L. (1988). *Evaluation report on the Unpuffables Pilot Project.* Unpublished manuscript, University of Minnesota.

Irvine, A. B., Biglan, A., Smolkowski, K., Metzler, C. W., & Ary, D. V. (1999). The effectiveness of a parenting skills program for parents of middle school students in small communities. *Journal of Consulting and Clinical Psychology, 67*, 811–825.

Kaslow, N. J., Deering, C. G., & Racusin, G. R. (1994). Depressed children and their families. *Clinical Psychology Review, 14*, 39–59.

Kazdin, A. D. (2000). Developing a research agenda for child and adolescent psychotherapy. *Archives of General Psychiatry, 57*, 829–835.

Kazdin, A. E., Esveldt-Dawson, K., French, N. H., & Unis, A. S. (1987). Effects of parent management training and problem-solving skills training combined in the treatment of antisocial child behavior. *Journal of the American Academy of Child and Adolescent Psychiatry, 26*, 416–424.

Kazdin, A., & Weisz, J. R. (1998). Identifying and developing empirically supported child and adolescent treatments. *Journal of Consulting and Clinical Psychology, 66*, 19–36.

Masten, A. S., & Coatsworth, J. D. (1998). The development of competence in favorable and unfavorable environments: Lessons from research on successful children. *American Psychologist, 53*, 205–220.

McGuire, W. J. (1985). Attitudes and attitude change. In G. Lindzey & E. Aronson (Eds.), *The handbook of social psychology* (pp. 233–246). New York: Random House.

Metzler, C. W., Taylor, T. K., Gunn, B. K., Fowler, R. C., Biglan, A., & Ary, D. V. (1998). A comprehensive approach to the prevention of behavior problems: Integrating effective practices to strengthen behavior management programs in schools. *Effective School Practices, 17*, 8–24.

Niensted, B. (1990). The policy effects of a DWI law and a publicity campaign. In R. Surette (Ed.), *The media and criminal justice policy: Recent research and social effects* (pp. 193–203). Springfield, IL: Charles C. Thomas.

O'Keefe, G., & Reid, K. (1990). Media public information campaigns and criminal justice policy—beyond "McGruff." In R. Surette (Ed.), *The media and criminal justice policy: Recent research and social effects* (pp. 209–223). Springfield, IL: Charles C. Thomas.

Offord, D. R., Kraemer, H. C., Kazdin, A. E., Jensen, P. S., & Harrington, R. (1998). Lowering the burden of suffering from child psychiatric disorder: Trade-offs among clinical, targeted, and universal interventions. *Journal of the American Academy of Child and Adolescent Psychiatry, 37*, 686–694.

Palmgreen, P., Donohew, L., Lorch, E. P., Hoyle, R. H., & Stephenson, M. T. (2001). Television campaigns and adolescent marijuana use: Tests of sensation seeking targeting. *American Journal of Public Health, 91*, 292–296.

Patterson, G. R., Chamberlain, P., & Reid, J. B. (1982). A comparative evaluation of parent training procedures. *Behavior Therapy, 13*, 638–650.

Pentz, M. A., Bonnie, R. J., & Shopland, D. R. (1996). Integrating supply and demand reduction strategies for drug abuse prevention. *American Behavioral Scientist, 39*, 897–910.

Perry, C. L., Finnegan, J. R., Forster, J. L., Wagenaar, A. C., & Wolfson, M. (1996). Project Northland: Outcomes of a community-wide alcohol use prevention program during early adolescence. *American Journal of Public Health, 86*, 956–965.

Prinz, R. J., Smith, E. P., Dumas, J. E., Laughlin, J. E., White, D. W., & Barron, R. (2001). Recruitment and retention of participants in prevention trials involving family-based interventions. *American Journal of Preventive Medicine, 20*, 31–37.

Reese, L. E., Vera, E. M., Simon, T. R., & Eda, R. M. (2000). The role of families and care givers as risk and protective factors in preventing youth violence. *Clinical Child and Family Psychology Review, 3*, 61–77.

Reid, J. B. (1991). Involving parents in the prevention of conduct disorders: Rationale, problems, and tactics. *Community Psychologist, 27*, 28–30.

Riley, D., & Meinhardt, G. (1991). How effective are age-paced newsletters for new parents? *Family Relations, 43*, 247–253.

Rogers, E. M. (1995). *Diffusion of innovations* (4th ed.). New York: Free Press.

Sanders, M. R. (1997). Commentary: Empirically validated treatments and child clinical interventions. *Behaviour Change, 14*, 15–17.

Sanders, M. R. (1999). Triple P–Positive Parenting Program: Towards an empirically validated multilevel parenting and family support strategy for the prevention of behavior and emotional problems in children. *Clinical Child and Family Psychology Review, 2*, 71–90.

Sanders, M. R., & Markie-Dadds, C. (1997). Managing common child behaviour problems. In M. R. Sanders, C. Mitchell & G. J. A. Byrne (Eds.), *Medical consultation skills: Behavioral and interpersonal dimensions of health care* (pp. 356–402). Melbourne, Australia: Addison-Wesley-Longman.

Sanders, M. R., Markie-Dadds, C., Tully, L. A., & Bor, W. (2000). The Triple P-Positive Parenting Program: A comparison of enhanced, standard, and self-directed behavioral family intervention for parents of children with early onset conduct problems. *Journal of Consulting and Clinical Psychology, 68*, 624–640.

Sanders, M. R., Montgomery, D. T., & Brechman-Toussaint, M. L. (2000). The mass media and the prevention of child behavior problems: The evaluation of a television series to promote positive outcomes for parents and their children. *Journal of Child Psychology and Psychiatry, 41*, 939–948.

Sheeber, L., Hops, H., & Davis, B. (2001). Family processes in adolescent depression. *Clinical Child Psychology and Family Review, 4*, 19–35.

Simpson, A. R. (1997). *The role of the mass media in parenting education.* Boston: Center for Health Communication, Harvard School of Public Health.

Spoth, R., & Redmond, C. (1995). Parent motivation to enroll in parenting skills programs: A model of family context and health belief predictors. *Journal of Family Psychology, 9*, 294–310.

Spoth, R., Redmond, C., Haggerty, K., & Ward, T. (1995). A controlled parenting skills outcome study examining individual difference and attendance effects. *Journal of Marriage and the Family, 57*, 449–464.

Taylor, T. K., & Biglan, A. (1998). Behavioral family interventions for improving childrearing: A review of the literature for clinicians and policy makers. *Clinical Child and Family Psychology Review, 1*, 41–60.

Taylor, T. K., Schmidt, F., Pepler, D., & Hodgkins, C. (1998). A comparison of eclectic treatment with Webster-Stratton's parents and children series in a children's mental health center: A randomized controlled trial. *Behavior Therapy, 29*, 221–240.

Warner, K. E. (1977). The effects of the anti-smoking campaign on cigarette consumption. *American Journal of Public Health, 67*, 645–650.

Warner, K. E. (1989). Implications of a nicotine-free society. *Journal of Substance Abuse, 1*, 359–368.

Webster-Stratton, C. (1994). Advancing videotape parent training: A comparison study. *Journal of Consulting and Clinical Psychology, 62*, 583–593.

Webster-Stratton, C. (1995). *The Teachers and Children Videotape Series.* Seattle, WA: Seth Enterprises.

Webster-Stratton, C., Kolpacoff, M., & Hollinsworth, T. (1988). Self-administered videotape therapy for families with conduct-problem children: Comparison with two cost-effective treatments and a control group. *Journal of Consulting and Clinical Psychology, 56*, 558–566.

Weisz, J. R. (2000). Agenda for child and adolescent psychotherapy research: On the need to put science into practice. *Archives of General Psychiatry, 57*, 837–838.

Weisz, J. R., Donenberg, G. R., Han, S. S., & Weiss, B. (1995). Bridging the gap between laboratory and clinic in child and adolescent psychotherapy. *Journal of Consulting and Clinical Psychology, 63*, 688–701.

Weisz, J. R., & Hawley, K. M. (1998). Finding, evaluating, refining, and applying empirically supported treatments for children and adolescents. *Journal of Clinical Child Psychology, 27*, 206–216.

Weisz, J. R., Weiss, B., & Donenberg, G. R. (1992). The lab versus the clinic: Effects of child and adolescent psychotherapy. *American Psychologist, 47*, 1578–1585.

CHAPTER 5

Preventing Physical and Sexual Abuse

John R. Lutzker and
Cynthia L. Boyle

DESCRIPTION OF THE PROBLEM

Child maltreatment is a serious and remarkably prevalent disorder affecting children and their families. Incidence studies conducted by the U.S. Department of Health and Human Services (USDHHS) indicated that 903,000 children were victims of child maltreatment in the United States in 1998, with physical abuse constituting 22.7 % and sexual abuse 11.5 % (USDHHS, 2000); neglected children constitutes the remaining cases. Physical abuse usually is defined as an act of commission that causes physical injury, including such intentional behaviors as punching, beating, kicking, or otherwise harming a child (Greene & Kilili, 1998). Physical abuse can be (a) repeated exposure of a chronic nature or (b) an acute, serious episode. Neglect generally is regarded as consisting of acts of omission, that is, the failure to provide for basic biological needs, abandonment, or lack of supervision resulting in emotional, physical, or educational harm to the child.

The definition of sexual abuse is problematic because state, federal, and community definitions vary widely. Under federal law sexual abuse is defined as (a) "the employment, use, persuasion, inducement, enticement, or coercion of any child to engage in, or assist any other person to engage in, any sexually explicit conduct or simulation of such conduct for the purpose of producing a visual depiction of such conduct" or (b) "the rape, and in cases of caretaker or interfamilial relationships, statutory rape, molestation, prostitution, or other form of sexual exploitation of children, or incest with children" (USDHHS, 1999, p. 1). These acts must be committed by a parent or a person responsible for the care of the child; otherwise, these acts constitute sexual assault rather than sexual abuse. Each state provides its own civil and criminal definitions of child maltreatment. Some states do not define sexual abuse separately from physical child abuse and neglect.

REVIEW AND CRITIQUE OF THE LITERATURE

In the history of research, intervention, and prevention of serious human mental health and related societal problems, child maltreatment represents a relatively short history in that it was only formally recognized in the 1960s with the publication of *The Battered Child Syndrome* (Kempe, Silverman, Steele, Drogemueller, & Silver, 1962). Early attempts to explain physical and sexual abuse came from the psychiatric literature, looking for intrapsychic explanations of why perpetrators would act in harmful ways toward children. The possibility that children were willful seducers was accepted by some psychoanalysts in the early 1900s (Bender & Blau, 1937). During that time, the dominant stereotype of child molesters was the "stranger" whose acts were explained as sexual deviance, thus minimizing the role of familial perpetrators (Olafson, Corwin, & Summit, 1993). Other theories have postulated that sexual abuse occurs as a result of the perpetrator's severe attachment deprivation (Parker & Parker, 1986), absence and noninvolvement during the child's early years (Parker & Parker, 1986), accepting belief systems (i.e., intergenerational sexual abuse; Faller, 1991), patriarchy (Solomon, 1992), and vulnerability factors (Trepper & Barrett, 1986).

Later came theories suggesting more complex reasons for child maltreatment, such as the social/ecological perspective (Belsky, 1980). Lutzker (1984) suggested that child maltreatment is a problem associated with multiple environmental, social, ecological, and intrapersonal issues. Wolfe (1999) has noted that child rearing represents a continuum of practices on which physical and sexual abuse are at one extreme. Additionally, different cultural practices play a role in how abuse may be defined in the continuum of child-rearing practices (Kapitanoff, Lutzker, & Bigelow, 2000). Thus, a contemporary perspective of child maltreatment is a comprehensive one that includes parent and child factors, the social ecology of the family, cultural variables, and consideration of biological variables that may drive some parents.

As theories of child maltreatment evolved from looking exclusively at the individual to looking at broader social/ecological contexts, so have interventions. For example, one of the earliest reported interventions was by Gilbert

(1976), who trained a mother reported for child abuse by modeling descriptive praise of child behaviors. Although there was some apparent behavior change, such a narrowly focused approach would seem simplistic today. Another set of strategies, described as cognitive-behavioral, have been combined with behavioral parent training to reduce recidivism in parents reported for child maltreatment (Peterson, Gable, Doyle, & Ewigman, 1997).

The ecobehavioral model was first described by Lutzker, Frame, and Rice (1982). They suggested that, because child maltreatment is a problem with multifaceted determinants, a multifaceted approach to assessment and intervention would seem to be the most fruitful way to address the problem. Thus, Project 12-Ways (Lutzker, 1984) was developed to provide parent-child training, stress reduction for the parents, basic skill training for the children, home safety training for the parents, social support, money management, health and nutrition, activity planning, multiple-setting behavior management, problem solving, relationship counseling, substance abuse referral, and a single-parent prevention program. Project 12-Ways has been ongoing since 1979. From 1994 to 1998, Project SafeCare, a systematic replication of Project 12-Ways, was developed in the Los Angeles area (Lutzker, Bigelow, Doctor, Gershater, & Greene, 1998). Project SafeCare attempted to prevent recidivistic child maltreatment in parents who had been reported and to prevent it in parents who were at high risk more succinctly than did Project 12-Ways. Thus, three of the most frequently used and effective Project 12-Ways services—bonding (parent-child training), home safety, and child health care—were "packaged" by Project SafeCare. Parents were taught in five sessions each (15 total intervention sessions) to engage their children in planned activities training (Bigelow & Lutzker, 1998) as a child management tool to make their homes safer and to properly attend to their children's health needs (e.g., by learning basic skills such as temperature taking and more sophisticated skills such as knowing when to seek medical attention) (Bigelow & Lutzker, 1998). Video was used as an adjunct to instruction by counselors in home safety and planned activities training.

Protocols on both projects have been empirically validated. For example, the Home Accident Prevention Inventory (HAPI; Tertinger, Greene, & Lutzker, 1984) was validated by safety experts, first in rural southern Illinois and subsequently in urban Los Angeles. The HAPI-R (Mandel, Bigelow, & Lutzker, 1998) is used to directly assess safety hazards that are accessible to young children in the home. After hazards are assessed, a safety education program is presented to the parents in which they are directly instructed on how to make their home safer for their children. Dramatic reductions in hazards have been shown when this program is effected (Mandel et al., 1998).

Problems of home safety are very common in child maltreatment families and are often the reason for a neglect referral. Also, if a child is injured as a result of a home safety hazard, a subsequent abuse or neglect report may be filed. Finally, if a child receives a disabling injury in a home safety accident, that child is at higher risk for subsequent abuse, because children with disabilities are at higher risk for abuse than children without disabilities. Thus, improving home safety can serve to deter existing or subsequent child maltreatment.

Giving child health care skills to young parents has been shown to be a very important intervention and prevention mechanism (Bigelow & Lutzker, 1998). Wasik (1998) has noted that early intervention programs help prevent child maltreatment and make for healthier children. She also has suggested that home visiting is a critical variable in the success of early intervention programs. Zigler (1995) demonstrated that children's IQs are positively affected by participation in early intervention programs. Olds, Henderson, Tatelbaum, and Chamberlain (1988) suggested that, in addition to child outcome measures such as IQ, parent outcome measures be used to evaluate early intervention programs. An underlying belief with respect to these types of interventions is that the more comprehensive the program, the more likely the success (Wasik, 1998).

Delgado and Lutzker (1988) developed and validated a set of protocols for teaching parents child health care skills. Bigelow and Lutzker (2000) revalidated these health protocols for Project SafeCare. The protocols also were developed in Spanish, because more than half of Project SafeCare's families were Spanish-speaking. Teaching strategies for these protocols involved having the parent read the protocols, take a quiz, have the counselor demonstrate the skill, ask the parent to imitate the model, and then provide feedback to the parent. A skill was considered to be acquired when a parent demonstrated it five consecutive times without a model. If a parent failed to meet the criterion, a massed practice session focused on that particular skill was conducted. Almost all parents who participated mastered the health care skills at a 100% criterion, with all parents reaching a criterion of at least 85%.

In the early to mid 1980s, child sexual abuse (CSA) prevention research focused on teaching elementary school children safety skills to avoid abduction (Kohl, 1993). In an early example, Poche, Brouwer, and Swearington (1981) taught three preschool children to avoid abduction using modeling, behavioral rehearsal, and social reinforcement. *In vivo* baseline observations were conducted of the children's responses to three abduction lures near the school and in the community by confederate males. All three children either went with or stayed near the confederate. Training took place on school grounds and near the school. Two trainers acted out an abduction scene, with one trainer presenting a lure and another modeling the target verbal and motor responses. Then the child was asked to rehearse the abduction scenario. Correct responses were followed by social reinforcement; incorrect responses were followed by additional modeling and rehearsal until the target responses occurred once.

The target verbal response was "No, I have to go ask my teacher," and the target motor response was to move 20 feet away within 3 seconds of the lure. When the target responses occurred across the three different types of lures, training ended and the children then were assessed in the community. During in vivo probes at posttraining, self-protective responses were generalized to novel suspects and locations. This research provided evidence that training could be effective in producing target responses without providing children with a rationale of potential danger.

In the past 10–15 years, lectures, discussions, written materials, plays, films/videos, books, puppet shows, and behavioral skills training programs have been developed to teach abduction and/or CSA prevention knowledge and skills (Carroll, Miltenberger, & O'Neill, 1992). The prototypal CSA prevention program teaches five-step training strategies including: (a) recognizing good and bad touches, (b) saying "no," (c) leaving the situation, (d) finding and telling an adult, and (e) accurately disclosing the abuse. Prevention programs typically take a behavioral or a cognitive approach to teaching prevention concepts. Behavioral skills training (BST) involves presentation of instructions, modeling by the trainer, rehearsal by the participant, reinforcement, and corrective feedback—and may or may not use some form of role playing. It is a rule-governed approach in which children are taught which body parts are private, as well as rules about touching. BST has been found to be the most effective method used to teach prevention knowledge and skills to children (Carroll-Rowan & Miltenberger, 1994; Gast, Collins, Wolery, & Jones, 1993; Holcombe, Wolery, & Katzanmayer, 1995). Cognitive approaches rely on a contingency-based approach in which children are taught to make discriminations about their "feelings" in identifying abuse. Children sometimes are taught what CSA is and/or information about a perpetrator's motivations (Wurtele, 1998). Children are taught to identify whether they are "feeling good," "feeling bad," or "feeling confused" about touch as a means to recognize potential abuse. Some children may not feel confused about touching when a context is already established, for example, with a parent. Likewise, sexual contact may "feel good" and will not be recognized by the child as "bad" or "uncomfortable" (Kraizer, 1986). Moreover, the very assumption that sexual contact can feel only "confusing" or "bad" allows the already abused child to misperceive that he or she has done something wrong. Misunderstanding of the touch continuum could lead to false reporting (Kraizer, 1986). The touch continuum also fails to address some common antecedents to CSA such as print, video, and electronic pornography (Kraizer, 1986). These limiting variables have been demonstrated in studies (e.g., Blumberg, Chadwick, Fogarty, Speth, & Chadwick, 1991) which found a "rule-based" approach to be more effective than a "feelings based" one in teaching inappropriate touching of the genitals.

Wurtele, Kast, Miller-Perrin, and Kondrick (1989) compared the Touch Continuum (TC), a cognitive approach, with BST to teach CSA prevention to children attending two Head Start preschools. In both conditions, children practiced discriminating between appropriate and inappropriate touch requests using instructions, modeling, rehearsal, praise, and feedback. The BST group was superior to the CT group in accurately recognizing inappropriate touch requests at posttest and at one-month follow-up.

Few of the books for parents, school curricula, videos, and films for CSA prevention training are empirically evaluated before they are placed on the market (Stilwell, Lutzker, & Greene, 1988). One commercially available work, however, the *Red Flag, Green Flag Prevention Book* (Rape and Abuse Crisis Center, 1986), was evaluated by Miltenberger and Thiesse-Duffy (1988), who compared it with a BST program. Prevention responses (saying "no," go, and tell) are illustrated through the presentation of 10 dangerous antecedent situations to CSA or abduction. BST consisted of one-to-one training using instructions, rehearsal, modeling, praise, and feedback. At 2 months, an *in vivo* probe was conducted in the natural environment in which a confederate presented an incentive lure to the child. The prevention book alone and also with instructions was not effective in producing criterion performance for any of the children. BST produced criterion performance for all participants; however, only children who were 6 and 7 years of age maintained these skills at 2-month follow-up.

Poche, Yoder, and Miltenberger (1988) compared the effectiveness of (a) a self-protective skills videotape training program alone, (b) the videotape training program plus behavioral rehearsal, (c) a standard program (i.e., one provided by the school), and (d) no training. The videotape plus rehearsal condition was found to be the most effective condition, followed by the videotape-only condition, the standard condition, and the no-training control condition at posttest. Responses to *in vivo* probes revealed that 75% of the children in the no-training control condition immediately went with the confederate or stayed near him. Approximately 90 % of the 5- to 7-year-old children in the standard safety program went with the confederate or stayed near him.

The efficacy of role-playing prevention skills in a BST program was investigated by Wurtele, Marrs, and Miller-Perrin (1987), who compared the effectiveness of children practicing versus children watching others perform prevention skills. Scores from children who actively practiced prevention skills significantly increased from pretest to posttest compared with those who watched others; only after the latter group was trained with active practice did its posttest scores increase significantly over pretest levels. The effectiveness of BST with role playing was replicated by Wurtele and her colleagues with 4-year-old children attending a YWCA preschool (Wurtele, 1990) and 4- and 5-year-old Head Start preschoolers, using parents and teachers as trainers (Wurtele, Gillispie, Currier, & Franklin, 1992).

Whether teachers and parents can effectively present CSA prevention topics was investigated further by Wurtele, Kast, and Melzer (1992). Preschoolers
were assigned to one of four personal safety training groups: BST teacher
alone, BST parent alone, BST teacher and parent, or a control group.
Preschoolers in the three treatment conditions scored higher than those in the
control group on levels of personal safety skills. The finding that parents can
effectively present the BST program was subsequently replicated with sexually abused and nonabused boys and girls (Currier & Wurtele, 1996).

The potential negative impact of CSA prevention programs remains controversial. Increased fear and anxiety have been found in a small percentage
of children (e.g., Hazzard, Webb, Kleemeier, Angert, & Pohl, 1991); "however,
no study has documented that such effects last beyond the period immediately
following the program" (Daro, 1991, p. 2). Others (e.g., Olsen-Woods,
Miltenberger, & Foreman, 1998) have found no evidence on measures of fear
or adverse reactions at home or school. Those who reported utilizing the concepts in their daily lives and rated the program as having an overall positive
effect were also more likely to report elevated levels of fear or anxiety
(Finkelhor, Asdigian, & Dziuba-Leatherman, 1993). Thus, the temporary fear
or anxiety experienced by participants may be a healthy response similar to
experiencing negative emotions after learning about any other dangers. Children
have responded negatively to questions about whether they are to blame if they
are sexually abused (e.g., Currier & Wurtele, 1996). Wurtele (1998) pointed
out that the fear of overgeneralization from inappropriate to appropriate touches
has not been demonstrated, in that appropriate touch scores have not decreased
as a result of training, and appropriate touch scores have increased in some
cases. Nonetheless, there is no extensive empirical evidence to suggest that
children will not suffer emotional disturbances.

Given these concerns, measurement is crucial in determining whether teaching CSA prevention is efficacious. Researchers have created their own measures or used established measures. Creating new measures has obvious
limitations. Although measures usually fail to meet replication criteria from
one study to the next, there are several common methods that have been used.
The most direct method has been the in vivo probe, in which a confederate
posing as a stranger presents a lure to a child in a prearranged setting. The
child's response is taken as an indicator of the probable response in the event
of a potential abusive incident. Because measuring behavioral change *in vivo*
for familial sexual abuse raises serious ethical considerations, research has
only directly measured responses *in vivo* to abduction lures (e.g., Holcombe,
Wolery, & Katzanmayer, 1995).

Role-playing evaluates how a child will respond when faced with a potential abusive situation. Demonstration that younger children can learn prevention skills more effectively through active practice than through instruction
alone has led many prevention programs to utilize this technique.

Self-report measures are the most prevalent type of assessment instrument. Common self-report dependent measures of knowledge and/or behavior concerning a response to a familial perpetrator lure are the 13-item Personal Safety Questionnaire (PSQ; Saslawsky & Wurtele, 1986), the 24-item Children's Knowledge of Abuse Questionnaire-Revised (Tutty, 1995), and the What I Know About Touching Scale (Hazzard, Webb, Kleemeier, Angert, & Pohl, 1991). These have had only limited psychometric analyses.

Vignettes that require children to state safety strategies have also been used to assess safety knowledge (e.g., Grober & Bogat, 1994). Hazzard et al. (1991) developed a video vignettes measure to evaluate the effectiveness of *Feeling Yes, Feeling No* (National Film Board of Canada, 1985), a curriculum that incorporates an affective component with concrete rules and behavioral rehearsal with 399 third- and fourth-grade elementary school children. After watching each of four vignettes, children were asked: (a) whether they thought the situation was safe or unsafe; (b) if unsafe, why this was so; (c) if this was happening to them, what they would say; and (d) what they would do in that situation. They also were asked to rate if they thought they would feel positive or negative feelings in those situations. Similarly, Johnson (2000) evaluated the effectiveness of a school-based prevention program, *Protective Behaviours* (Flandreau West, 1984; 1989), via three video vignettes that depicted child actors experiencing physical, emotional, and sexual abuse. The participants were from 5 to 14 years old. Adverse reactions to the video vignettes were not reported by interviewers, teachers, or parents of children who participated.

A commonly used psychometrically sophisticated measure of prevention knowledge and skills is the What if Situations Test (WIST; Saslawsky & Wurtele, 1986), designed so that individual prevention skills could be analyzed. The WIST presents six scenarios which probe children's knowledge of responses to: (a) appropriate touch by parents and medical personnel because of injury, (b) inappropriate removal of clothes with a known person, (c) inappropriate touching of a known person, and (d) inappropriate touching of a child by a familiar person. Several studies have analyzed separate WIST components; however, the results have varied (e.g., Wurtele, Gillispie, Currier, & Franklin, 1992). Liang, Bogat, and McGrath (1993) empirically established that each component in CSA prevention training is a discrete skill. Their hypothesis was that correct performance of action skills (saying no, go, tell who, tell what) is contingent on correct performance of the first step in prevention training—recognizing that an interaction is potentially unsafe, and that the action skills are ordered in a sequence of least to most in difficulty. More than half of the children responded according to this pattern, falling slightly below statistical significance.

Numerous studies (e.g., Tutty, 2000) have found that older children learn more than younger children from prevention programs. This has been used to spur the debate that CSA prevention for younger children may be less efficacious because they are cognitively unprepared to learn safety concepts. Rispens, Aleman, and Goudena's (1997) meta-analysis of school-based CSA programs, however, revealed that younger children have greater knowledge gains than older children. Contingency-based approaches, that is, those dependent on discriminating feelings, such as the Touch Continuum, are less concrete than rule-governed approaches and may prove more difficult for younger children to grasp. Some of the same studies that found that younger children learn less were contingency-based (e.g., Tutty, 2000). Programs that have been successful with younger children are often rule-based (e.g., Miltenberger & Thiesse-Duffy, 1988; Wurtele, 1990; Wurtele et al., 1989; Wurtele, Currier, Gillispie, & Franklin, 1991; Wurtele & Sarno Owens, 1997). Although younger children benefit from training initially, gains tend to decrease over time (Rispens, Aleman, & Goudena, 1997). Providing subsequent booster sessions has been tried with success (Olsen-Woods, Miltenberger, & Foreman, 1998) and is commonly suggested by researchers (e.g., Rispens, Aleman, & Goudena, 1997; Wurtele, Kast, & Melzer, 1992; Wurtele & Sarno-Owens, 1997).

Unfortunately, to date there is no empirical evidence that CSA prevention programs have reduced the incidence of CSA. One retrospective study (Gibson & Leitenberg, 2000), however, found that a sample of college females who recalled participating in a CSA prevention program were significantly less likely to report experiencing CSA. Those who had not participated were twice as likely to report experiencing CSA. Moreover, a trend toward earlier disclosure and shorter duration of CSA was found in the CSA prevention program participants. No differences in sexual development or adjustment were found between the two groups.

Vermont developed the first public health campaign designed to target adults for prevention (Chasan-Taber & Tabachnick, 1999). Baseline data on attitudes, awareness, knowledge, and policies were collected from the residents of Vermont through random-digit dialing. Sexual abuser, family member, and friend focus groups were interviewed regarding strategies to promote self-disclosure by sexual abusers and action by family members who suspect abuse. A broad media campaign, a one-to-one outreach, and a systems change strategy were designed and implemented as a statewide prevention initiative. Followup was conducted 2 years later. Although the reported results were equivocal, the ability to define CSA increased by 20% and the belief that abusers live in one's community increased by 10%. Calls received (241) by a help line over the 2-year period found that 23% of callers identified themselves as abusers. The majority of 19 key decision makers and leaders in Vermont who were interviewed expressed a change in attitude from skepticism to support regarding the campaign. This approach serves as a promising complement to prevention efforts directed at children.

CASE EXAMPLES

Physical Abuse Case Example

Claudia was an 18-year-old Latina mother of a 1-month-old boy, referred from the child maternity center of a major local hospital for prevention. She spoke some English, but Project SafeCare sent a fluent Spanish-speaking female graduate assistant as the counselor. Claudia had completed her junior year of high school when she became pregnant. At the time, she was living at home, but she dropped out of school and moved into an apartment with her boyfriend, the father of the child. Shortly before she gave birth, the boyfriend left Claudia. At the time of the referral, Claudia was living alone with the child and was receiving public assistance. She was considered to be at risk for committing abuse because basic risk factors such as her being a poor young parent and socially isolated were present.

Project SafeCare assessed Claudia with the Beck Depression Inventory (BDI; Beck & Steer, 1993), the Parenting Stress Index (PSI; Abidin, 1990), and the Child Abuse Potential Inventory (CAPI; Milner 1986). The BDI indicated moderate depression, the PSI stress, and the CAPI that the child was at risk for abuse. By her own admission, Claudia did not have good child-rearing knowledge or skills. Baseline data collection on her parenting skills indicated few requisite parent/infant interaction skills. Her apartment had more than 150 accessible hazards to a young child, and she was able to meet only 30% of the skills assessed for child health care.

Because the child was an infant, the first skill package taught was child health care. In five sessions, Claudia was provided training to identify illnesses and to decide which could be treated by her and which should receive medical attention; additionally, she was asked to show what behaviors were required in emergency situations. Any skill on which criterion performance was not shown required positive practice of that skill. After five sessions, Claudia mastered the health care protocols to a 100% criterion and showed 100% performance on the generalization scenarios. Follow-up at 3 and 6 months demonstrated continued mastery.

After five successful training sessions in child health care, Claudia was taught parent-infant stimulation (PCI) and planned activities training (PAT). This was chosen over home safety because the child was so young that most of the safety hazards in the home would only be accessible once the child began to crawl and walk. Direct counselor intervention was supplemented by videos. The PCI videos stress the importance of attending to infants' needs and the importance of talking with young children so that language becomes a soothing stimulus event and a stimulus that promotes language in the young child.

The video, manual, and practice exercise also show simple stretching and other play activities for parents to do with infants. PAT stresses planning activities in advance, using incidental teaching strategies, stating rules of activities, and providing children with feedback about the performance during activities. Although infants will not understand the components of PAT, it is important to imbed these skills in the young parent, so that when the child becomes verbal, the parent can enhance language skills and prevent disruptive behaviors through PAT.

Claudia showed enthusiasm about PCI and PAT. Baseline indicated that she had few of these skills. After five intervention sessions, she demonstrated the requisite skills. Generalization to untrained activity settings and situations was nearly 100%. Follow-up at 3 and 6 months showed mastery not only of the trained skills, but also those assessed in all generalization settings.

After the completion of PCI/PAT in five sessions, home safety was taught. Using the Spanish-speaking counselor and the Spanish safety videos, Claudia was guided through the home safety program. First, the Home Accident Prevention Inventory-Revised (HAPI-R; Mandel, Bigelow, & Lutzker, 1998) was conducted. Claudia gave permission for observers to conduct this direct assessment of accessible home safety hazards in all rooms of her apartment. Next, she was provided with safety devices such as cabinet locks and electric socket plugs. Then, each session focused on a different room in which the counselor modeled how to install safety devices and then referred Claudia to the safety video, which showed how to make hazards inaccessible. After each segment of the protocol was provided to Claudia over five sessions, she had removed all of the hazards, in each room and made them inaccessible to the child. Follow-up data at 3 and 6 months showed that the reduction in accessible hazards had been maintained.

The BDI, the CAPI, and the PSI were administered after all training had been completed. Claudia's BDI scored moved from the moderate range of depression to below the clinical cut-off. Thus, no notable depression was reported after services were rendered. The CAPI scores and the PSI scores after services also went from stressed levels to below cut-off levels. Therefore, as with the majority of families who completed Project SafeCare services, Claudia went from a parent who was moderately depressed, stressed, and at risk of harming her child to a parent who no longer expressed depression, was less stressed, and was at much less risk of harming her child. Additionally, feeling more comfortable and confident with her skills and life situation, Claudia was able to arrange child care and begin a community college vocational program. Claudia's responses to the social validation questionnaire indicated that she was quite satisfied with Project SafeCare services and would readily recommend them to a friend. Of considerable significance, Claudia was never reported for child maltreatment.

This case example is representative of the 41 families who completed the Project SafeCare interventions services. That is, the program evaluation data indicated that there were significant pretest to posttest increases in parents' interaction skills with their children, decreases in accessible hazards in their homes, and increases in child health care skills. There were also clinically and statistically significant improvements in PSI, CAP-I, and BDI scores. Finally, analyses have shown large differences between Project SafeCare families and comparison families with regard to recidivism. Two years after intervention, 85% of the families served by Project SafeCare had no reports of child maltreatment, whereas only 56% of the comparison group had no reports.

Sexual Abuse Case Example

Taking the lead of Rothbaum et al. (1995), who conducted the first controlled study of virtual reality exposure therapy for the treatment of phobia, and the current state of the CSA literature, the following is a hypothetical example which comprises components of an ideal CSA prevention program.

As children enter preschool, training specific to CSA would be conducted as part of a multicomponent curriculum. CSA training and assessment for typically developing preschoolers would be conducted using a three-dimensional virtual world accessed through a head-mounted display providing visual and audio input. The CSA prevention program would begin with a pretest for knowledge of the names and locations of body parts. Children would wear the head-mounted display and see anatomically correct three-dimensional images of male and female human anatomy. First, children would *verbalize* the names of body parts highlighted by the computer on either the male or female anatomy. Second, they would *point* to body parts verbally prompted by a computer-generated male or female voice. Inability to verbalize and/or point to a body part would indicate that one or the other repertoire was deficient, thus requiring that response class to be taught directly. The presentation for identification of body parts would be similar to the pretest with the exception that the computer would generate an interactive learning experience. Correct answers would be reinforced with points and delivered in a manner similar to video games or pinball machines (e.g., flashing lights, engaging graphics, and applause). After a repertoire of correct labeling was established, a baseline for responses to validated scenarios that require children to discriminate whether or not the situation is appropriate or inappropriate would be presented. The scenario would be interactive in that the child would be immersed in the virtual environment specific to each scenario. For example, a scenario might play out as follows:

A doctor standing in a examining room beckons the child into the office. The child complies and the doctor remarks, "Looks like you have been hurt." The child looks down and sees a big band aid on his pants area over his private part. The doctor asks, "May I take a look at your (private part) to make sure you are OK?" The child must then respond to the request. With the child's response, the trial would end.

The participants would be taught, via presentation of an anatomically correct male and female, that private parts are the parts of the body beneath the underwear or swimsuit. With male and female models wearing swimsuits as cues, the participants would be prompted to verbally state and point to private parts once. Rules about appropriate and inappropriate touching would be presented verbally and visually. For example, with the rule that "it is not OK for anyone to touch you with their private parts," the child would be standing by a girl sitting on a ledge of a swimming pool and an adult nearby in his bathing suit. Much like a "cut and paste," the adult's bathing suit region would be "cut and pasted" from his body to contact the girl's arm with an immediate red circle and slash mark covering the touch. Thereafter, rules and visuals would be presented twice in discrete trial format (e.g., "Is it OK for anyone to touch you with their private parts?") until correct responses to rules occurred on three occasions.

After rules were taught, adaptive training tailored to the performance level of the child, established during baseline, would be presented. If a particular concept was clear to the child, that type of scenario would be eliminated, and those with which the child was having difficulty would be increased. The training would consist of a pool of 100 or more interactive scenarios similar to those used in baseline. The characters in the scenarios would need to depict strangers; familiar, but unknown persons, the child had previously encountered; family friends and known adults; and relatives or people within the family. However, the latter characters would not be identifiable or named (e.g., "mommy" or "daddy"). Types of scenarios would include: (a) antecedents to abuse (e.g., removal of child or adult clothing at inappropriate times, verbalizations regarding secret keeping or threats, unsupervised time with an adult without parent approval); (b) nonantecedents to abuse (e.g., appropriate interactions between children and others); (c) appropriate touch of private parts; (d) inappropriate touch of private parts; (e) inappropriate touch of others; and (f) appropriate touch of others. A typical scenario might proceed as follows:

A child is standing in what looks like a child's bedroom and sees that he is in his pajamas. A voice from another room says, "Get into bed and I'll read you a story." The child gets into bed and under the covers. A man who might be someone's grandfather enters the room with a book in his hand. He looks at the child and asks, "You don't mind if I sit here on the edge of your bed while I read you the story, do you?" The child responds "no," and the trial ends.

Correct responses would be reinforced with points. Incorrect responses would be immediately followed by a verbalization describing why that response was incorrect and then the correct response. The child would be presented with the scenario again and reinforced with points for the correct response. After the child responded to all scenarios without error, the training would end. Booster sessions could be conducted at 6-month intervals thereafter. The absence of error after three consecutive booster sessions would conclude training.

FUTURE DIRECTIONS

Dissemination is a critical step in expanding the ecobehavioral model. What distinguishes this model from large national programs such as Healthy Start are its empirical focus, emphasis on criterion performance for staff and families, and fidelity measures of intervention. Staff must show that they meet skill levels at predetermined criteria. Furthermore, the fidelity of their skills are observed in family homes. The participating families also must show criterion skills before advancing to other intervention components. Additionally, the skills expected from the families are skills that are measured directly, rather than evaluated by ratings or questionnaires.

CSA prevention models are limited by their inability to directly measure the efficacy of the independent variable and the validity of the dependent variable. Efforts to measure children's actual responses to potentially unsafe situations by staging abduction scenarios have brought the field closer to a true measure of safety skills; however, further investigation of these methods has not been conducted due to ethical considerations (Wurtele, 1998). CSA prevention models and measures that specifically target the most frequently occurring kind of sexual abuse (i.e., that perpetrated by familiar, known, or related persons) have yet to be sufficiently developed. Practical suggestions, such as using anatomical dolls in role plays to demonstrate prevention skills (Miltenberger, Thiesse-Duffy, Suda, Kozac, & Bruellman, 1990), are often difficult to initiate given the process of consent by institutional review boards, educators, and parents. Future research should investigate what factors have influenced well-received CSA programs by educators and parents. Teachers may play a key role in influencing whether a CSA program will be accepted by a school. Offering education in training techniques might thus lead to receptive responses from teachers. Longitudinal studies that assess whether pre-school children subsequently avoid abuse after prevention training compared with children who did not receive such training could provide valuable information to disseminate to educational decision makers who believe that younger children are incapable of learning or would be too shocked by prevention content. Wurtele (1993) described emerging and optimistic support for behavioral approaches to CSA prevention. Since then, the efficacy of the behavioral approach as a training method has been established (see Wurtele, 1998); however, lack of evidence for primary prevention has lead to dwindling acceptance of CSA prevention programs by critics. Wurtele (1998) recently addressed this trend, passionately concluding that these programs should not be abolished but merely challenged with more questions.

Wurtele (1993) made a number of excellent suggestions concerning what could be improved in the prevention of physical child maltreatment. Little has changed since those suggestions were made. For example, she suggested that a broader demographic than low socioeconomic status might be worth examining. This has generally not been implemented. Similarly, she opined that child victims should receive attention via empirically validated services. This, too, has largely not been implemented. Finally, a particularly cogent suggestion is the examination of "best fit" practices. That, is we need to be able to identify which strategies from our armamentarium are the most effective for various kinds of families.

Three areas of prevention deserve additional attention. First, Wurtele (1998) has suggested that a human development curriculum should be required in schools. The best of all worlds would have a curriculum that is skill-based and competency-based from preschool through college. This curriculum would have developmentally appropriate modules teaching positive relationships: problem solving, conflict resolution, CSA prevention, date rape prevention, and parenting/child care skills. Second, providing intervention for child victims of maltreatment aids in the prevention of subsequent posttraumatic stress disorder and other sequelae associated with child maltreatment. Only a handful of interventions have been employed with child victims, and most of them have little empirical support. This is an area of future fertile possibilities. Finally, the media, particularly the visual media, could contribute greatly to prevention efforts. If the media could be convinced by parents and other consumer advocates to present less violence and portray appropriate models for parenting and childcare, and even sex abuse awareness, further prevention might well occur.

Intervention and research in child maltreatment has a short history compared with more established fields such as medicine, psychology, and social work. Work in child maltreatment is also most often interdisciplinary, creating some challenges not found in a single discipline. Thus, a well-established prevention model has not yet been developed. Nonetheless, as seen in this chapter, some clear progress has been made which, we hope, will continue in the coming decade.

REFERENCES

Abidin, R. R. (1990). *Parenting Stress Index* (2nd ed.). Charlottesville, VA: Pediatric Psychology Press.

Beck, A. T., & Steer, R. A. (1993). *Beck Depression Inventory: Manual.* San Antonio, TX: Psychological Corporation.

Belsky, J. (1980). Child maltreatment: An ecological integration. *American Psychologist, 35,* 320–335.

Bender, L., & Blau, A. (1937). The reaction of children to sexual relations with adults. *American Journal of Orthopsychiatry, 7,* 500–518.

Bigelow, K. M., & Lutzker, J. R. (2000). Training parents reported for or at risk for child abuse and neglect to identify and treat their children's illnesses. *Journal of Family Violence, 15,* 311–330.

Bigelow, K. M., & Lutzker, J. R. (1998). Using video to teach planned activities to parents reported for child abuse. *Child & Family Behavior Therapy, 20,* 1–14.

Blumberg, E., Chadwick, M., Fogarty, L., Speth, T., & Chadwick, D. (1991). The touch discrimination component of sexual abuse prevention training: Unanticipated positive consequences. *Journal of Interpersonal Violence, 6,* 12–28.

Carroll, L., Miltenberger, R., & O'Neill, K. (1992). A review and critique of research evaluating child sexual abuse prevention programs. *Education and Treatment of Children, 15,* 335–354.

Carroll-Rowan, L. A., & Miltenberger, R. G. (1994). A comparison of procedures for teaching abduction prevention to preschoolers. *Education and Treatment of Children, 17,* 113–128.

Chasan-Taber, L., & Tabachnick, J. (1999). Evaluation of a child sexual abuse prevention program. *Sexual Abuse, 11,* 279–292.

Currier, L. L., & Wurtele, S. K. (1996). A pilot study of previously abused and non-sexually abused children's responses to a personal safety program. *Journal of Child Sexual Abuse, 5,* 71–87.

Daro, D. (1991). Child sexual abuse prevention: Separating fact from fiction. *Child Abuse and Neglect, 15,* 1–4.

Delgado, L. E., & Lutzker, J. R. (1988). Training young parents to identify and report their children's illnesses. *Journal of Applied Behavior Analysis, 21,* 311–319.

Erickson, W. D., Luxenburg, M. G., Walbek, N. H., & Seely, R. K. (1987). Frequency of MMPI two-point code types among sex offenders. *Journal of Consulting and Clinical Psychology, 55*, 566–570.

Faller, K. (1991). Polyincestuous families: An exploratory study. *Journal of Interpersonal Violence, 6*, 310–322.

Finkelhor, D., Asdigian, N., & Dziuba-Leatherman, J. (1993). *Victimization prevention training in action: A national survey of children's experiences coping with actual threats and assaults and reactions.* Final report of the National Youth Victimization Prevention Study, funded by the Boy Scouts of America.

Flandreau West, P. (1989). *The basic essentials: Protective behaviours antivictimization and empowerment process.* Adelaide, Australia: Essence Publications.

Flandreau West, P. (1984). *Protective behaviours—An anti-victimization program.* Madison, WI: Protective Behaviours.

Gast, D. L., Collins, B. C., Wolery, M., & Jones, R. (1993). Teaching preschool children with disabilities to respond to the lures of strangers. *Exceptional Children, 59*, 301–311.

Greene, B. F., & Kilili, S. (1998). How good does a parent have to be? Issues and examples associated with empirical assessments of parenting adequacy in cases of child abuse and neglect. In J. R. Lutzker (Ed.), *Handbook of child abuse research and treatment* (pp. 53–72). New York: Plenum.

Gibson, L. E., & Leitenberg, H. (2000). Child sexual abuse prevention programs: Do they decrease the occurrence of child sexual abuse? *Child Abuse & Neglect, 24*, 1115–1125.

Grober, J. S., & Bogat, G. A. (1994). Social problem solving in unsafe situations: Implications for sexual abuse education programs. *American Journal of Community Psychology, 22*, 399–414.

Hall, G. C., Maiuro, R. D., Vitaliano, P. P., & Procter, W. D. (1986). The utility of the MMPI with men who have sexually assaulted children. *Journal of Consulting and Clinical Psychology, 54*, 493–496.

Hazzard, A., Webb, C., Kleemeier, C., Angert, L., & Pohl, J. (1991). Child sexual abuse prevention: Evaluation and one-year follow-up. *Child Abuse and Neglect, 15*, 123–138.

Holcombe, A., Wolery, M., & Katzanmayer, J. (1995). Teaching preschoolers to avoid abduction by strangers: Evaluation of maintenance strategies. *Journal of Child and Family Studies, 4*, 177–191.

Johnson, B. (2000). Using video vignettes to evaluate children's personal safety knowledge: Methodological and ethical issues. *Child Abuse & Neglect, 24*, 811–827.

Kapitanoff, S., Lutzker, J. R., & Bigelow, K. M. (2000). Cross-cultural issues in disabilities and abuse. *Aggression and Violent Behavior, 5*, 227–244.

Kraizer, S. K. (1986). Rethinking prevention. *Child Abuse & Neglect, 10,* 259–261.

Kraizer, S., Witte, S., & Fryer, G. (1989). Child sexual abuse prevention programs: What makes them effective in protecting children? *Children Today, 18,* 23–27.

Kaufman, I., Peck, A. L., Tagiuri, C. K. (1954). The family constellation and overt incestuous relations between father and daughter. *American Journal of Orthopsychiatry, 24,* 266–279.

Kempe, C. H., Silverman, F. N., Steele, B. F., Droegemueller, N., & Silver, H. K. (1962). The battered child syndrome. *Journal of the American Medical Association, 181,* 17–24.

Kohl, J. (1993). School-based child sexual abuse prevention programs. *Journal of Family Violence, 8,* 137–150.

Liang, B., Bogat, G. A., & McGrath, M. P. (1993). Differential understanding of sexual abuse prevention concepts among preschoolers. *Child Abuse and Neglect, 17,* 641–650.

Lutzker, J. R. (1984). Project 12-Ways: Treating child abuse and neglect from an ecobehavioral perspective. In R. F. Dangel & R. A. Polster (Eds.), *Parent training: Foundations of research and practice* (pp. 260–291). New York: Guilford.

Lutzker, J. R., Frame, R. E., & Rice, J. M. (1982). Project 12-Ways: An ecobehavioral approach to the treatment and prevention of child abuse and neglect. *Eduction & Treatment of Children, 5,* 141–155.

Lutzker, J. R., Bigelow, K. M., Doctor, R. M., Gershater, R. M., & Greene, B. F. (1998). An ecobehavioral model for the prevention and treatment of child abuse and neglect: History and applications. In J. R. Lutzker (Ed.), *A handbook of child abuse research and treatment* (pp. 239–266). New York: Plenum.

Malcolm, P. B., Andrews, D. A., & Quinsey, V. L. (1993). Discriminant and predictive validity of phallometrically measured sexual age and gender preference. *Journal of Interpersonal Violence, 8,* 486–501.

Mandel, U., Bigelow, K. M., & Lutzker, J. R. (1998). Using video to reduce home safety hazards with parents reported for child abuse or neglect. *Journal of Family Violence, 13,* 147–162.

Milner, J. S. (1986). *The child abuse potential inventory: Manual (2nd ed.).* Webster, NC: Psytec.

Miltenberger, R. G., & Thiesse-Duffy, E. (1988). Evaluation of home-based programs for teaching personal safety skills to children. *Journal of Applied Behavior Analysis, 21,* 81–87.

Miltenberger, R. G., Thiesse-Duffy, E., Suda, K. T., Kozak, C., & Bruellman, J. (1990). Teaching prevention skills to children: The use of multiple measures to evaluate parent versus expert instruction. *Child and Family Behavior Therapy, 12,* 65–87.

National Clearinghouse on Child Abuse and Neglect Information. (1999). *Child abuse and neglect state statutes elements: Reporting laws, number 1, definitions of child abuse and neglect.* Washington, DC: U.S. Department of Health and Human Services.

National Film Board of Canada. (1985). *Feeling yes, feeling no* [video]. Available from Perennial Education, 930 Pitner, Evanston, Illinois 60620.

Olafson, E., Corwin, D. L., & Summit, R. C. (1993). Modern history of child sexual abuse awareness: Cycles of discovery and suppression. *Child Abuse & Neglect, 17,* 7–24.

Olds, D. L., Henderson, C. R., Tatelbaum, R., & Chamberlain, R. (1988). Improving the delivery of prenatal care and outcomes of pregnancy: A random trial of nurse home visitation. *American Journal of Public Health, 78,* 1436–1445.

Olsen-Woods, L. A., Miltenberger, R. G., & Foreman, G. (1998). Effects of correspondence training in an abduction prevention training program. *Child & Family Behavior Therapy, 20,* 15–34.

Parker, H., & Parker, S. (1986). Father-daughter sexual abuse: An emerging perspective. *American Journal of Orthopsychiatry, 56,* 531–549.

Peterson, L., Gable, S., Doyle, C., & Ewigman, B. (1997). Beyond parenting skills: Battling barriers and building bonds to prevent child abuse and neglect. *Cognitive & Behavioral Practice, 4,* 53–74.

Poche, C., Brouwer, R., & Swearingen, M. (1981). Teaching self-protection to young children. *Journal of Applied Behavior Analysis, 14,* 169–176.

Poche, C., Yoder, P., & Miltenberger, R. (1988). Teaching self-protection to children using television techniques. *Journal of Applied Behavior Analysis, 21,* 253–261.

Rape and Abuse Crisis Center (1986). *Red flag, green flag prevention book.* Fargo, ND: Author.

Rispens, J., Aleman, A., & Goudena, P. P. (1997). Prevention of child sexual abuse victimization: A meta-analysis of school programs. *Child Abuse & Neglect, 21,* 975–987.

Rothbaum, B. O., Hodges, L. F., Kooper, R., Opdyke, D., Williford, J., & North, M. M. (1995). Effectiveness of computer-generated (virtual reality) graded exposure in the treatment of acrophobia. *American Journal of Psychiatry, 152,* 626–628.

Saslawsky, D. A., & Wurtele, S. K. (1986). Educating children about sexual abuse: Implications for pediatric intervention and possible prevention. *Journal of Pediatric Psychology, 11,* 235–245.

Solomon, J. C., (1992). Child sexual abuse by family members: A radical feminist perspective. *Sex Roles, 27,* 473–485.

Stilwell, S. L., Lutzker, J. R., & Greene, B. F. (1988). Evaluation of a sexual abuse prevention program for preschoolers. *Journal of Family Violence, 13,* 269–280.

Tertinger, Greene, & Lutzker (1984). Home safety: Development and validation of one component of an ecobehavioral treatment for abused and neglected children. *Journal of Applied Behavior Analysis, 13*, 159–174.
Trepper, T. S., & Barrett, M. (1986). Vulnerability to incest: A framework for
  assessment. *Journal of Psychotherapy & the Family, 2*, 13–25.
Tutty, L. M. (1995). The revised Children's Knowledge of Abuse Questionnaire:
  Development of a measure of children's understanding of sexual abuse
  prevention concepts. *Social Work Research, 19*, 112–120.
Tutty, L. M. (2000). What children learn from sexual abuse prevention pro-
  grams: Difficult concepts and developmental issues. *Research on Social
  Work Practice, 10*, 275–300.
U. S. Department of Health and Human Services, Administration on Children,
  Youth, and Families (2000). *Child maltreatment 1998: Reports from the
  states to the National Child Abuse and Neglect Data System.* Washington,
  DC: U. S. Government Printing Office.
Wasik, B. H. (1998). Implications for child abuse and neglect: Interventions
  from early education interventions. In J. R. Lutzker (Ed.), *Handbook of
  child abuse research and treatment* (pp. 75–115). New York: Plenum.
Wolfe, D. A. (1999). *Child abuse* (2nd edition). Thousand Oaks, CA: Sage.
Wurtele, S. K. (1998). School-based child sexual abuse prevention programs:
  Questions, answers, and more questions. In J. R. Lutzker (Ed.), *Handbook
  of child abuse research and treatment* (pp. 501–516). New York: Plenum.
Wurtele, S. K. (1993). Prevention of child physical and sexual abuse. In D. S.
  Glenwick & L. A. Jason (Eds.), *Promoting health and mental health in
  children, youth, and families* (pp. 33–49). New York: Springer Publishing.
Wurtele, S. K. (1990). Teaching personal safety skills to four-year-old children: A behavioral approach. *Behavior Therapy, 21*, 25–32.
Wurtele, S. K., Currier, L. L., Gillispie, E. I., & Franklin, C. F. (1991). The
  efficacy of a parent implemented program for teaching preschoolers personal safety skills. *Behavior Therapy, 22*, 69–83.
Wurtele, S. K., Gillispie, E. I., Currier, L. L., & Franklin, C. F. (1992). A comparison of teachers vs. parents as instructors of a personal safety program
  for preschoolers. *Child Abuse and Neglect, 16*, 127–137.
Wurtele, S. K., Kast, L. C., & Melzer, A. M. (1992). Sexual abuse prevention
  education for young children: A comparison of teachers and parents as
  instructors. *Child Abuse and Neglect, 16*, 865–876.
Wurtele, S. K., Kast, L. C., Miller-Perrin, C. L., & Kondrick, P.A. (1989).
  Comparison of programs for teaching personal safety skills to preschoolers. *Journal of Consulting and Clinical Psychology, 57*, 505–511.
Wurtele, S. K., Marrs, S. R., & Miller-Perrin, C. L. (1987). Practice makes
  perfect? The role of participant modeling in sexual abuse prevention programs. *Journal of Consulting and Clinical Psychology, 55*, 599–602.

Wurtele, S. K., & Miller-Perrin, C. L. (1987). An evaluation of side-effects associated with participation in a child sexual abuse prevention program. *Journal of School Health, 57*, 228–231.

Wurtele, S. K., & Sarno-Owens, J. (1997). Teaching personal safety skills to young children: An investigation of age and gender across five studies. *Child Abuse and Neglect, 21*, 805–814.

Zigler, E. F. (1995). Can we "cure" mental retardation among individuals in the lower socioeconomic stratum? *American Journal of Public Health, 85*, 302–304.

CHAPTER 6

Preventing School Failure and Promoting Positive Outcomes

Lisa Machoian,

Jean E. Rhodes,

Nancy Rappaport, and

Ranjini Reddy

DESCRIPTION OF THE PROBLEM

Despite the trend toward high-school completion, about 5% of American high-school students drop out of school each year (Kaufman, Kwon, Klein, & Chapman, 1999; Rumberger, 2001). High-school dropouts face greater risks for unemployment, reliance on public assistance, low wages, and incarceration than their peers (Finn, 1989; Rossi & Montgomery, 1994; Rumberger, 1987). Learning disabilities, untreated attention deficit hyperactivity disorder, early parenthood, emotional reactions to family stressors, and chronic illnesses have all been implicated in school failure (Mattison, 2001; Steinberg, Brown, & Dornbusch 1997). Other factors, which are the focus of this chapter, are best described as problems in the structure and organizational culture of American schools. Irrespective of the reasons, however, the cost to society of these poor outcomes is tremendous. Clearly, there is a need to intervene early to prevent school failure.

What can be done to prevent failure and to ensure that all students achieve to the best of their abilities in school? Educational reformers have wrestled with this question for decades and have attempted countless strategies with varying degrees of success. These have included instructional changes (e.g., curricular improvements, more rigorous standards, better textbooks), grouping strategies (e.g., ability tracking, cooperative learning), improvements in teaching (e.g., professionalizing teaching, improving salaries), enhancing support (e.g., facilitating teacher-student relationships, mentoring programs), structural reforms (e.g., smaller groupings, fewer transitions), alternatives to the public schools (e.g., charter schools, vouchers, contracting), improving attendance and reducing attrition (e.g., dropout prevention), and home-school partnerships (e.g., building connections between parents and schools). Although a complete review of the rationale for and effectiveness of these approaches is beyond this chapter's scope, we will highlight some of the more commonly advocated strategies for preventing school failure and promoting achievement.

REVIEW AND CRITIQUE OF THE LITERATURE

Instructional Changes

Educators and policy makers often focus on modifying classroom learning and curricula as a means of preventing school failure and improving students' performance. Experts (e.g., Murnane & Levy, 1996) argued that American students do poorly in comparison with students from other industrialized countries because American schools provide relatively fewer opportunities for in-depth, thorough learning. Along these lines, Darling-Hammond (1997) has advocated more meaningful and relevant school experiences that promote critical thinking and deeper engagement of students in the learning process rather than rote memory of decontextualized information.

Early experience with school-to-work programs and other applied learning activities often are advocated as strategies for more fully engaging some students in school. With academic learning complementing the work experience, students improve their proficiency and are better prepared for employment (Eccles & Midgley, 1989). For instance, the Work Experience Program was designed for students in grades 7 through 10 who have been identified as being at risk for school dropout by virtue of their economic disadvantage and lack of motivation to perform in school (Fernandez, 1991). The Work Experience Program offers these students planned learning experiences with job shadowing, student internships, and exposure to employment opportunities. Work Experience programs and other school-to-work experiences can engage students in the learning process. By taking abstract concepts to the workplace, initially reluctant learners can have the opportunity to discover the relevance and applicability of information to real life (Fernandez, 1991).

Other researchers (e.g., Chall, 2000; Ravitch, 2000) have argued for a return to basics in curricula. They emphasize standards and the mastery of core concepts on the grounds that all students, irrespective of race or class, need to have a common knowledge base. Chall (2000), for example, has argued that many educational innovations do little more than dilute learning and undermine academic achievement. This criticism has prompted districts to adopt tightly stipulated curricula, standardized across settings. Critics of this core base of knowledge perspective are cautious about gaining a superficial exposure to a large number of concepts from different disciplines (e.g., Perkins, 1992). Their premise is that knowledge is accumulated over many years as a consequence of students engaging school content thoughtfully.

Grouping Strategies

Another approach to preventing school failure is to design a more customized educational plan for each individual student. Proponents (e.g., Levine, 2000) of this approach have argued that, because students are diverse in their abilities, they need curricula that are more directly tailored to their abilities. This, in turn, can lead to greater precision in how students are grouped. As Levine (2000) predicted, "We are heading to an era in which schooling will change profoundly.... Children will no longer be grouped by age. Each student will advance at his or her own pace in each subject area through individualized tutorials, student-centered group learning, and a cornucopia of new technology and software" (p. 24).

Other researchers (e.g., McEwin, Dickenson, & Jenkins, 1996) have argued for more heterogeneous ability tracking as a way to redress the fact that students from the dominant culture often are overly represented in the higher-performing academic sections. Within this context, cooperative learning and interdisciplinary teaming have become popular reforms, aimed at achieving educational equity and reducing school failure among students at greatest risk (Jackson & Davis, 2000). In cooperative learning, for example, students work in small groups that encourage peer interaction and cooperation. There is a subtle shift from a teacher-led classroom to more student-driven learning. This approach is seen as particularly important to minority students, who often respond to the covert struggles of domination by asserting their resistance and establishing their identity as uninterested and disruptive students (Fordham, 1996; Gibson & Ogbu, 1991). The underachievement pattern of minority students is expected to shift as cooperative learning fosters greater autonomy and responsibility for pursuing knowledge (Delpit, 1995).

Another approach, interdisciplinary teaming, involves the assignment of a common group of students to a team of two or more teachers. This allows teachers to work more closely with a group of students and offers opportunities for increasing teacher-student bonds. In addition, by working together, teachers develop a sense of community and can work more effectively to address common student problems. Empirical research (Arhar & Kromrey, 1995) has indeed found positive benefits to the continuity that interdisciplinary teaming provides, including increased emotional connectedness between teachers and students.

It should be noted, however, that interdisciplinary teaming has not always resulted in positive gains, particularly since the formation of small groups does not prevent the development of ability status comparisons among students (Cohen & Lotan, 1995). Arhar (1997) echoed these concerns, suggesting that interdisciplinary teaming can sometimes lead to time conflicts in the scheduling needs of the team and the school as a whole and competition among teams. Therefore, it is important to implement teams with adequate teacher training and ongoing support. In their review of the literature, Jackson and Davis (2000) concluded that effective teams are those teams that plan and focus on their goals (e.g., student learning), develop specific strategies for sustaining staff and student involvement and energy, are flexible and continually tuned to the cultural and social values of students' context, and continuously assess their progress.

Improvements in Teaching

Other strategies for preventing school failure have focused on teacher competence and the relationships that teachers forge with their students. Research (Delpit, 1995) indicates that a key element in predicting students' success in school is their exposure to effective teachers. Ferguson (1991), for example, found that teachers' expertise (as measured by advanced educational degrees, high licensing examination scores, and experience) accounted for considerable variance in students' achievement, even when compensating for family and socioeconomic disadvantage. In a comprehensive review by Greenwald, Hedges, and Lain (1996) of 60 studies, similar findings emerged. Greenwald et al. (1996) concluded that teacher' competence (as measured by classroom management and pedagogical rigor) and advanced education were associated with significant increases in student achievement.

In light of these and related findings, researchers and policy makers (e.g., Darling-Hammond, 1997) have increasingly advocated strategies that enhance the teaching profession by improving and standardizing teacher educational requirements, offering professional development, and hiring better-paid, well-educated teachers (Darling-Hammond, 1997). Also, good teaching is fostered by schools where the structure of the school allows teachers to build on each other's strengths and compensate for weaknesses (Oakes, Quartz, Ryan, & Lipton, 2000). As Meier (1995) reflected, "School change of the depth and breath required, change that breaks within the tradition of our own schooling, cannot be undertaken by a faculty that is not convinced and involved" (p. 109).

Structural Reforms

Reforms that seek to change the school environment play a prominent role in efforts to prevent failure and promote better student outcomes. These efforts often focus on the creation of smaller schools and class sizes, advising programs, school-within-school programs, and transition programs. Many of these programs are initiated as a means of helping students as they make transitions to new schools or into middle or high school, when students are more vulnerable to declining school performance (Felner, Primavera, & Cauce, 1981; Jason et al., 1992; MacIver, 1990). Such programs attempt to redress some of the problems that emerge as a function of the changing structure of middle and high schools. For example, supportive bonds with teachers often become less practical as students move into middle and high school and no longer have a primary teacher with whom they spend most of the day (Eccles, Lord, & Buchanan, 1996). These changes, unfortunately, often lead to declining teacher-student closeness. Midgley, Feldlaufer, and Eccles (1989) found that students perceived middle-school teachers as more remote and impersonal than elementary-school teachers. This growing distance decreases the likelihood that teachers can intervene with problems at an early stage. Indeed, researchers (Cauce, Mason, Gonzales, Hiraga, & Liu, 1994; Lynch & Cicchetti, 1997) have noted that middle-school students tend to have few positive interactions with teachers outside of instruction and feel less secure with their teachers than do elementary school children. The growing emphasis on standardized testing in middle and high school often gives rise to rigid curricular demands that constrain teachers and leave little room for the kinds of activities that typically draw them closer to their students. These trends have created obstacles to the formation of genuine, trusting relationships between teachers and students (Evans, 1996; Freedman, 1993; McDonald, 1996; Oakes et al., 2000). Moreover, cuts in school budgets have resulted in larger teacher-to-student ratios, making it more difficult or challenging for teachers to give students individual attention.

To address these obstacles, some structural school reform efforts have focused on reducing the barriers to positive student-teacher relationships. Practices such as homeroom assignments, advising, multiyear teacher assignments (i.e., maintaining the same teacher for more than 1 year), and smaller groupings of students have all been employed (Noddings, 1992; Oakes et al., 2000; Pianta, 2000; Sergiovannl, 1994). Homeroom teachers' roles may be modified to include counseling and tracking student absences and grades; in this way, they can serve as a key link between the students, their parents, and the rest of the school (Felner & Adan, 1988). There appears to be considerable variation in the extent to which these efforts have led to meaningful change in schools, particularly when the reforms have the unintended impact of over-burdening teachers or undermining their sense of autonomy over classroom practices (Oakes et al., 2000; Phillips, 1997). A major challenge for schools is to create settings that can maximize teachers' and other staff members' caring potential, while maintaining academic rigor and some degree of teacher autonomy.

Unfortunately, many programs involving structural changes never get off the ground and are difficult to sustain in public schools. Teachers and administrators sometimes resist efforts that are seen as being too big a drain on resources or as destabilizing to the system (Oakes et al., 2000). Advising programs, for example, require a significant reallocation of resources, time, and staff professional development to expand teachers' roles (Rappaport, 1999). Faced with competing demands on resources and teachers' time, many schools do not make the investment necessary to sustain school reforms (Ravitch, 2000).

Alternative Settings

Beyond the changes that have been implemented in the public school system, a major trend in recent years has been the emergence of charter schools. Charter schools are independent public schools that operate with greater autonomy than traditional public schools (Darling-Hammond, 1997). They are established with performance contracts or "charters," which stipulate the schools' missions, approaches, goals, and evaluation criteria. Charter schools reflect a movement to create small, intimate school communities with stringent forms of accountability, and, often, heterogeneous grouping (Fine, 1994). Although not conclusive, several studies report improved academic achievement, better attendance, increased parent involvement, and fewer discipline problems (Darling-Hammond, 1997).

A major impetus for such alternatives is the recognition that there is often resistance to innovation within public schools. For example, the Edison Project, which enlists public school districts and charter school boards for the right to manage their elementary, middle, and high schools, reflects the vision that many reformers propose for restructured schools. Edison Project schools typically feature a decentralized structure of teams, standardized curricula and assessment, access to technology, professional development and improved compensation for teachers, parent and community involvement, and a national system of supports (Edison Schools, Inc., 2000). However, the student improvement that occurs in such schools may be due to a redistribution of students with poorer-performing students being forced out of the school (Wyatt, 2001). As another alternative to public schools or charter schools, parochial schools typically provide traditional academic curricula in small-scale settings and sometimes can succeed in educating students where public schools have failed (Ravitch, 2000).

Reducing Attrition and Improving Attendance: Dropout Prevention

Research (Rumberger, 1995; Rumberger & Larson, 1998; Rumberger & Thomas, 2000) suggests that poor attendance or absenteeism is a strong predictor of attrition or dropping out. Low test scores, poor attendance, and disengagement from school are risk factors for dropping out (Newmann, 1992; Rumberger, 1995; Rumberger & Thomas, 2000; Wehlage, Rutter, Smith, & Lesko, 1989). Dropout rates are higher for students of low socioeconomic (SES) status; members of racial, ethnic, and language minorities; and men (Rumberger, 1987). Hispanic youth have the highest dropout rate of all the racial/ethnic groups in American schools (Velez, 1989). Low-SES high schools have dropout rates 60 percent higher than average-SES high schools (Rumberger & Thomas, 2000).

School factors may affect attendance and attrition (Rumberger, 1995, 2001; Rumberger & Thomas, 2000). For example, school resources such as teacher/student ratios have a significant effect on middle-school and high-school dropout rates (McNeal, 1997; Rumberger, 1995; Rumberger & Thomas, 2000). Rumberger and Thomas (2000) found that the higher the quality of the teachers, as perceived by students, the lower the dropout rates; however, the higher the quality of teachers, as perceived by the principal, the higher the dropout rates. This discrepancy between students and principals may indicate differing ideas regarding high-quality teaching. For example, for students, good teachers may be teachers who are supportive and understanding which helps students stay in school, whereas for principals, "good" teachers may use strict discipline and very tough academic standards that may actually contribute to student dropout (Rumberger & Thomas, 2000). Structural factors, such as class size and school size, may affect attrition (Lee, 2000; Lee & Smith, 1995; Rumberger, 2001). Students in Catholic and other private schools tend to have lower dropout rates than do students in public schools (Bryk, Lee, & Holland, 1993; Bryk & Thum, 1989; Coleman, 1987; Goldschmidt & Wang, 1999; Rumberger, 1995; Rumberger & Thomas, 2000). School policies and practices also influence attendance and attrition, and the perception of discipline has been associated with attrition. Schools in which students perceive that the discipline is fair have lower dropout rates than schools in which students perceive the discipline to be unfair (Rumberger, 1995; Wehlage & Rutter, 1986). The single most important predictor of dropping out is grade retention (i.e., having students repeat a grade). This effect is consistent for both early and late dropouts (Goldschmidt & Wang, 1999), indicating the need for early intervention (e.g., the High/Scope Perry Preschool Program; see page 116).

Fashola and Slavin (1998) reviewed programs focused on reducing attrition among at-risk middle-school and high-school students and reported on two rigorously evaluated dropout prevention programs designed to increase high school graduation (for a review of elementary-school and middle-school programs, see Fashola & Slavin, 1997). These two were the Coca-Cola Valued Youth Program (VYP) and Achievement for Latinos through Academic Success (ALAS).

Developed by the Intercultural Development and Research Association in San Antonio, Texas, and initially funded by Coca-Cola, the Coca-Cola Valued Youth Program (VYP) was implemented in five high-school districts between 1984 and 1988 (Fashola and Slavin, 1998). VYP uses cross-age tutoring aimed at reducing the dropout rare and increasing the school success and self-esteem of at-risk middle-school and high-school students by providing them with positions of responsibility as tutors of younger elementary age students. Students' academic skills are addressed when they agree to serve as tutors and are required to enroll in a class that focuses on helping them develop and improve their own basic academic skills and their tutoring skills. The tutors work a total of about four hours per week with three elementary school students at a time and are paid a minimum wage stipend. They are recognized and honored as role models at functions given on their behalf, awarded certificates of merit for their efforts, and given caps and T-shirts (Fashola & Slavin, 1998).

An evaluation of VYP by Cardenas, Montecel, Supik, and Harris, (1992) comparing 63 VYP tutors with 70 comparison students who did not receive the program, found that 2 years after the program started, 1% percent of the VYP students had dropped out, compared with 12 % of the comparison group. The students in the VYP group had significantly higher reading grades and scored higher on measures of self-esteem and attitudes toward school than did the students in the control group. VYP has been replicated across the southwest and is currently being extended to other parts of the United States (Fashola & Slavin, 1998).

Achievement for Latinos through Academic Success (ALAS) was developed as a dropout prevention program for low SES, at-risk, middle-school Latino students in Los Angeles (see Fashola & Slavin, 1998; Larson & Rumberger, 1995; Rumberger, 2001). The program specifically targeted special education students and students who were at risk of dropping out because of low income, poor academic performance, and behavior problems. ALAS is based on the foundation and premise that intervention should address the three major forces influencing adolescent lives: family, community, and school. Students in ALAS were provided with counseling, training in social problem solving, and recognition for academic success. In addition, participants' attendance was closely monitored, with daily follow-up with parents. Bonding activities and recognition were provided for the students, as well as frequent feedback from teachers to parents and students. Strategies for the family included workshops on parent training in guiding and monitoring adolescents, school participation, and the use of community resources. Specific community strategies focused on facilitating collaboration among agencies serving youth and families, and on developing and enhancing skills of agency personnel.

Students who participated received the intervention for all 3 years they remained in the target school. Evaluation data revealed that by the end of the ninth grade (the final year of the program) students not in the ALAS group had twice the number of failed classes, were twice as likely to be lagging in high-school graduation credits, and were four times more likely to have excessive absences than ALAS participants. However, once the ALAS program ended, these effects were not sustained throughout the following high school years, indicating that drop-out prevention programs must continue throughout the secondary school years (Fashola & Slavin, 1998; Rumberger, 2001).

Given that grade retention is an important predictor of school dropout, programs that focus on reducing grade retention should be of help in reducing attrition. This raises the question as to whether early childhood and elementary school intervention programs have long-term positive effects (Rumberger, 2001). One program that has empirically documented long-term success is the High/Scope Perry Preschool Project (Barnett, 1985, 1995) which took place from 1962 to 1967. This program targeted 123 low-SES African American children; at ages 3 and 4, one subgroup received a quality preschool program based upon High/Scope's active learning approach and home visits (CITE), while a comparison subgroup did not. Follow-up research found that the program members subsequently graduated from high school at significantly higher rates (67%) than did nonmembers (49%) and also had higher achievement test scores, higher grades, and lower rates of special education and grade retention (Barnett, 1995). These findings suggest early intervention programs for those at risk for dropping out can be successful.

Home-School Partnerships

With parental involvement being seen as an important venue through which schools can accomplish their goals, efforts to engage parents in their children's education have been increasingly advocated (Steinberg et al., 1997). Home-school partnerships are an important component of preventing school failure, and parental involvement is connected to school success (Lareau, 1989). Lareau (1989) noted that SES exerts a strong influence on parental involvement, with lower SES parents tending to be less involved than middle-class and upper-class parents. Implementing a large-scale school transition program, Weine, Kuraski, Jason, Danner, and Johnson (1993) found that, when parents were encouraged and trained to consistently tutor their children in their homes, their children adjusted to their new school's academic requirements significantly better than children who were not tutored. In this review of the literature Coleman (1987; Coleman & Hoffer, 1987) also concluded that parental involvement improved school performance and decreased drop-out rates (Coleman & Hoffer, 1987). Likewise, Miedel and Reynolds (1999) found that parent involvement in urban schools was correlated with lower rates of high-school dropout. Opening channels of communication between parents and schools can empower parents in the education process and also help the school administration understand the sociocultural and economic realities of students' families.

The Comer School Development Project (SDP) has been particularly successful in this regard and is different from other programs because it focuses on the total parent population (Comer, 1993; Drake, 1995). SDP was developed in New Haven, Connecticut, during the 1968–69 school year and was based on the premise that the home, the parents, the neighborhood, the teacher, the school, and the school program need to work together (Comer, 1993). SDP has nine components, the Parents' Program being one of them. The SDP sees relationships between school personnel and parents as based on a foundation of mutual respect, trust, and shared power in order to develop a positive climate in which children's growth is supported (Comer, 1993; Drake, 1995). The Parent's Program is designed for broad-based participation in order for all parents to be involved in their children's education. SDP has three levels of parental participation. Level Three parents participate in many activities such as general business meetings, fundraising, special events and potluck dinners, drama and musical performances, Halloween parades, and conferences with the staff. Level Two parents are involved in parent-staff workshops and room-mother activities; volunteer in the lunchroom, classroom, library, playground, and attend field trips. They may also work with the school's Mental Health Team. SDP Level Two parents developed many committees, such as the Parent Interest Group, the Parent Advisory Board, the Parent-Teacher Association, and the Parent-Teacher Power Team. Parents often go from Level Two to Level One. Level One parents are decision-makers and are involved in school governance, management, and curriculum and operation policy determinations. Planning, implementing, and evaluating school activities is an area of focus for the governance committee, as is working with staff. Through these arrangements, parents can participate to the extent to which they are comfortable and capable and can change as they desire (Comer, 1993). Meaningful parental involvement in the daily and ongoing activities of a school benefits students, families, and communities (see Henderson, 1987), and as the Comer model suggests, home-school connections help foster student success in school (Drake, 1995).

CASE EXAMPLE

As outlined in this chapter, wide ranges of strategies have been employed to prevent school failure and promote academic achievement. In this section, we focus on one such strategy—advising programs. In doing so, we highlight some of the issues that arise when a school attempts to institutionalize an intervention that changes the school structure in order to strengthen the student-teacher relationship.

Background   •

Teachers and administrators who are searching for effective ways to motivate students to care about their education sometimes implement advising programs. In small alternative high schools, well-planned advising programs have made a difference in outcomes for at-risk students (Meier, 1995; Oakes et al., 2000). However, in larger public high schools, advising programs have not been consistently executed or sufficiently evaluated. In most cases, they have not been tried at all (Rappaport, 1999).

This makes what is happening at Cambridge Rindge and Latin High School (CRLS), a large public high school in Cambridge, Massachusetts,. For the past 6 years, CRLS has made a concerted effort to provide an advising program for its students based on the premise that constructive relationships between students and adults at school can enhance learning. The impetus for this effort stemmed from recognition of the vulnerabilities of the diverse body of students attending the high school. A district-wide analysis of school performance revealed that approximately one-third of the students fail at least one course every semester. The failure rate for minorities was even higher—41% for African American students and 43% for Latino students. Of the more than 2,000 students who attend Rindge, approximately 60% are racial or ethnic minorities, more than half are eligible to receive free lunches, and one third speak a first language other than English.

The advising program at CRLS is being phased in as part of ongoing restructuring, which includes heterogeneous student grouping, interdisciplinary teaming, and time structured for staff to collaborate. The advising is currently limited to 9th and 10th graders, who see their advisors 1 or 2 days a week during a regular class period, but it will eventually expand to all four grades. Evaluations of the CRLS program have revealed promising preliminary findings, including high satisfaction ratings from teachers and students alike (Rappaport, 2001). Eighty percent of the students have reported that their advisers are strong advocates for them in the school. Preliminary analyses of a broad range of indices (e.g., grade point average, suspensions, detentions) also indicate positive effects (Rappaport, 2001).

Implementation Issues

As with many reform efforts, implementing an advising program involves several issues, including finding time in the schedule, determining which students to include, deciding curriculum content, and defining staff support (Rappaport, 2000). In this section, we discuss some of these issues and ways to resolve them.

At a very basic level, schools must identify staff members who should (and should not) engage in advising relationships with students. When programs are mandatory, they may enlist teachers who are reluctant to participate and unwilling to make the necessary effort to establish successful relationships. For example, some teachers may prefer to maintain their professional distance with their students and focus only on academic goals. When participation is voluntary, as is the case at CRLS, there is a greater likelihood of including teachers who are comfortable, enthusiastic, and engaged in the advising role. The disadvantage of voluntary enrollment is that some of the most dedicated and conscientious teachers in the school may not volunteer for fear that they will overextend themselves. CRLS has addressed such concerns by offering reduced workloads (i.e., release from a course), a costly strategy that implies the full support of school administrators and parents. Unfortunately, teachers of core subjects cannot always be released and sometimes feel resentful of those who obtain reduced workloads.

Along similar lines, schools must decide whether to involve all students in the advisory program or to select only those students who are at greatest risk for academic failure. Some administrators believe that advising should be reserved for high-risk students, whereas others have suggested that all students can benefit. The proponents of including all students in the advising program at CRLS advanced several arguments. They saw advising as a preventive intervention; to preselect students would defeat this purpose. Furthermore, many of the students who most need to examine their attitudes toward learning and their investment in school might choose not to participate. Finally, selecting only underachieving students for the advising program would create the risk of stigmatizing them and making them feel more inadequate. On the other hand, there were some concerns that students might not feel comfortable making disclosures to certain teachers and that they should not be forced into such relationships. CRLS resolved this conflict by making a reasonable compromise. All students were expected to participate, but students could opt out in consultation with a school administrator. Although some administrators anticipated a mass exodus of students, only two students chose not to participate in the advising program.

Beyond these selection issues, there is a need to consider the integration of the program into the overall school setting. Understanding internal and external power structures is a crucial step in facilitating the successful implementation of advisory programs or other innovations. For example, an important element of success for introducing any sort of change in a school is the establishment of positive collaborative relationships with individuals serving as "gatekeepers"—those who oversee and sanction changes in the school. Some individuals have been assigned to this role formally, while others adopt it more informally (Glidewell, 1959). At CRLS, the guidance counselors serve as the key gatekeepers in the implementation process, presenting concrete information about graduation requirements, transcripts, goal setting, and course selection three times a year to each advising group. They have welcomed access to the advising groups because they see it as an efficient way to deliver information and therefore present it to teachers in a positive light.

In addition to understanding internal power structures, program implementers must be familiar with external factors that might bear on program functioning (Caplan, 1974). If, in the past, many other programs have been tried and failed, school personnel might be reluctant to attempt another intervention (Rhodes & Englund, 1993). In the past 10 years, there had been four different failed efforts to institutionalize reform efforts at CRLS. Although there has been cautious optimism because the external personnel such as the school districts, the superintendent, and the school board have endorsed the present intervention, the current advising program often has been vulnerable to the vicissitudes of the political climate and shifting educational pedagogy.

Irrespective of context, efforts to prevent student failure are often difficult to implement. Moreover, not all interventions are equally effective across school contexts. Adolescents with a higher probability of failure and dropout are a psychosocially heterogeneous group (Janosz, LeBlanc, Boulerice, & Tremblay, 2000). Practices that seem perfect in theory may result in negative consequences if they fail to target the underlying problems or are insensitive to the ecological context (Battistich, Solomon, Watson, & Schaps, 1997; Schensul, 1998).

Moreover, successful school change depends on the readiness and willingness of school staff, parents, and students to actively engage in reform efforts. Reforms can be rendered effective or ineffective by the knowledge, skills, and commitments of those stakeholders in school. Without administrative and teacher acceptance and appropriate support, school-based advising programs and other innovations cannot succeed. Indeed, school systems (like many administrative structures) tend to seek a state of equilibrium, and innovative practices may be seen as a drain on resources and a threat to the system's stability (Evans, 1996).

Although our preliminary findings suggest that effective relationships emerge through a combination of structure, activity, and emotional support, these observations need to be further refined. There is also a need for empirically validated guidelines to identify the needed infrastructure and training techniques in order to maximize advisers' impact. Additional understanding of the processes involved in creating trustworthy and consistent advising relationships is likely to lead to enhanced student competencies and reduced school failure.

FUTURE DIRECTIONS

To date, much of the research on intervention and funding priorities has concentrated on the student, ignoring the crucial contributing roles of the teacher and contextual variables. The multidetermined nature of school failure, however, makes it necessary to expand, and even alter, traditional approaches. As noted throughout this chapter, relationships that transpire within school settings, school resources, and structural characteristics (such as class size) can shape students' experiences in school. We have suggested strategies for transforming schools, and carefully implemented research and program evaluation will be required to assess and refine these strategies across settings.

Several promising trends have emerged in recent years that provide some hope that this work will be accomplished. For example, the growing number of university-school collaborations is likely to result in more program evaluations that can identify and address the factors that underlie school failure. Within this context, systematic comparisons of strategies that vary by type and intensity should be conducted in order to provide a sound basis for comparisons and decision making. Of course, evaluations of treatment effects in school settings are complicated by the fact that the relationships do not exist in a vacuum and programs are often linked to a broader array of services.

In addition to comparing programs and specifying outcomes, a deeper understanding of the reasons for school failure is needed. Qualitative studies may shed additional light on both the circumstances that give rise to school failure and the most appropriate means of redressing these problems within various contexts. Lightfoot (1983), based on her qualitative inquiry, suggested that in "good" high schools, "students feel visible and accountable" (p. 26). School leaders express a need for nurturance and partnership—"they do not want to go it alone" (Lightfoot, 1983, p. 333)—and teachers' needs are carefully attended to, with their work supported and rewarded. Given the importance of student-teacher ties, scholarly attention also should be directed to the processes that give rise to and govern these relationships. As Pianta (2000), concluded, "Relationships with adults are a cornerstone of development—they are responsible for a large proportion of school success. Too often the role of the adult-child relationship is underestimated either because it is not well understood, or because the role of the context is not understood or emphasized in prevailing models for understanding development" (p. 188). Developing and testing conceptual models of teacher support will be an important challenge in the coming years.

Students' experiences with teachers and, more generally, in school shape their appraisals of the school "climate." Because students' perceptions of school climate are considered to be key mediators between contextual variables (e.g., family and school characteristics) and academic, emotional, and behavioral outcomes (Roeser, Eccles, & Sameroff, 2000), school climate represents a promising variable for expanding researchers' attention beyond measures of individual student adjustment.

Taken together, the range of preventive approaches considered in this chapter has the potential to reverse school failure. Such approaches, combined with careful program evaluations that are anchored in theory and scientific evidence, can contribute to more theoretically informed and practically applicable prevention efforts.

REFERENCES

Arhar, J. M. (1997). The effects of interdisciplinary teaming on teachers and students. In J. Irvine (Ed.), *What current research says to the middle level practitioner* (pp. 49–56). Columbus, OH: National Middle School Association.

Arhar, J. M., & Kromrey, J. (1995). Interdiscplinary teaming and the demographics of membership: A comparison of students belonging in high SES and low SES middle-level schools. *Research in Middle Level Education, 18*, 71–88.

Barnett, W. S. (1985). *The Perry Preschool Program and its long-term effects: A benefit-cost analysis.* Ypsilanti, MI: High/Scope Educational Research Foundation.

Barnett, W. S. (1995). Long-term effects of early childhood programs on cognitive and school outcomes. *The Future of Children, 5*, 25–50.

Battistich, V., Solomon, D., Watson, M., & Schaps, E. (1997). Caring school communities. *Educational Psychologist, 32*, 137–151.

Bryk, A. S., Lee, V. E., & Holland, P. B. (1993). *Catholic schools and the common good.* Cambridge, MA: Harvard University Press

Bryk, A. S., & Thum, Y. M. (1989). The effects of high-school organization on dropping out: An exploratory investigation. *American Educational Research Journal, 26*, 353–383.

Caplan, G. (1974). *Support systems and community mental health.* New York: Behavioral Sciences Press.

Cardenas, J. A., Montecel, M. R., Supik,, J. D., & Harris, J. R. (1992). The Coca-Cola Valued Youth Program: Dropout prevention strategies for at-risk students. *Texas Researcher, 3*, 111–130.

Cauce, A. M., Mason, C., Gonzales, N., Hiraga, Y., & Liu, G. (1994). Social support during adolescence: Methodological and theoretical considerations. In F. Nestmann & K. Hurrelmann (Eds.), *Social networks and social support in childhood and adolescence: Prevention and intervention in childhood and adolescence* (pp. 89–108). Berlin, Germany: Walter De Gruyter.

Chall, J. (2000). *The academic achievement challenge: What really works in the classroom?* New York: Random House.

Cohen, E. G., & Lotan, R. A. (1995). Producing equal-status interaction in the heterogeneous classroom. *American Educational Research Journal, 32*, 99–120.

Coleman, J.S. (1987). Families and schools. *Educational Researcher, 16*, 32–38.

Coleman, J.S., & Hoffer, T. (1987). *Public and private high schools: The impact of communities.* New York: Basic Books.

Comer, J. P. (1993). *School power: Implications of an intervention project.* New York: The Free Press.

Darling-Hammond, L. (1997). *The right to learn: A blueprint for creating schools that work.* San Francisco, CA: Jossey-Bass.

Delpit, L. (1995). *Other people's children: Cultural conflict in the classroom.* New York: The Free Press.

Drake, D. D. (1995). Student success and the family: Using the Comer model for home-school connections. *The Clearing House, 68*, 313–316.

Eccles, J. S., Lord, S., & Buchanan, C. M. (1996). School transitions in early adolescence: What are we doing to our young people? In J. A. Graber, J. Brooks-Gunn & A.C. Peterson (Eds.), *Transitions through adolescence interpersonal domains and context.* (pp. 251–284). Hillside, NJ: Erlbaum.

Eccles, J. S., & Midgley, C. (1989). Stage-environment fit: Developmentally appropriate classrooms for young adolescents. In C. Ames & R. Ames

(Eds.), *Advances in motivation in education: Vol 3. Goals and cognitions* (pp. 13–44). New York: Academic Press.

Edison Schools, Inc. (2000). Annual report. New York: Author.

Evans, R. (1996). *The human side of school change: Reform, resistance, and the real-life problems of innovation.* San Francisco: Jossey Bass.

Fashola, O. S., & Slavin, R. E. (1997). Promising programs for elementary and middle schools: Evidence of effectiveness and replicability. *Journal of Education for Students Placed at Risk, 2,* 251–307.

Fashola, O. S., & Slavin, R. E. (1998). Effective dropout prevention and college attendance programs for students placed at risk. *Journal of Education for Students Placed at Risk, 3,* 159–183.

Felner, R. D., & Adan, A. M. (1988). The school transition environment project: An ecological intervention and evaluation. In R. H. Price, E. L. Cowen, R. P. Lorion, & J. Ramos-McKay (Eds.), *Fourteen ounces of prevention: A casebook for practitioners.* Washington, DC: American Psychological Association Press.

Felner, R. D., Primavera, J. S., & Cauce, A. M. (1981). The impact of school transitions: A focus for preventive efforts. *American Journal of Community Psychology, 9,* 449–459.

Ferguson, R. F. (1991). Paying for public education: New evidence of how and why money matters. *Harvard Journal on Legislation, 28,* 465–98.

Fernandez, J. (1991). Restructuring schools to guarantee education success for at-risk students. In C.C.S.S. Officers (Ed.), *Restructuring schools: Potential for students at risk* (pp. 11–26). Washington, DC: Editor.

Fine, M. (Ed.) (1994). *Chartering urban school reform reflections on public high schools in the midst of change.* New York: Teachers College Press.

Finn, J. D. (1989). Withdrawing from school. *Review of Educational Research, 59,* 117–142.

Fordham, S. (1996). *Blacked out dilemmas of race, identity and success at Capital High.* Chicago: University of Chicago.

Freedman, M. (1993). *The kindness of strangers: Adult mentors, urban youth, and the new volunteerism.* San Francisco: Jossey-Bass.

Gibson, M., & Ogbu, J. (1991). *Minority status and schooling a comparative study of immgrant and involuntary minorities.* New York: Garland.

Glidewell, J. (1959). The entry problem in consultation. *Journal of Social Issues, 15,* 51–59.

Goldschmidt, P., & Wang, J. (1999). When can schools affect dropout behavior? A longitudinal multilevel analysis. *American Educational Research Journal, 36,* 715–738.

Greenwald, R., Hedges, L. V., & Laine, R. D. (1996). The effect of school resources on student achievement. *Review of Educational Research, 66,* 361–396.

Henderson, A. (1987). *The evidence continues to grow: Parental involvement improves student achievement.* Columbia, MD: National Committee for Citizens in Education.

Jackson, A. W., & Davis, G. A. (2000). *Turning points 2000: Educating adolescents in the 21st century.* New York: Carnegie Cooperation.

Janosz, M., Le Blanc, M., Boulerice, B., & Tremblay, R. E. (2000). Predicting different types of school dropouts: A typological approach with two longitudinal samples. *Journal of Educational Psychology, 92,* 171–190.

Jason, L. A., Weine, A. M., Johnson, J. H., Warren-Sohlberg, L., Filippelli, L. A., Turner, E. Y., & Lardon, C. (1992). *Helping transfer students: Strategies for educational and social readjustment.* San Francisco: Jossey-Bass.

Kaufman, P., Kwon, J. Y., Klein, S., & Chapman, C. D. (1999). *Dropout rates in the United States: 1998.* Washington, DC: U.S. Department of Education.

Lareau, A. (1989). *Home advantage: Social class and parental intervention in elementary education.* New York: The Falmer Press.

Larson, K., & Rumberger, R. (1995). Doubling school success in highest-risk Latino youth: Results from a middle school intervention study. In R. F. Macias & R. Garcia Ramos (Eds.), *Changing schools for changing students* (pp. 157–179). Santa Barbara, CA: University of California, Santa Barbara.

Lee, V. E. (2000). Using hierarchical linear modeling to study social contexts: The case of school effects. *Educational Psychologist, 35,* 125–141.

Lee, V. E., & Smith, J. B. (1995). Effects of high school restructuring and size on early gains in achievement and engagement. *Sociology of Education, 68,* 241–270.

Levine, A. (2000). Next, an education revolution? *New York Times* (December 29), p. 24.

Lighfoot, L. S. (1983). *The good high school.* New York: Basic Books.

Lynch, M., & Cicchetti, D. (1997). Children's relationships with adults and peers: An examination of elementary and junior high-school students. *Journal of School Psychology, 35,* 81–99.

MacIver, D. (1990). Meeting the needs of young adolescents: Advisory groups, interdisciplinary teaching teams, and school transition programs. *Phi Delta Kappan, 71,* 458–464.

Mattison, R. (2001). School consultation: A review of research on issues unique to school environment. *Journal of American Academy Child Adolescent Psychology, 39,* 402–413.

McDonald, J. (1996) *Redesigning school lessons for the 21st Century.* San Francisco: Jossey-Bass.

McEwin, K. C., Dickinson, T. S., & Jenkins, D. M. (1996). *America's middle schools: Practices and progress. A 25-year perspective.* Columbus, OH: National Middle School Association.

McNeal, R. B. (1997). High-school drop outs: A closer examination of school effects. *Social Science Quarterly, 78*, 209–22.

Meier, D. (1995). *Power of their ideas.* Boston: Beacon Press.

Midgley, C., Feldlaufer, H., & Eccles, J. S. (1989). Student/teacher relations and attitudes toward mathematics before and after the transition to junior high school. *Child Development, 60*, 981–992.

Miedel, W. T., & Reynolds, A. J. (1999, April). *Parent involvement in elementary-school and high-school success: Is there a connection?* Paper presented at the Society for Research in Child Development biannual meeting, Albuquerque, New Mexico.

Murnane, R. J., & Levy, F. (1996). *Teaching the new basic skills: Principles for educating children to thrive in a changing economy.* New York: Martin Kessler Books.

Newmann, F. M. (Ed.). (1992). *Student engagement and achievement in American secondary schools.* New York: Teachers College Press.

Noddings, N. (1992). *The challenges to care in schools: An alternative approach to education.* New York: Teachers College Press.

Oakes, J., Quartz, K. H., Ryan, S., & Lipton, M. (2000). *Becoming good American schools: The struggle for civic virtue in education reform.* San Francisco: Jossey-Bass.

Perkins, D. (1992). *Smart schools, better thinking and learning for every child.* New York: Free Press.

Phillips, M. (1997). What makes school effective? A comparison of the relationships of communitarian climate and academic climate to achievement and attendance during middle school. *American Educational Research Journal, 34*, 633–662.

Pianta, R. C. (2000). *Enhancing relationships between children and teachers.* Washington, DC: American Psychological Association.

Rappaport, N. (1999). An advising program in a large urban high school: The magic match. In A. H. Esman, L. Flaherty, & H. Horowitz (Eds). *Adolescent psychiatry* (Vol. 24, pp. 207–231). London: The Analytic Press.

Rappaport, N. (2000). Small advising groups: Relationships for success. *The High School Magazine, 7*, 45–48.

Rappaport, N. (2001). *Institutionalizing care in schools through advising.* Unpublished manuscript.

Ravitch, D. (2000). *Left back: A century of failed school reforms.* New York: Simon & Schuster.

Rhodes, J. E. (in press). *Stand by me: Risks and rewards in youth mentoring.* Cambridge, MA: Harvard University Press.

Roeser, R. W., Eccles, J. S., & Sameroff, A. J. (2000). School as a context of early adolescents' academic and social-emotional development: A summary of research findings. *Elementary School Journal, 100*, 443–471.

Rossi, R., & Montgomery, A. (1994). *Educational reforms and students at risk: A review of the current state of the art.* Available: http://www.ed.gov/ pubs/EdReformStudies/EdReforms/[2000, November 09].

Rumberger, R. W. (1987). High school dropouts: A review of issues and evidence. *Review of Educational Research, 57*, 101–122.

Rumberger, R. W. (1995). Dropping out of middle school: A multilevel analysis of students and schools. *American Educational Research Journal, 32*, 583–625.

Rumberger, R. W. (2001, January). *Why students drop out and what can be done.* Paper presented at the conference, Dropouts in America: How Severe Is the Problem? What Do We Know About Intervention and Prevention?, Sponsored by Harvard University Graduate School of Education, Civil Rights Project, Cambridge, Massachusetts.

Rumberger, R. W., & Larson, K. A. (1998). Student mobility and the increased risk of high-school dropout. *American Journal of Education, 107*, 1–35.

Rumberger, R. W., & Thomas, S. L. (2000). The distribution of dropout and turnover rates among urban and suburban high schools. *Sociology of Education, 73*, 39–67.

Schensul, J. J. (1998). Community-based risk prevention with urban youth. *School Psychology Review, 27*, 233–245.

Sergiovannl, T. (1994). *Building community in schools.* San Francisco: Jossey-Bass.

Steinberg, L., Brown, B. B., & Dornbusch, S. M. (1997). *Beyond the classroom: Why school reform has failed and what parents need to do.* New York: Random House.

Velez, W. (1989). High-school attrition among Hispanic and non-Hispanic white youths. *Sociology of Education, 62*, 119–133.

Wehlage, G. G., & Rutter, R. (1986). Dropping out: How much do schools contribute to the problem? *Teachers College Record, 87*, 374–392.

Wehlage, G. G., Rutter, R. A., Smith, G. A., & Lesko, N. (1989). *Reducing the risk: Schools as communities of support.* New York: Falmer Press.

Weine, A. M., Kurasaki, K. S., Jason, L. A., Danner, K. E., & Johnson, J. (1993). An evaluation of preventive tutoring programs for transfer students. *Child Study Journal, 23*, 135–152.

Wyatt, E. (2001). Higher scores aren't cure-all, school run for profit learns. *New York Times*, March, 13, p. 1.

CHAPTER 7

Preventing Delinquency and Antisocial Behavior

Jennifer J. Treuting,
Tamara M. Haegerich, and
Patrick H. Tolan

DESCRIPTION OF THE PROBLEM

Although rates of antisocial and violent behavior have decreased among young people in recent years, they remain at very high levels (Snyder & Sickmund, 1999). Violent Crime Index juvenile arrests increased by 60% in the 1980s (Snyder & Sickmund, 1999) and, compared with other industrialized nations, levels of antisocial and violent behavior are elevated in the United States (Rosenberg, 1991). Stark and dramatic examples of youth violence also have increased concern about youth violence (Tolan, in press). In response to this growing public concern, policy makers and others have advocated for punitive measures. Metal detectors are becoming commonplace in schools; youths are beginning to be charged, tried, and sentenced as adults; and legislative measures are being enacted to curtail opportunities for treatment and supportive intervention with youthful offenders. Although appealing to the sentiment to "do something," these efforts often are poorly formulated and highly unlikely to improve safety (Tolan, 2000; Tolan & Gorman-Smith, 1998).

In recognition of these circumstances, a number of panels and reports, including the American Psychological Association's Commission on Youth Violence (1993) and the National Research Council (1993), have convened to examine the current state of knowledge about youth delinquency. Furthermore, research on delinquency and other forms of antisocial behavior has burgeoned over the last two decades (see Farrington & Loeber, 1999, for a recent summary), in no small part due to the support and initiative of the Office of Juvenile Justice and Delinquency Prevention (OJJDP) and the Center for Substance Abuse Prevention (CSAP), a division of the Substance Abuse and Mental Health Services Administration (SAMHSA). Important risk factors for youth antisocial behavior have been clarified, processes linking risk and outcomes are being described, and promising strategies for prevention and treatment have emerged.

Risk and Protective Factors for Delinquency

Understanding the key risk factors for delinquency is a complex matter. Most research has moved toward a perspective that incorporates multiple factors within a social-ecological perspective and that emphasizes the role of these factors in developmental trajectories for multiple patterns of involvement (Elliott & Tolan, 1999; Tolan, Guerra, & Kendall, 1995). Tolan and Guerra (1994) suggested applying an ecological model, based on Bronfenbrenner's (1988) work, that organizes risk factors by system level, from individual to close interpersonal relationships (e.g., family and peers), to less proximal developmental microsystems (such as neighborhood conditions), to macrosystem influences. The following summary of the most promising risk factors to target for intervention is based on the most rigorous longitudinal studies and meta-analyses to date (see Hawkins et al., 1998; Lipsy & Wilson, 1998; Loeber & Farrington, 1998; and Tolan & Loeber, 1993, for more comprehensive reviews).

Over the last two decades, researchers (e.g., Coie et al., 1993; Howell, Krisberg, Hawkins, & Wilson, 1996; Kellam & Rebok, 1992) have increasingly adopted a risk-focused approach to the study of childhood problems, including antisocial and delinquent behavior. According to this framework, risk for disorder is not uniformly distributed across individuals. Rather, particular risk factors are associated with a relatively greater chance of developing a particular problem. Protective factors, in contrast, counter risk or improve the chances that one will develop in a healthy manner in the face of otherwise increased risk. Both risk and protective factors interact over time and with development to influence outcomes, and they exist at every level of the biopsychosocial system, from the most micro (e.g., individual) to the most macro (e.g., societal) level, and every level in between (e.g., familial, peer group, and setting-related influences). In this framework, epidemiologic data are used to build models of risk, these models are tested empirically, and results are used to inform intervention design.

Individual Risk Factors

These factors include demographic characteristics, such as male gender and adolescent age. Adolescent boys, for example, are more likely than others to become involved in criminal activities. Similarly, the kinds of attention and behavioral regulation difficulties that are characterized by attention deficit hyperactivity disorder (ADHD) are associated with increased risk for involvement in antisocial behaviors (Hinshaw, 1987; Pliszka, 2000). Other identified risk factors at the individual level include poor peer relations and problem-solving skills (Agnew, 1990; Dodge, 1993); deficient and distinct patterns of social information processing (e.g., hostile attributional biases, inaccuracy in detecting intention cues, poor evaluation of response outcomes) (Crick & Dodge, 1994; Huesmann, 1998); academic underachievement and impaired cognitive functioning (Moffitt, 1993); and, in the early grades, poor reading skills and a lack of bonding to school and to teachers (Hawkins et al., 1992).

Family Factors

Factors related to family functioning also emerge as critical to delinquent and antisocial behavior patterns among youth. Poor parent management practices (e.g., inconsistent use of consequences, overly harsh discipline practices, poor supervision and monitoring), low emotional cohesion, family conflict, and difficulties in family problem-solving and coping have been found to increase risk (Gorman-Smith, Tolan, Zelli, & Huesmann, 1996; Hawkins et al., 1992; Yoshikawa, 1994). Children whose parents engage in antisocial activities are likely to do so as well (Lahey et al., 1995).

Peer Factors

The impact of peers is also important, since association with antisocial peers increases one's risk for involvement (Farrington & Hawkins, 1991; Wright, Caspi, Moffit, & Silva, 2001). Processes accounting for peer influence have not been explored fully, but among those clearly identified are peer deviancy, peer rejection, and social norms that support antisocial behavior (Coie et al., 1999; Dodge, Coie, Pettit, & Price 1996; Henry, Tolan, & Gorman-Smith, in press).

Community-Level Factors

The role of community-level influences in delinquency and antisocial behavior is suggested by the markedly uneven distribution of delinquent, antisocial, and violent behavior across neighborhood and community contexts. Children who live in impoverished neighborhoods, particularly those characterized by high rates of unemployment and mobility, are at higher risk of both participating in and being victimized by crime and other antisocial activities. Likewise, children residing in highly disorganized neighborhoods (i.e., those with high crime rates, marked violence, and a lack of informal child supervision by adults) are more likely than children from other neighborhoods to commit delinquent acts (Farrington, 1991; Sampson, 2000). Community characteristics increase risk in several different ways, both direct and indirect. For example, chronic community problems often disrupt family functioning, subsequently placing children at risk for poor outcomes (Gorman-Smith, Tolan, & Henry, in press). Likewise, life in a chaotic and violent neighborhood also appears to leave children particularly vulnerable to the effects of other risk factors (Tolan & Gorman-Smith, 1997).

Societal Factors

Risk factors at a societal level can help explain the markedly higher rates of violence in the United States compared with other industrialized nations (Rosenberg, 1991). For example, widespread availability of handguns, tolerance of youth alcohol use, and societal norms that support media violence all have been associated with relatively higher rates of violent behavior in U.S. society (Baron, Straus, & Jaffee, 1990; Mercy & Rosenberg, 1998; National Research Council, 1993).

Protective Factors

In addition to risk factors, there has been increasing interest in focusing on protective factors—those developmental influences that are associated with lower-than-expected risk. However, most of the research in this area is merely an examination of risk factors rescaled (e.g., high family cohesion relates to low delinquency, while low cohesion relates to high delinquency). As the methodological and theoretical complexities are refined, it is likely that this area of work will provide important advances (Tolan, Sherrod, Gorman-Smith, & Henry, in press).

It must be stressed that risk and protective factors reflect complex, dynamic, and reciprocal processes that unfold as the individual interacts with his or her environment over time, and that lead to varied developmental outcomes (Elliot & Tolan, 1999). Risk factors are not independent and tend to co-occur, cluster, and interact to compound risk. For example, children facing multiple risks are substantially more likely to engage in problem behavior than would be predicted by each individual risk factor alone (Thornberry, Huizinga, & Loeber, 1995). Also, many of the risk factors cited in this chapter are not specific to delinquency, but predict risk for many problems of childhood and adolescence. Therefore, interventions that target and decrease risk factors for delinquency may decrease risk for several problem outcomes.

REVIEW AND CRITIQUE OF THE LITERATURE

Interventions That Work

As the literature on delinquency risk has grown, so, too, has research on the effectiveness of programs aimed at preventing, or encouraging desistance from, participation in antisocial activities. The quality of the research varies widely, as does the quality of the programs and efforts tested; meta-analyses (Lipsey & Wilson, 1998) suggest that research characteristics account for as large a proportion of effect sizes as does the approach used. Also, what is considered evidence can vary widely. Often proxies for delinquency or behaviors linked as risk factors to delinquency are what have been affected, leaving open the question of impact on actual delinquency. It should be noted that how these indicators, including delinquency, are measured varies widely. Program efficacy often is measured in terms of proximal outcomes (i.e., decreasing the presence of risk factors or increasing the presence of protective factors). Distal outcomes, including prevention of delinquency itself, are more difficult to study because these effects may not be seen until many years after the intervention is implemented. All of these factors can affect research results that, in turn, affect what is deemed promising or effective. Fortunately, the last decade has seen great progress in this area, prompting a number of detailed reviews of the topic (Guerra, Tolan, & Hammond, 1994; Lipsey & Wilson, 1998; Mulvey, Arthur, & Reppucci, 1993; Tolan & Guerra, 1994). Much is still to be learned, however, particularly given that the effects of many of the most popular and widely used prevention approaches (e.g., mentoring programs, youth alternative programs) have not yet been evaluated rigorously or have not fared well in these investigations (Tolan, in press).

Prevention efforts can be broadly grouped into three categories, based on the level of population targeted (Mrazek & Haggerty, 1994; Offord, Kramer, Kazdin, Peter, & Harrington, 1998). *Universal programs* are offered to all individuals within a given population, often chosen based on exposure to broad-based risk factors (e.g., inner-city residence). These programs typically are focused on enriching and enhancing developmental processes (e.g., social problem-solving skills) or inoculating against or buffering the negative effects of broad-based risk (e.g., improving the reading skills of children in underperforming schools). *Selected programs*, in contrast, serve children, adolescents, or families who are exposed to risk factors related to delinquency or have evidenced an earlier or related behavior (e.g., children displaying aggressive behavior). Finally, *indicated programs* target youths who have shown early delinquent or antisocial behavior, with the goal of limiting or halting their involvement in delinquent, antisocial, or violent behavior and preventing more devastating subsequent outcomes.

Despite the utility of this schema, few studies or programs have organized their work along these dimensions, and evaluations are seldom grounded in this approach. Instead, intervention approaches typically are differentiated by their targets for change. Some focus exclusively on the individual's cognition, motivation, or behavior. Others, including family-, peer-, and school-focused approaches, are geared toward various ecological systems in which children spend their time. Finally, broad-based community initiatives and policy efforts aim at decreasing risk by changing norms or behavioral options in larger social groups.

Among individual-level approaches, programs focusing on social-cognitive processes, including applied problem-solving skills and moral reasoning, have shown the greatest promise in achieving positive outcomes, at least in the short term (Guerra & Slaby, 1990). These programs have been used with preschool to high-school children, with content and implementation methods varying as a function of developmental level. Many are universal and classroom-based (Shure, 1997; Greenberg, Kusche, Cook, & Quamma, 1995). Others have been used with children deemed at risk by virtue of early aggressive or antisocial behavior (Conduct Problems Prevention Research Group, 1999). Programs that foster opportunities for youth involvement in legitimate school and community activities and that encourage adult recognition of the contributions made by youth also appear promising in forestalling youth involvement in criminal activities (Bry, 1982; Gottfredson, Gottfredson, & Skroban, 1996).

Peer-group approaches have targeted high-risk youths and usually use a group format to change norms. However, evidence is accumulating that such groups can have significant negative effects (Dishion, McCord, & Poulin, 1999).

What is less clear is whether social-cognitive programs, offered in groups, also have these negative effects (Tolan et al., 2002). Few studies have evaluated how peer relation and peer skill development might be used to modify risk.

Family-focused approaches, whether focused on selected or indicated populations or implemented universally, have repeatedly demonstrated efficacy in reducing youth antisocial behavior (Tolan, in press; Tolan & Guerra, 1994) and may be among the most useful prevention strategies. Such interventions include parenting groups, family groups, and more traditional family therapy. The most common strategy, behavioral parent training, has shown success in improving parents' ability to manage children's behavior, increasing parental monitoring of youth, and altering the patterns of family interaction that contribute to youth antisocial behavior and subsequent delinquency (Patterson, Reid, & Dishion, 1992). However, evidence (Henggeler, Borduin, & Mann, 1993) is emerging that the success of such programs in *preventing* antisocial behavior rests on expanding the focus to help families improve their problem-solving and relationship-management skills as well. Family-focused programs grounded in structural and strategic family therapy traditions extend the goals of intervention to include improvements in familial relationships (e.g., closeness, emotional warmth and cohesion, improved communication). Such approaches have shown efficacy in preventing significant antisocial behavior among children (Conduct Problems Prevention Research Group, 1999; Metropolitan Area Child Study Research Group, 2000; Reid, Eddy, Fetrow, & Stoolmiller, 1999) and in curtailing adolescent involvement once it has occurred (Henggeler, Melton, Smith, Schoenwald, & Hanley, 1993). This expansion of intervention goals appears particularly important, and such programs have garnered the most consistent empirical support in addressing family-level risk and, in some cases, in decreasing youth antisocial behavior, even among families in high-risk situations (Henggeler, Melton, Smith, Schoenwald, & Hanley, 1993; Tolan, McKay, Hanish, & Dickey, 2000).

Perhaps what most clearly emerges from the research is that no single intervention targeting a single domain of interest holds the key for preventing antisocial behavior in youths (Elliot & Tolan, 1999). Instead, a combination of approaches is needed (Tolan, 1998), including large-scale universal (primary prevention) interventions focused on changing the norms and practices of youth behavior and supervision in key social settings; selective interventions targeting at-risk youths and families; and more intensive, indicated interventions to support the families of children with emerging antisocial behavior. Prevention models are already, and will continue to grow even more, sophisticated and complex.

Current Issues and Challenges

Definition of Delinquency and Scope of the Problem

The term *antisocial youth* encompasses a wide variety of behaviors as well as individuals. As an umbrella term, antisocial behavior refers to actions that are socially unacceptable, whereas delinquency, aggression, and violence are classes or categories of antisocial behavior. The broader term encompasses a range of related behaviors spanning the developmental spectrum; the narrower terms differentiate behaviors that may result from somewhat distinct developmental pathways or constellations of risk.

Youth who are considered at risk for antisocial or delinquent behavior are a far from homogeneous group. Perhaps because of the public outcry over recent violent incidents involving youth, the focus on delinquent youth who are frequent, serious, and violent offenders has intensified. In fact, a small portion of the population commits a relatively large percentage of crimes (see Loeber, Farrington, & Waschbusch, 1998), and, among those who commit criminal acts, an even smaller portion commits most of the serious offenses, including violent crime (Moffitt, 1993; White, Moffitt, Earls, Robins, & Silva, 1990). Clearly, prevention efforts targeting these children are important and are likely to require involvement in multiple systems, including family, school, peer group, and neighborhood.

However, the vast majority of children who commit delinquent and antisocial acts are not violent, serious, repeat offenders. Various forms of antisocial behaviors can be placed along a continuum from less to more severe. Serious forms of behavior rarely emerge without prior antisocial involvement (Nagin & Tremblay, 1999), but the pathways to involvement in more extreme forms of behavior are diverse. Loeber and his colleagues (Loeber & Hay, 1997; Loeber, Keenan, & Zhang, 1997) described three such pathways of increasingly serious antisocial behavior. An overt pathway is characterized by acts of increasingly serious aggression including bullying and physical fighting, and culminating in acts such as rape and assault. A covert pathway begins with minor acts such as shoplifting and lying, which lead to more serious acts, such as fire-setting or vandalism, and culminate in serious covert behaviors such as fraud and burglary. Finally, an authority conflict pathway is marked by early argumentative and defiant behavior, leading to serious forms of defiance toward authority such as truancy, running away, and chronic and serious rulebreaking. The earlier the onset of the problem behavior, the greater the likelihood that more than one pathway will be followed and that serious and chronic behavior will ensue. Evidence across studies suggests that these pathways capture the behavior of many antisocial youth (Gorman-Smith, Tolan, Loeber, & Henry, 1998; Tolan & Gorman-Smith, 1998).

Similarly, antisocial behavior can be described by age of onset. Youths who show early onset tend to be male, more aggressive and hyperactive than their peers, and often characterized by learning difficulties and a history of family problems (Moffitt, 1993). Their antisocial behavior tends to be particularly severe and persistent (Farrington, Loeber, & Van Kammen, 1990; Tolan & Thomas, 1995), leading Moffitt (1993) to deem them the *life course persistent* group. In contrast, youths who first initiate antisocial involvement in adolescence tend to associate with other antisocial adolescents and tend to show fewer individual or familial risks. The term *adolescent-limited* has been used to describe them, based on the hypothesis that this form of antisocial behavior is more self-limiting (Moffitt, 1993). More recently, trajectories of involvement in various forms of antisocial behavior have been delineated by their relative persistence over the course of development (Nagin & Tremblay, 1999).

Efforts to describe various courses of antisocial involvement serve several goals. First, they highlight the evolving, rather than static, nature of trajectories involving antisocial behavior. Second, they offer the opportunity to develop more accurate models of risk based on meaningful subsets of youth behavior. Third, they may provide important information about the most promising targets for preventive interventions. Thus, this research represents a significant step in our growing understanding of the conditions and types of antisocial behaviors that lead to particularly problematic courses of behavior.

Theoretical Framework for Delinquency Prevention Research

Delinquency prevention research has long been criticized (Hawkins & Weis, 1985; Lorion, Tolan, & Wahler, 1987) for its lack of grounding in a coherent theoretical framework or conceptual foundation. Consistent with previous reviews and commission recommendations (American Psychological Association Commission on Youth Violence, 1993; National Research Council, 1993; Tolan, Guerra, & Kendall, 1995), we believe that the key to progress in delinquency prevention lies in establishing a solid empirical base via research that is theoretically grounded. In fact, however, many widespread interventions continue to be implemented because they have gained public appeal and acceptance rather than because they are empirically justified based on the population characteristics and risk factors. This method of implementation is likely to severely compromise the effectiveness of such programs (Garbarino, 1993). It is hard to imagine that a good idea put into action by well-meaning and thoughtful people may not have the intended effect, and, given the social importance of the problem of delinquency, it may seem that any effort is better than nothing. Yet, reviews of the literature and several of the more long-term, sophisticated analyses suggest that both of these assumptions can be dangerously wrong. Not only have such programs been ineffective, but some efforts have exacerbated the behavior of intervention participants (for critiques, see Lorion et al., 1987; Dishion, McCord, & Poulin, 1999). Thus, there is a need to design theory-driven interventions to gather more specific and extensive data on delinquency, which will, in turn, make future interventions more successful.

In their current state, models of antisocial behavior and delinquency often fall short of their intended goals. These models appropriately identify correlates and risk factors of delinquency, but they do not always elucidate mechanisms by which risk factors and outcomes might be related. This is a particularly imposing task, given that these theoretical models must retain sufficient complexity to reflect the fact that children, parents, peers, neighborhoods, and larger communities and cultures are all influential in determining risk for antisocial and delinquent behavior; that these levels of risk are not independent, but rather are "nested" in one another (i.e., children are located within family and peer networks that, in turn, are nested within ecological settings that influence the availability of opportunities and constraints); and that models must have a temporal perspective that describes how developmental challenges shift over time. Clearly, complex and multidimensional models of development are needed to capture these interactions.

For these reasons, a developmental-ecological framework has gained widespread use. This approach incorporates both life-course development (Jessor, 1993; Sampson & Laub, 1992) and social-ecological approaches (Bronfenbrenner, 1988) and highlights interactions among multiple risk factors that vary in importance over the course of development (Reid & Eddy, 1997). Successful prevention efforts are thought to be those that alter key risk processes, as well as those that delay the onset, or decrease the severity, of antisocial behavior. This framework also emphasizes the dynamic relationships among individuals and the various social systems (e.g., families, peer groups), settings (e.g., schools, workplaces), and contexts (e.g., neighborhoods, communities, cultural contexts) in which they live. Societal-level events and culture influence interactions in these more local settings as well.

This framework allows for the creation of more specific models of risk. A number of developmental-ecological risk models have been proposed and tested in recent years (Tolan et al., 1995). However, considerable refinement of these models is still needed. First, relations between multiple risk factors and various outcomes must be explicitly proposed and tested. For example, we must determine the risks that are necessary and sufficient to produce a given outcome, the variables that predispose certain conditions, and the mediators and moderators of more central risk factors.

Second, we must better understand the roles that gender, social class, community context, and culture play in risk models (Cauce, Ryan, & Grove, 1998). For example, evidence suggests that processes leading to delinquency may differ between boys and girls (Wangby, Bergman, & Magnusson, 1999). In our own research (Gorman-Smith, Tolan, Henry, & Florsheim, 2000), we have found that the relationships between adolescents' beliefs about family and their involvement in antisocial behavior differ distinctly between Mexican American and African American families. Clearly, beliefs about family are related to risk in both groups, but the mechanisms of risk appear dependent on cultural context. We also have found that relationships among family functioning, stress, and delinquent behavior vary distinctly as a function of community of residence (inner-city poor vs. other urban poor) (Gorman-Smith, Tolan, & Henry, 1999; Gorman-Smith, Tolan, & Henry, in press). Explanations for moderated findings of this kind may emerge through closer consideration of the unique experiences of different groups of children and families (Tolan & Guerra, 1994). For example, participation in crime is likely to hold different meaning for youth growing up in different contexts. Young, urban children witness, and are victims of, violence at alarmingly high rates (Garbarino, 1999; Garbarino, Kostelny & Dubrow, 1991; Shakoor & Chalmers, 1991), and delinquent or antisocial behavior may serve utilitarian purposes under some conditions, including securing material goods and respect from peers (Fagan & Wilkinson, 1998). Urban children who are poor, most of whom are also of color, are likely to face much harsher consequences for their delinquent behavior if caught than are their nonurban, White peers (Snyder & Sickmund, 1999). Unfortunately, most risk models have not begun to address the ways in which such aspects of experience affect risk for participation in delinquent behavior. In fact, as with most other areas of psychological research, our assumptions about antisocial behavior and delinquency are largely based on research with White, middle-class children and their families (Rogoff & Morelli, 1989). Even when considerable numbers of ethnic minority youth are included in research, the role of ethnic or cultural background in the developmental processes rarely is considered. As a consequence, important aspects of their experience may be conspicuously absent from mainstream models of development and risk, perhaps necessitating new, more comprehensive, and more ecologically sensitive models (Garcia Coll et al., 1996).

A number of innovative interventions, solidly grounded in developmental-ecological theory, have emerged recently. These programs take into account both the ecological context of the problem and the socioecological level at which the intervention should optimally be targeted to reach a given aim. A program that clearly stands out as a universal approach to the prevention of delinquency and other antisocial behaviors (e.g., substance abuse) is the Seattle Social Development Project (SSDP; Hawkins et al., 1992). This multicomponent program focuses on encouraging prosocial behavior and decreasing antisocial behavior through intervention components aimed at both school and family functioning. The classroom-based intervention is grounded on the premise that, through improved teaching and classroom management practices, children's bonds to school and societal conventions will be strengthened. Likewise, through parent training and support, opportunities for prosocial responses in the home will increase. The intervention program proceeds in developmentally sequenced steps delivered through the early elementary school years. At follow-up, violence and arrests for crime among the youth involved in the SSDP had declined and other academic and prosocial behavior benefits were evident as well. Notably, short-term or immediate effects were much less consistent and substantial than longer-term ones.

Also securely grounded within a developmental-ecological framework is the Linking the Interests of Families and Teachers (LIFT) program, designed by Reid and his colleagues (Reid, Eddy, Fetrow, & Stoolmiller, 1999). This program targets children growing up in neighborhoods with particularly elevated rates of juvenile delinquency and focuses on a clearly defined set of proximal risks for the development of conduct problems. LIFT includes a set of intervention components that target family management practice, classroom-based social skills, and behavior management on school playgrounds. The program also explicitly focuses on strengthening links between parents and teachers as a way to promote positive youth behavior in a more uniform manner. Importantly, the research design also investigates the optimal developmental timing for the intervention by delivering the program to both first and fifth graders and their families. Preliminary results appear promising.

An innovative approach to targeted intervention also has been undertaken by Henggeler and his colleagues in their multisystemic therapy (MST; Brown et al., 1997; Henggeler, 1999). MST interventions have been used to prevent psychiatric hospitalization and incarceration among youth with serious clinical problems. This approach recognizes the multidetermined nature of significant clinical difficulties and targets for change those areas of functioning that are known predictors of such problems (e.g., poor family functioning, academic difficulties, association with delinquent peers). Although the model is characterized by flexibility in the clinical options that might be used in a given case, the primary goals of MST include improving internal family functioning and helping youth and their families develop more adaptive and supportive interactions with their larger social environments (e.g., neighborhood, community, school). This form of intervention has evidenced quite strong results in terms of both clinical outcome and cost-effectiveness in dealing with problems that have often been considered intractable.

Correspondence of Intervention Characteristics, Societal Context, and Population Characteristics

As discussed, there is great heterogeneity among youth who offend, the patterns of delinquency they exhibit over time, and the contexts within which such youth engage in antisocial behavior. Thus, there is a need to identify how risk factors for delinquency vary by the population, social context, and developmental stage of interest. Correspondingly, it is necessary to determine whether and how intervention effects vary along these same lines. In other words, we must think in terms of "what works for whom and under what conditions" and how intervention effects may depend on ethnicity, gender, developmental phase, socioeconomic status, or other subgroup differences (Tolan, 2000).

Clearly, this is easier said than done. However, we have tackled this issue in our own research in several ways. For example, in the Metropolitan Area Child Study (MACS; Metropolitan Area Child Study Research Group, in press), participating schools not only were assigned to receive different intervention "packages" (i.e., universal classroom-based vs. universal plus peer group intervention vs. the latter plus family group intervention), but schools also were assigned to receive the intervention at one of two distinct developmental phases (either early or late elementary grades). Schools also had been specifically recruited so that they varied in school and community resources and community risk. By including these population, school, and community characteristics in our intervention planning, we were able to examine the relative utility of the intervention when implemented in different settings and under different circumstances. These analyses were critical in elucidating the nature of our treatment effects. For example, the intervention showed benefits on aggression only for young children in moderate-resource schools, and actually showed some iatrogenic effects on aggression for younger children in low-resource schools and among older children regardless of school resources. This can be understood in terms of intervention fit, which can involve both individual and contextual characteristics (Metropolitan Area Child Study Research Group, in press). In other words, the intervention must fit the developmental needs and capacities of children, families, and schools. Similarly, an organization must be "ready" to integrate an intervention into its setting, including having sufficient resources to support it (Elias, 1997). When a particular intervention is found to be ineffective under given circumstances or within a given population, it does not mean that the intervention is ineffective or that risk cannot be lowered among the population targeted. It may only mean that the characteristics of intervention, as implemented, do not meet the needs of the population or the demands of setting, and, thus, a different type of intervention is warranted.

CASE EXAMPLE

In our own research programs, including the MACS (Metropolitan Area Child Study Research Group, in press) and the SAFEChildren Program (Tolan, Gorman-Smith, & Henry, 2001), we have tried to ground the intervention in a developmental-ecological perspective on risk for aggression (Guerra, Eron, Huesmann, Tolan, & VanAcker, 1998; Tolan et al., 1995). In these trials, we test the relative utility of promising intervention formats, attempting to organize these to be developmentally appropriate, with a strong family emphasis, and focused on empirically identified risk factors for later delinquency and antisocial behavior. In the MACS, for example, we randomly assigned 16 schools located in two different types of urban communities (inner-city vs. urban poor) to one of four intervention conditions: no-treatment control; general enhancement classroom program; general enhancement plus small-group, peer-skills training; or general enhancement plus small-group, peer-skills training plus family intervention. The general enhancement classroom program was a universal intervention that focused on social-cognitive skills training for the children and on classroom management and child development principles training for the teachers. It was conducted over 2 years. This program was provided to all students, while the small-group and family interventions were provided only to high-risk children. The small-group program emphasized the same social-cognitive skills as the general enhancement program but also focused on peer skills. The family intervention focused on parenting skills, management of family relationship, life stressors, and neighborhood issues and worked to build support networks among the families (see Eargle, Guerra, & Tolan, 1994; Metropolitan Area Child Study Research Group, in press; and Tolan & McKay, 1996, for more in-depth description of program design and components).

   This comparison and program development was based on research suggesting each approach might mitigate aggression and school failure, two of the best predictors of later delinquency. We wanted to determine if these promising approaches would work in these challenging environments, where school and community resources are limited, and impediments and risk-inducing circumstances are high. We also wanted to understand the extent of intervention that was necessary to affect risk and whether just affecting the school ecology (the social skills of the children, the teacher's approach to classroom management, and the norms in the classrooms about aggression and on-task behavior) would reduce aggression and improve achievement, thereby reducing risk for later delinquency. We expected, though, that universal general interventions based solely in the classroom would be inadequate to prevent or mitigate aggression among high-risk youth. The tiered intervention design was used to test the viability of the underlying theoretical model(s) regarding the etiology and prevention of aggression, thus increasing the potential for long-term and generalized effects. During the 10 years of this study, over 8000 students in eight cohorts participated. Although designed to be implemented with the careful control that is important for valid experimental study, the project also was required to be immediately valuable and responsive to the real needs of the schools. For example, schools would change administrators, and the new principal might not have been as supportive of the project. Similarly, in the middle of the intervention program, Chicago began a process of school reform that put greater emphasis on academic achievement. There were many lessons in the mismatch between (a) the dynamic and shifting nature of the social ecology and the intervention setting and (b) the values of firm control and careful manipulation of interventions that are scientifically valued. This scientific study within a given social ecology had its value not in identifying the basic elements of effective prevention but in identifying how the setting influences preventive benefits and in helping to develop more interesting and utilitarian questions (Tolan, Chertok, Keys, & Jason, 1990).

The initial outcome test of the proximal effects showed that effects depend on what aspect of functioning is measured (e.g., aggression vs. school achievement), when the intervention is applied, whether or not the school and community setting has adequate resources to support the intervention, and which intervention method(s) are used. Interested readers are referred to the article by the Metropolitan Area Child Study Group (in press) for details of the proximal effects. Summarily, the prevention efforts were effective but only when applied early in the elementary years; they did not show benefits for older children. However, a second dose in the later years magnified the effects (positive and negative) found from the early intervention. For aggression, the full intervention (all three components) was necessary and the benefits were seen only in noninner-city schools. In fact, in the inner-city schools there appeared to be a negative effect of applying the small-group program for high-risk youth, if applied late in the elementary years; the group involvement seemed to block a developmentally normal diminishment of aggression. Notably, this small-group effect seemed to be for the portion of the high-risk group with less initial aggression. For those children with "clinical level" aggression, the program was more beneficial across settings and did not have any negative effects. The overall results concur with many others in advising against small-group approaches for preventing/treating delinquency risk and in favor of the critical role of family intervention in finding benefits. Academic functioning was affected positively across settings, but the effect was much greater in the noninner-city schools. Also, this academic boost was found only from early intervention and was not enhanced by additional later intervention. The small-group and family interventions did not enhance this effect. Thus, these results suggest that approaches found to be promising elsewhere can have benefits in these more difficult social ecologies, but when school and community effects are measured they reveal that results vary substantially by setting characteristics. In addition, these results point to the value of early intervention but do not definitively argue against later intervention, particularly to enhance early benefits.

The MACS was one of the first studies of school-level assignment to intervention condition that incorporated consideration of this critical developmental setting. The results reveal that schools vary substantially in how they affect prevention and development. The study also demonstrates the tension between maintaining the degree of internal consistency of intervention needed for scientific clarity and recognizing the complex factors and necessary adaptations involved in work in real settings. This decade of work revealed many of the limitations of the then-current designs but also illuminated much about what future work should incorporate.

FUTURE DIRECTIONS

Policy makers and prevention researchers exist in quite different worlds and are forced to contend with the quite different demands of the systems in which they work. Nonetheless, the larger aims of many prevention researchers are vitally linked to the actions of those in the policy arena. For this reason alone, we would argue that more mutually beneficial links should be forged between these two groups. Researchers must understand the political climate within which an intervention will be introduced and the resulting implications for social policy. For example, research on delinquency prevention indicates that developmentally oriented, multisystemic intervention programs—both universal and more targeted in nature—are necessary to effect meaningful change, particularly in high-risk settings. Unfortunately, it benefits policy makers to support short-term, intensive programs that have quick, proximal effects. Because politicians often focus on alternatives that are likely to have an impact before the next election, it is difficult to persuade them that long-term prevention efforts are the best alternative, given that results may not be seen for years to come. Policy makers' biases, often contrary to what research supports, provide sobering knowledge that prevention advocates must take into consideration in planning and implementing interventions.

Another emerging and related trend is to support policies based on specific incidents and political expedience rather than strategies based on empirical findings (Tolan, 2000). Social policy often grows out of "fireside inductions" (i.e., common sense, anecdotal beliefs) (Sechrest & Bootzin, 1996) and catch phrases that seem to characterize the problem in some palatable way, such as the seriously misleading term "superpredators" (DiIulio, 1995) and unsupported assertions such as Bennett, DiIulio, and Walters' (1996, p. 26) claim that we are about to encounter the "youngest, biggest, and baddest generation any society has every known." Policy also often relies on ideas about delinquency that, although appealing and popular, have been proven either ineffective or harmful, or certainly do not offer the solutions implied in their promotion. For example, evidence is accumulating that punitive, legalistic approaches have no substantial impact on youth violence (Tolan & Gorman-Smith, 1998). On the other hand, graduated legal sanctions may help if they are thoughtfully integrated into policies that focus most funding and efforts on prevention (Krisberg & Howell, 1998).

We urge that those conducting delinquency prevention research and programs continue to argue that laws and policies should follow what evidence indicates is necessary and effective. This evidence can be formulated into a coherent approach. There is now an accumulated set of studies that provide consistent, generalizable findings, and many methods exist to determine what should be done, where, and with whom. For example, most youth are not violent, and very few are repeatedly violent. However, there is a group of young people who show early aggression and increasingly antisocial behavior into and beyond adolescence. This group is also at high risk for other social problems, such as drug and alcohol abuse, academic and employment failure, and poor relationship stability (Moffitt, 1993). Thus, accurate, early identification of this group and strong intervention can have positive effects not only for violence but also for many associated social problems.

These youths are currently identified by many service systems, including school, child welfare, police, and health care. These diverse identification systems also operate disjunctively as service systems, particularly for children and families with needs that cross service systems. Strategies to develop service funding, program development, service delivery, and collaborations across current systems are critical. We must do more to encourage integrated responses in identifying at-risk youths and providing services so they are no longer bound to the happenstance of what system first becomes aware of them. Such integrated services, particularly if family-focused, have been shown to be quite effective (Henggeler, Cunningham, Pickrel, Schoenwald, & Brondino, 1996). Initiatives that identify the most effective financial and administrative approaches for promoting and maintaining integrated and sound interventions for these high-risk youths are needed. Models for legislation that are based on both cost management and program quality must be developed.

We agree with Sechrest and Bootzin (1996, p. 381), who state that "policy may be better formed out of the best evidence available than out of the prejudices of individual decision makers or out of thin air." However, we also believe that it is incumbent on prevention researchers to arm themselves with the tools necessary to communicate effectively with those who make decisions of policy and practice. Prevention researchers must go beyond the mores of common academic practice and disseminate their research findings in such a manner that they will affect public policy. In line with Grisso and Melton's (1987) suggestions to child law researchers, we suggest that prevention researchers pursue dissemination outlets that policy makers often access, such as the popular media, law reviews, books, newsletters, newspapers, and magazines. Some (e.g., Grisso & Melton, 1987) would even argue that researchers have an ethical obligation to promote social welfare by disseminating research finds through such outlets.

In our own experience, we have worked to provide basic information about empirical findings to both local and federal policy makers. For example, in his recent testimony before the United States House of Representatives Subcommittee on Crime regarding the effectiveness of existing violence prevention programs, Tolan provided basic information about empirically supported strategies for violence prevention. Tolan's (2000) testimony provides a fitting summary regarding what we know and what we need to do: Effects depend on both the content and the quality of implementation of a given program; prevention is more effective and less costly than punishment and incarceration; objective evaluations with sound scientific controls are necessary to provide information about valuable approaches; and, despite its promise, prevention often is set aside in favor of treatment because treatment effects are often more immediately and blatantly observable. Thus, we would concur with the statement of Bottoms, Reppucci, Tweed, and Nysse (in press, p. 2) that research that "advances psychological theory *and* results in concrete, beneficial changes in policies, laws, and/or practices" should be considered as constituting an outstanding achievement.

REFERENCES

Agnew, R. (1990). Adolescent resources and delinquency. *Criminology, 28,* 535–566.

American Psychological Association Commission on Youth Violence (1993). *Violence and youth: Psychology's response.* Washington, DC: Author.

Bennett, W. J., DiIulio, J. J., & Walters, J. P. (1996). *Body count: Moral poverty—and how to win America's war against crime and drugs.* New York: Simon & Schuster.

Baron, L., Straus, M. A., & Jaffee, D. (1990). Legitimate violence, violent attitudes, and rape: A test of the cultural spillover theory. *Annals of New York Academy of Sciences, 528,* 79–110.

Bottoms, B. L., Reppucci, N. D., Tweed, J. A., & Nysse, K. L. (in press). Children, psychology, and the law: Reflections on past and future contributions to science and policy. In J. Ogloff (Ed.), *Psychology and law in the 21st century.* New York: Kluwer.

Bronfenbrenner, U. (1988). Interacting systems in human development: Research paradigms: Present and future. In N. Bolger, A. Caspi, G. Downey & M. Moorehouse (Eds.), *Persons in context: Developmental processes* (pp. 25–49). New York: Cambridge University Press.

Brown, T. L., Swenson, C. C., Cunningham, P. B., Henggeler, S. W., Schoenwald, S., & Rowland, M. D. (1997). Multisystemic treatment of violent and chronic juvenile offenders: Bridging the gap between research and practice. *Administration and Policy in Mental Health, 25,* 221–238.

Bry, B. H. (1982). Reducing the incidence of adolescent problems through preventive intervention: One- and five-year follow up. *American Journal of Community Psychology, 10,* 265–276.

Cauce, A. M., Ryan, K. D., & Grove, K. (1998). Children and adolescents of color, where are you? Participation, selection, recruitment, and retention in developmental research. In V. C. McLoyd & L. Steinberg (Eds.), *Studying minority adolescents: Conceptual, methodological, and theoretical issues* (pp. 147–166). Mahwah, NJ: Erlbaum.

Coie, J. D., Cillessen, A. H. N., Dodge, K. A., Hubbard, J. A., Schwartz, D., Lemerise, E. A., & Bateman, H. (1999). It takes two to fight: A test of relational factors and a method for assessing aggressive dyads. *Developmental Psychology, 35,* 1179–1188.

Coie, J. D., Watt, N. F., West, S. G., Hawkins, J. D., Asarnow, J. R., Markman, H. J., Ramey, S. L., Shure, M. B., & Long, B. (1993). The science of prevention: A conceptual framework and some directions for a national research program. *American Psychologist, 48,* 1013–1022.

Conduct Problems Prevention Research Group (1999). Initial impact of the fast track prevention trial for conduct problems: I. The high risk sample. *Journal of Consulting and Clinical Psychology, 67,* 631–647.

Crick, N., & Dodge, K. (1994). A review and reformulation of social information processing mechanisms in children's adjustment. *Psychological Bulletin, 115,* 74–101.

DiIulio, J. J., Jr. (1995). Moral poverty: The coming of the superpredators should scare us into wanting to get to the root causes of crime a lot faster. *Chicago Tribune,* December, 15, Section 1, p. 31.

Dishion, T. J., McCord, J., & Poulin, F. (1999). When interventions harm: Peer groups and problem behavior. *American Psychologist, 54,* 755–764.

Dodge, K. A. (1993). Social-cognitive mechanisms in the development of conduct disorder and depression. *Annual Review of Psychology, 44*, 559–584.

Dodge, K. A., Coie, J. D., Pettit, G. S., & Price, J. M. (1996). Peer status and aggression in boys' groups: Developmental and contextual analyses. *Child Development, 61*, 1289–1309.

Eargle, A. E., Guerra, N. G., & Tolan, P. H. (1994). Preventing aggression in inner-city children: Small group training to change cognitions, social skills, and behavior. *Journal of Child and Adolescent Group Therapy, 4*, 229–242.

Eddy, J. M., Reid, J. B., & Fetrow, R. A. (2000). An elementary school-based prevention program targeting modifiable antecedents of youth delinquency and violence: Linking the Interests of Families and Teachers (LIFT). *Journal of Emotional & Behavioral Disorders, 8*, 165–176.

Elias, M. J. (1997). Reinterpreting dissemination of prevention programs as widespread implementation with effectiveness and fidelity. In R. P. Weissberg, T. P. Gullotta, R. L. Hampton, B. A. Ryan, & G. A. Adams (Eds.), *Establishing preventive services* (pp. 253–289). Thousand Oaks, CA: Sage.

Elliot, D. S., & Tolan, P. H. (1999). Youth violence prevention, intervention, and social policy: An overview. In D. Flannery & R. Hoff (Eds.), *Youth violence: Prevention, intervention, and social policy* (pp. 3–46). Washington, DC: American Psychiatric Association.

Fagan, J., & Wilkinson, D. L. (1998). Social contexts and functions of adolescent violence. In D. S. Elliott, B. A. Hamburg, & K. R. Williams (Eds.), *Violence in American schools: A new perspective* (pp. 55–93). New York: Cambridge University Press.

Farrington, D. P. (1991). Childhood aggression and adult violence. In D. Pepler & K. H. Rubin (Eds.), *The development and treatment of childhood aggression* (pp. 5–29). Hillsdale, NJ: Erlbaum.

Farrington, D. P., & Hawkins, J. D. (1991). Predicting participation, early onset, and later persistence in officially recorded offending. *Criminal Behavior and Mental Health, 1*, 1–33.

Farrington, D. P., & Loeber, R. (1999). Transatlantic replicability of risk factors in the development of delinquency. In P. Cohen, C. Slomkowski, & L. N. Robins (Eds.), *Historical and geographical influences on psychopathology* (pp. 299–329). Mahwah, NJ: Erlbaum.

Farrington, D. P., Loeber, R., & Van Kammen, W. B. (1990). Long-term criminal outcomes of hyperactivity-impulsivity-attention deficit and conduct problems in childhood. In L. N. Robins & M. Rutter (Eds.), *Straight and devious pathways from childhood to adulthood* (pp. 62–81). Cambridge, England: Cambridge University Press.

Garbarino, J. (1993). Enhancing adolescent development through social policy. In P. H. Tolan & B. J. Cohler (Eds.), *Handbook of clinical research and practice with adolescents* (pp. 469–488). New York: Wiley.

Garbarino, J. (1999). The effects of community violence on children. In L. Balter & C. S. Tamis-LeMonda (Eds.), *Child psychology: A handbook of contemporary issues* (pp. 412–425). Philadelphia, PA: Psychology Press/Taylor-Francis.

Garbarino, J., Kostelny, K., & Dubrow, N. (1991). What children can tell us about living in danger. *American Psychologist, 46*, 376–383.

Garcia Coll, C., Lamberty, G., Jenkins, R., McAdoo, H. P., Crnic, K., Wasik, B. H., & Vasquez Garcia, H. (1996). An integrative model for the study of developmental competencies in minority children. *Child Development, 67*, 1891–1914.

Gorman-Smith, D., Tolan, P. H., & Henry, D. B. (1999). The relation of community and family to risk among urban poor adolescents. In P. Cohen, L. Robins & C. Slomkowski (Eds.), *Where and when: Influence of historical time and place on aspects of psychopathology* (pp. 349–367). Hillsdale, NJ: Earlbaum.

Gorman-Smith, D., Tolan, P. H., & Henry, D. B. (2000). A developmental-ecological model of the relation of family functioning to patterns of delinquency. *Journal of Quantitative Criminology, 16*, 169–198.

Gorman-Smith, D., Tolan, P. H., Henry, D. B., & Florsheim, P. (2000). Patterns of family functioning and adolescent outcomes among urban African American and Mexican American families. *Journal of Family Psychology, 14*, 436–457.

Gorman-Smith, D., Tolan, P. H., Loeber, R. & Henry, D. B. (1998). The relation of family problems to patterns of delinquent involvement among urban youth. *Journal of Abnormal Child Psychology, 26*, 319–333.

Gorman-Smith, D., Tolan, P. H., Zelli, A., & Huesmann, L. R. (1996). The relation of family functioning to violence among inner-city minority youth. *Journal of Family Psychology, 10*, 115–119.

Gottfredson, D. C., Gottfredson, G. D., & Skroban, S. (1996). A multimodal school based prevention demonstration. *Journal of Adolescent Research, 11*, 97–115.

Greenberg, M. T., Kusche, C. A., Cook, E. T., & Quamma, J. P. (1995). Promoting emotional competence in school-aged children: The effects of the PATHS curriculum. *Development and Psychopathology, 7*, 117–136.

Grisso, T., & Melton, G. B. (1987). Getting child development research to legal practitioners: Which way to the trenches? In G. B. Melton (Ed.), *Reforming the law* (pp. 146–176). New York: Guilford.

Guerra, N. G., Eron, L. D., Huesmann, L. R., Tolan, P. H., & VanAcker, R. (1998). A cognitive-ecological approach to the prevention and mitigation of violence and aggression in inner-city youth. In K. Bijorkquist & D. P. Fry (Eds.), *Styles and conflict resolution: Models and applications from around the world* (pp. 199–213). Orlando, FL: Academic Press.

Guerra, N. G., & Slaby, R. G. (1990). Cognitive mediators of aggression in adolescent offenders: 2. Intervention. *Developmental Psychology, 26,* 269–277.

Guerra, N. G., Tolan, P. H., & Hammond, W. R. (1994). Prevention and treatment of adolescent violence. In L. D. Eron, J. H. Gentry, & P. Schlegel (Eds.), *Reason to hope: A psychological perspective on violence and youth* (pp. 383–403). Washington, DC: American Psychological Association.

Hawkins, J. D., Catalano, R. F., Morrison, D. M., O'Donnell, J., Abbot, R. D., & Day, L. E. (1992). Seattle Social Development Project: Effects of the first four years on protective factors and problem behaviors. In J. McCord & R. E. Tremblay (Eds.), *Preventing antisocial behavior: Interventions from birth through adolescence* (pp. 139–161). New York: Guilford.

Hawkins, J. D., Herrenkohl, T., Farrington, D. P., Brewer, D., Catalano, R. F., & Harachi, T. W. (1998). A review of predictors of youth violence. In R. Loeber & D. P. Farrington (Eds.), *Serious and violent juvenile offenders: Risk factors and successful interventions* (pp. 106–146). Thousand Oaks, CA: Sage.

Hawkins, J. D., & Weis, J. G. (1985). The social development model: An integrated approach to delinquency prevention. *Journal of Primary Prevention, 6,* 73–97.

Henggeler, S. W. (1999). Multisystemic therapy: An overview of clinical procedures, outcomes, and policy implications. *Child Psychology and Psychiatry Review, 4,* 2–10.

Henggeler, S. W., Borduin, C. M., & Mann, B. J. (1993). Advances in family therapy: Empirical foundations. *Advances in Clinical Child Psychology, 15,* 207–241.

Henggeler, S. W., Cunningham, P. B., Pickrel, S. G., Schoenwald, S. K., & Brondino, M. J. (1996). Multisystemic therapy: An effective violence prevention approach for serious juvenile offenders. *Journal of Adolescence, 19,* 47–61.

Henggeler, S. W., Melton, G. B., Smith, L. A., Schoenwald, S. K., & Hanley, J. H. (1993). Family preservation using multisystemic treatment: Long-term follow-up to a clinical trial with serious juvenile offenders. *Journal of Child & Family Studies, 2,* 283–293.

Henry, D. B., Tolan, P. H., & Gorman-Smith, D. (2001). Longitudinal family and peer group effects on violent and non-violent delinquency. *Journal of Clinical Child Psychology, 30,* 172–186.

Hinshaw, S. P. (1987). On the distinction between attentional deficits/hyperactivity and conduct problems/aggression in child psychopathology. *Psychological Bulletin, 101,* 443–463.

Howell, J. C., Krisberg, B., Hawkins, J. D., & Wilson, J. J. (1996). *A sourcebook:*

Serious, violent, and chronic juvenile offenders. Thousand Oaks, CA: Sage.

Huesmann, L. R. (1998). The role of social information processing and cognitive schemas in the acquisition and maintenance of habitual aggressive behavior. In R G. Geen & E. Donnerstein (Eds.), *Human aggression: Theories, research, and implications for policy* (pp. 73–109). New York: Academic Press.

Jessor, R. (1993). Successful adolescent development among youth in high-risk settings. *American Psychologist, 48*, 117–126.

Kellam, S. G., & Rebok, G. W. (1992). Building developmental and etiological theory through epidemiologically based preventive intervention trials. In J. McCord & R. E. Tremblay (Eds.), *Preventing antisocial behavior: Interventions from birth through adolescence* (pp. 162–195). New York: Guilford.

Krisberg, B., & Howell, J. C. (1998). The impact of the juvenile justice system and prospects for graduated sanctions in a comprehensive strategy. In R. Loeber & D. P. Farrington (Eds.), *Serious and violent juvenile offenders: Risk factors and successful interventions* (pp. 346–366).Thousand Oaks, CA: Sage.

Lahey, B. B., Loeber, R., Hart, E. L., Frick, P. J., Applegate, B., Zhang, Q., Green, S. M., & Russo, M. F. (1995). Four-year longitudinal study of conduct disorder in boys: Patterns and predictors of persistence. *Journal of Abnormal Psychology, 104*, 83–93.

Lipsey, M. W., & Wilson, D. B. (1998). Effective intervention for serious juvenile offenders: A synthesis of research. In R. Loeber & D. P. Farrington (Eds.), *Serious and violent juvenile offenders: Risk factors and successful interventions* (pp. 313–345). Thousand Oaks, CA: Sage.

Loeber, R., & Farrington, D. P. (Eds.) (1998). *Serious and violent juvenile offenders: Risk factors and successful interventions.* Thousand Oaks, CA: Sage.

Loeber, R., Farrington, D. P., & Waschbusch, D. A. (1998). Serious and violent juvenile offenders. In R. Loeber & D. Farrington (Eds.), *Serious and violent juvenile offenders: Risk factors and successful interventions* (pp. 13–29). Thousand Oaks, CA: Sage.

Loeber, R., & Hay, D. (1997). Key issues in the development of aggression and violence from childhood to early adulthood. *Annual Review of Psychology, 48*, 371–410.

Loeber, R., Keenan, K., & Zhang, Q. (1997). Boys' experimentation and persistence in developmental pathways toward serious delinquency. *Journal of Child and Family Studies, 6*, 321–357.

Loeber, R., Wung, P., Keenan, K., Giroux, B., Stouthamer-Loeber, M., van Kammen, W. B., & Maughan, B. (1993). Developmental pathways in disruptive child behavior. *Development and Psychopathology, 5*, 103–133.

Lorion, R. P., Tolan, P. H., & Wahler, R. G. (1987). Prevention. In H. C. Quay (Ed.), *Handbook of juvenile delinquency* (pp. 383–416). New York: Wiley.

Mercy, J., & Rosenberg, M. (1998). Preventing firearm violence in and around the schools. In E. D. Elliott, B. Hamburg, & K. Williams (Eds.), *Violence in American schools: New perspectives and solutions* (pp. 159–187). New York: Cambridge University Press.

Metropolitan Area Child Study Research Group (2002). A cognitive-ecological approach to preventing aggression in urban settings: Initial outcomes for high-risk children. *Journal of Consulting and Clinical Psychology, 70* 179–194.

Moffitt, T. (1993). Adolescence-limited and life-course-persistent antisocial behavior: A developmental taxonomy. *Psychological Review, 100*, 674–701.

Mrazek, P. J., & Haggerty, R. J. (1994). *Reducing risks for mental disorders: Frontiers for preventive intervention research*. Washington DC: National Academy Press.

Mulvey, E. P., Arthur, M. W., & Reppucci, N. D. (1993). The prevention and treatment of juvenile delinquency: A review of the research. *Clinical Psychology Review, 13*, 133–167.

Nagin, D., & Tremblay, R. E. (1999). Trajectories of boys' physical aggression, opposition and hyperactivity on the path to psychically violent and non-violent juvenile delinquency. *Child Development, 70*, 1181–1196.

National Research Council (1993). *Understanding and preventing violence*. Washington, DC: National Academy Press.

Offord, D. R., Kraemer, H. C., Kazdin, A. J., Peter, S., & Harrington, R. (1998) Lowering the burden of suffering from child psychiatric disorder: Trade-offs among clinical, targeted, and universal interventions. *Journal of the American Academy of Child & Adolescent Psychiatry, 37*, 686–694.

Patterson, G. R., Reid, J. B., & Dishion, T. J. (1992). *Antisocial boys: A social interaction approach*. Eugene, OR: Castalia.

Pliszka, S. R. (2000). Patterns of psychiatric comorbidity with attention-deficit/hyperactivity disorder. *Child and Adolescent Psychiatric Clinics of North America, 9*, 525–540.

Reid, J. B., & Eddy, J. M. (1997). The prevention of antisocial behavior: Some considerations in the search for effective interventions. In D. M. Stoff, J. Breiling, & J. D. Maser (Eds.), *Handbook of antisocial behavior* (pp. 343–356). New York: Wiley.

Reid, J. B., Eddy, J. M., Fetrow, R. A., & Stoolmiller, M. (1999). Description and immediate impacts of a preventive intervention for conduct problems. *American Journal of Community Psychology, 27*, 483–517.

Rogoff, B., & Morelli, G. (1989). Perspectives on children's development from cultural psychology. *American Psychologist, 44*, 343–348.

Rosenberg, M. L. (1991). *Violence in America*. New York: Oxford University Press.

Sampson, R. J. (2000). A neighborhood-level perspective on social change and the social control of adolescent delinquency. In L. J. Crocket & R. K. Silbereisen (Eds.), *Negotiating adolescence in times of social change* (pp. 178–188). New York: Cambridge University Press.

Sampson, R. J., & Laub, J. H. (1992). Crime and deviance in the life course. *Annual Review of Sociology, 18*, 63–84.

Sechrest, L. B., & Bootzin, R. R. (1996). Psychology and inferences about public policy. *Psychology, Public Policy, and the Law, 2*, 377–392.

Shakoor, B. H., & Chalmers, D. (1991). Co-victimization of African-American children who witness violence and the theoretical implications of its effects on their cognitive, emotional, and behavioral development. *Journal of the National Medical Association, 83*, 233–238.

Shure, M. B. (1997). Interpersonal cognitive problem solving: Primary prevention of early high-risk behaviors in the preschool and primary years. In G. W. Albee & T. P. Gullotta (Eds.), *Primary prevention works: Issues in children's and families' lives* (Vol. 6, pp. 167–188). Thousand Oaks, CA: Sage.

Snyder, H. N., & Sickmund, M. (1999). *Juvenile offenders and victims: 1999 national report*. Washington, DC: National Center for Juvenile Justice, Office of Juvenile Justice and Delinquency Prevention.

Thornberry, T. P., Huizinga, D., & Loeber, R. (1995). The prevention of serious delinquency and violence: Implications from the Program of Research on the Causes and Correlates of Delinquency. In J. C. Howel, B. Krisberg, J. D. Hawkins, & J. J. Wilson (Eds.), Source book on serious, violent, and chronic offenders (pp. 213–237). Thousand Oaks, CA: Sage.

Tolan, P. H. (1998). Research methods in community-based treatment and prevention. In P. Kendall, J. Butcher, & G. Holmbeck (Eds.), *Handbook of research methods in clinical psychology* (2nd ed., pp. 403–418). New York: Wiley.

Tolan, P. H. (1999, February). *Youth violence prevention*. Paper presented at the Packard Foundation/Family Violence Consortium Meeting on Integrating Violence Research, San Francisco, CA.

Tolan, P. H. (2000), *What We Know About What Works in Preventing Youth Crime and Violence: Hearings Before the Subcommittee on Crime, Oversight Hearing on Preventing and Fighting Crime: What Works*, Testimony before the 106th Cong., 2d Sess. 74 (2000).

Tolan, P. H., Chertok, F., Keys, C., & Jason, L. (1990). Conversing about theories, methods, and community research. In P. Tolan, C. Keys, F. Chertok, & L. Jason (Eds.), *Researching community psychology: Issues of theory and methods* (pp. 3–8). Washington, DC: American Psychological Association.

Tolan, P. H., & Gorman-Smith, D. (1997). Families and the development of urban children. In H. J. Walberg, O. Reyes, & R. P. Weissberg (Eds.), *Children and youth: Interdisciplinary perspectives. Issues in children's and families' lives* (Vol. 7, pp. 67–91). Thousand Oaks, CA: Sage.

Tolan, P. H., & Gorman-Smith, D. (1998). Development of serious, violent, and chronic offenders. In R. Loeber & D. P. Farrington (Eds.), *Serious, violent, and chronic juvenile offenders: Risk factors and successful interventions* (pp. 68–85). Beverly Hills, CA: Sage.

Tolan, P. H., Gorman-Smith, D., & Henry, D. H. (2001). *Proximal effects of the SAFEChildren Program.* Manuscript submitted for publication.

Tolan, P. H., & Guerra, N. (1994). *What works in reducing adolescent violence: An empirical review of the field.* Boulder, CO: Center for the Study of Prevention and Violence.

Tolan, P. H., Guerra, N., & Kendall, P. C. (1995). A developmental-ecological perspective on antisocial behavior in children and adolescents: Toward a unified risk and intervention framework. *Journal of Consulting and Clinical Psychology, 63*, 579–584.

Tolan, P. H., & Loeber, R. (1993). Antisocial behavior. In P. H. Tolan & B. J. Cohler (Eds.), *Handbook of clinical research and practice with adolescents* (pp. 307–331). New York: Wiley.

Tolan, P. H., & McKay, M. M. (1996). Preventing serious antisocial behavior in inner-city children: An empirically based family intervention program. *Family Relations: Journal of Applied Family and Child Studies, 45*, 148–155.

Tolan, P. H., McKay, M. M., Hanish, L. D., & Dickey, M. H. (2000). *Measures for evaluating process in child and family interventions: An example in the prevention of aggression.* Manuscript submitted for publication.

Tolan, P. H., Sherrod, L., Gorman-Smith, D., & Henry, D. B. (in press). A developmental-ecological approach to positive youth development in the inner city. In K. Maton, B. Ledheather, & A. Solarz (Eds.), *Positive youth development: Research and policy.* Washington, DC: American Psychological Association.

Tolan, P. H., & Thomas, P. (1995). The implications of age of onset for delinquency risk: II. Longitudinal data. *Journal of Abnormal Child Psychology, 23*, 157–181.

Wangby, M., Bergman, L. R., & Magnusson, D. (1999). Development of adjustment problems in girls: What syndromes emerge? *Child Development, 70*, 678–699.

White, J. L., Moffitt, T. E., Earls, F., Robins, L., & Silva, P. A. (1990). How early can we tell? Predictors of childhood conduct disorder and adolescent delinquency. *Criminology, 28*, 507–533.

Wright, B. R. E., Caspi, A., Moffit, T. E., & Silva, P. A. (2001). The effects of social ties on crime vary by criminal propensity: A life-course model of interdependence. *Criminology, 39*, 321–351.

Yoshikawa, H. (1994). Prevention as cumulative protection: Effects of early family support and education on chronic delinquency and its risks. *Psychological Bulletin, 115*, 28–54.

CHAPTER 8

Preventing Depression in Youth

W. LaVome Robinson and
Mary H. Case

DESCRIPTION OF THE PROBLEM

Depression poses significant and enduring risk to the well-being, productivity, and survival of children and adolescents alike. The occurrence of depression during childhood and adolescence is neither a normal developmental episode nor a transient difficulty that desists with time (Kovacs, 1989; Lewinsohn, Rohde, Klein, & Seeley, 1999). Furthermore, a diagnosis of depression during childhood or adolescence increases the likelihood that youths will suffer from depressive symptoms or disorders throughout their childhood and into adulthood (Kessler, Avenevoli, & Merikangas, 2001; Lewinsohn, Hops, Roberts, Seeley, & Andrews, 1993; Rao, Hammen, & Daley, 1999), leaving the individual vulnerable to a broad spectrum of lifelong psychosocial risks (Geller, Zimerman, Williams, Bolhofner, & Craney, 2001; Kovacs et al., 1984; Weissman et al., 1999). The associated concomitant factors and comorbid disorders of childhood and adolescent depression cannot be minimized and warrant effective prevention efforts at optimal stages of development.

Further complicating the clinical picture of childhood and adolescent depression is the bleak social and economic climate surrounding issues of mental health services. Available resources for mental health services within the United States remain inadequate to handle the needs of its citizens. The costs of depression are far-reaching. Indeed, Hirschfeld, Keller, Pamico, and Arons (1997) estimated the annual cost of depression at $43 billion, including the expense of treatment, lost productivity, and premature death. Despite increasing evidence for the efficacy of intervention strategies targeting depressed youths, many children and adolescents lack access to, or knowledge of, such services (Keller, Lavori, Beardslee, & Wunder, 1991). As a result, children and adolescents suffering from depression are even less likely to receive treatment than adults with similar disorders (Beardslee, Keller, Lavori, Staley, & Sacks, 1993; Hirschfeld et al., 1997; Robins & Regier, 1991). Estimates suggest that approximately 70% to 80% of depressed teenagers never receive treatment for depressive symptoms and disorders (Keller et al., 1991; Rohde, Lewinsohn, & Seeley, 1991).

Prevalence

Prevalence rates of depression among children and adolescents highlight the frequency of these concerns among youths. Recent studies suggest that the lifetime prevalence for depressive disorders by the end of adolescence is close to 25% (Kessler, Avenevoli, & Merikangas, 2001). Approximately 5% of children ages 9 to 17 will suffer from a major depressive disorder, with an average episode lasting seven to nine months (Birmaher et al., 1996). Estimates of the prevalence rates of major depressive disorder, characterized by severe depressive symptomatology that interferes with functioning, range from 0.4% to 2.5% for children and from 0.4% to 8.3% for adolescents (Birmaher et al., 1996). Alarmingly, 20% to 40% of these youths likely will relapse within a two-year period (Harrington, Fudge, Rutter, Pickles, & Hill, 1990; Lewinsohn, Clarke, Seeley, & Rohde, 1994), underscoring the need for more effective secondary prevention programs.

Onset of dysthymia, a more chronic condition, is most common during childhood or adolescence, with an estimated rate of 3% (Garrison, Waller, Cuffee, McKeown, Addy, & Jackson, 1997) and an average duration of approximately four years (Kovacs, Akiskal, Gatsonis, & Parrone, 1994). Prevalence rates of dysthymia have ranged from 0.6% to 1.7% in children and from 1.6% to 8.0% in adolescents (Birmaher et al., 1996). Unfortunately, for those individuals suffering from dysthymic disorder, impairment is frequently greater than those diagnosed with major depressive disorder (Klein, Lewinsohn, & Seeley, 1997). This elevated impairment may reflect the longer duration and chronicity of dysthymia. Not surprisingly, given (a) the longstanding nature of this disorder, (b) its typical initial onset during childhood or adolescence, and (c) the 70% likelihood of later episodes of major depressive disorder (Akiskal,

1983; Klein et al., 1997), dysthymic disorder poses a significant threat to normal adjustment. The long-term prognosis for dysthymia is particularly bleak, since most individuals continue to report varying levels of symptoms and social limitations throughout their lives. Moreover, when dysthymia occurs prior to major depressive disorder among children and adolescents, a greater risk exists for developing subsequent mood disorders (Kovacs et al., 1994). Ultimately, concurrent diagnoses of dysthymia and major depressive disorder pose the most severe risk to youths, leaving children and adolescents most vulnerable to future mental health risks and difficulties in social functioning (Kovacs ert al., 1994).

Depressive symptomatology and its related disorders are precarious not only because of the negative and disabling aspects inherent in depression itself, but also because other comorbid conditions are frequently found to be correlated with childhood and adolescent depression. In fact, children and adolescents are consistently more likely than adults to develop comorbid disorders that accompany depression (Cantwell, 1992; Hammen & Compas, 1994). Two-thirds of youths with major depressive disorder also have another diagnosable psychiatric disorder (Anderson & McGee, 1994; Angold & Costello, 1993). Specifically, studies have found that 30% to 75% of clinically depressed youths also meet the criteria for an anxiety disorder (Kovacs, 1989). In another study, 33% of youths with depression received a conduct disorder diagnosis, and 50% were diagnosed with oppositional defiant disorder (Kashani et al., 1987). Other disorders, such as attention deficit with hyperactivity disorder (ADHD), eating disorders, and substance abuse disorders, also frequently occur along with depression (Angold & Costello, 1993; Attie, Brooks-Gunn, & Petersen, 1990; Kashani et al., 1987; Katon, Kleinman, & Rosen, 1982; Rivinus et al., 1984). In brief, depressive mood, depressive syndromes, and depressive disorders are all related to a wide array of comorbid psychiatric disorders in childhood and adolescence. Whether depression represents the underlying factor associated with these disorders or the resultant condition remains to be clarified.

Gender Differences

Researchers examining gender differences in depression have found an interactive effect between gender and age. Prepubertal investigations yield conflicting findings, suggesting higher rates of depression among prepubertal boys than girls, (Anderson, Williams, McGee, & Silva, 1987) or equal rates of prepubertal depression among both boys and girls (Rutter, 1986). At and beyond puberty, studies consistently report greater rates of depression among girls than boys (Kandel & Davies, 1982; Kashani et al., 1987; Lewinsohn, Rohde, Klein, & Seeley, 1999). Of additional concern is the finding that after age 15 girls are twice as likely to experience concomitant dysthymia and major depressive disorder (Linehan, Heard, & Armstrong, 1993; Weissman & Klerman, 1977) than their male counterparts.

These trends among boys and girls appear to persist into adulthood, yet there is no consensus as to why they occur. Some researchers maintain that these apparent gender differences reflect differing styles of communication and comfort in responding to questions on research measures and do not represent true differences in depression. Nonetheless, substantial research (Gove & Tudor, 1973; Nolen-Hoeksema, 1987; Nolen-Hoeksema, Girgus, & Seligman, 1991; Weissman & Klerman, 1977) supports distinct levels and experiences of depression among males and females. Studies further support hypotheses that girls' levels of depression is related to more intense challenges in early adolescence compared with boys (e.g., Petersen, Sarigiani, & Kennedy, 1991), such as earlier incidence of puberty (Ge, Conger, & Elder, 2001; Petersen, Kennedy, & Sullivan, 1991; Simmons & Blyth, 1987) and increased likelihood of parental divorce during early adolescence (Block, Block, & Gjerde, 1986; Petersen, Kennedy, & Sullivan, 1991), the latter due perhaps to fathers being more involved with their sons than with their daughters, and thus less likely to leave the marriage. These challenges faced by adolescent girls may be further complicated by girls being more socially oriented, more dependent on social relationships, and thus more vulnerable and sensitive to the loss of these relationships than boys (Allgood-Merten, Lewinsohn, & Hops, 1990). Furthermore, Nolen-Hoeksema and Girgus (1994) suggested that girls utilize denial as a coping mechanism far less commonly than boys, instead often using a ruminating style when handling difficult life experiences. Such styles of managing stressful life events may leave these young women more vulnerable to depressive disorders. Future research is needed to determine the specific trajectories among girls and boys that lead to the development of depression and how social expectations of females shape the use of particular defense mechanisms and the expression of depression.

Ethnic Differences in Depression

The research literature suggests that rates of depression and depressed mood exist more frequently in some ethnic groups than in others. In a review of community samples, Fleming and Offord (1990) reported that in two of five studies African-American adolescents had higher rates of depression and depressed mood than White adolescents. Research consistently has indicated that inner-city African-American adolescents stand at exceptionally high risk for elevated levels of stress (Baldwin, Harris, & Chambliss, 1997; Henry et al., 1995; Jonen, 1999) and depressive symptomatology and clinical depression (Garrison, Jackson, Marsteller, & McKeown, 1990; Robinson, 2000). A cross-sectional study (Robinson, 2000) of inner-city Chicago African-American adolescents found that 99% of the youths reported one or more indicators of poverty *and* were scored as high risk for clinical depression, with 46.6% of the participants scoring above the clinical cut-off on the Center for Epidemiologic Studies–Depression Scale (CES-D; Radloff, 1977). This finding suggests a sizable, nonignorable level of elevated depressive symptomatology within the population. The picture is even more bleak when considering observations that African-American youths may express their feelings of depression in nontraditional ways, such as aggressiveness (Gibbs & Moskowitz-Sweet, 1991). Thus, the prevalence of depression may pose an ominous threat to the well being of African-American youths, a threat even greater than these and similar statistics reveal.

Risk of Suicide

Researchers have found that as many as 90% of children and adolescents who commit suicide suffer from psychological disorders before their death (Shaffer & Craft, 1999), with children and particularly adolescents who suffer from depression being at much greater risk of committing suicide relative to youths not reporting depressive symptoms (Shaffer, Fisher et al., 1996). Girls and boys suffering from major depression are approximately 12 times as likely to commit suicide than their nondepressed peers (Shaffer, Gould et al., 1996).

Etiology of Depression

Although the cause of depression remains a point of debate, many theories have been proposed. Single-risk factors seldom account for the development of depression. Instead, interrelated biological, psychosocial, and cultural systems must be considered when examining the development of depression. Hammen (1992) proposed that we move beyond identifying isolated cognitive, affective, interpersonal, and biological elements of depressive patterns, and instead attempt to understand the development of these qualities and their interactive impact on the individual's biological and psychological well-being.

The considerable literature on adult depression largely supports both biological and psychological theories of development (Kendler, 1995). Unfortunately, research targeting youth populations has been less extensive (Digdon & Gotlib, 1985) and represents a still nascent, though sharply increasing, area of inquiry. Furthermore, available research with children and adolescents suffering from depression is largely drawn from mental health clinic patients. Such individuals frequently suffer more severe and recurrent forms of depression than youths either not seeking out services or receiving privatized care, and the generalizability of these findings is questionable.

Research findings (Kovacs, Devlin, Pollock, Richards, & Mukerji, 1997; Puig-Antich et al., 1989) suggest that between 20% and 50% of youths suffering from depression also have a family history of depression. Potentially the most convincing evidence for familial transmission is found in studies where monozygotic twins are four to five times more likely than dizygotic twins to show concordance for major depressive disorder (Kendler, Heath, Martin, & Eaves, 1986; Wender, Kety, Rosenthal, & Schulsinger, 1986), suggesting a strong genetic link. On the other hand, the lack of perfect concordance between monozygotic twins highlights the existence of additional factors in the development of depression. Several factors in addition to genetic influences may account for the apparent relationship between parental and childhood depression (Weissman, 1990). These include lack of emotional concern from parental figures (Lee & Gotlib, 1991), parent-child conflict (Burge & Hammen, 1991), marital conflict (Downey & Coyne, 1990), and lower socioeconomic status (Asamarov & Horton, 1990). Parental divorce also may contribute to behavioral problems and symptoms of depression among youths (Block, Block, Gjerde, 1986; Cherlin, Furstenberg, Chase-Lansdale, & Kiernan, 1991).

Cognitive aspects of development also have been linked to depression (Graber & Petersen, 1991; Keating, 1990), with significant attention being directed to the relationship between cognitive functioning and depression. Children and adolescents who attribute negative events to internal, stable, and global causes demonstrate higher levels of depressive symptomatology (Kaslow, Rehm, & Siegel, 1984). Interestingly, a recent longitudinal study (Nolen-Hoeksema, Girgus, & Seligman, 1992) indicated that individuals who adopt this attributional style are at greater risk of depressive symptoms later in childhood and early adolescence but not during early childhood. This type of thinking may precede depression, represent a symptom of depression, or be a consequence of previous depressive episodes (Lewinsohn, Steinmetz, Larson, & Franklin, 1981). Indeed, some research suggests that children having suffered from depression learn to interpret their life experiences in this manner, leaving them at greater risk for future depressive episodes (Nolen-Hoeksema et al., 1992). Similarly, Lewinsohn, Joiner, and Rohde (2001) in a longitudinal study found support for a diathesis-stress model of depression among adolescents. The authors found that among adolescents faced with negative life-events, it was those exhibiting a high level of dysfunctional attitudes that were most vulnerable 1 year later to depressive symptoms.

Other factors, too (either as causes, correlates, and/or consequences), have been linked to the development of childhood and adolescent depression, including low self-esteem (Harter, 1990; Renouf & Harter, 1990); anxiety (Finch, Lipovsky, & Casat, 1989; Kovacs, 1990; Suomi, 1991); negative body image and eating disorders, particularly among females (Attie & Brooks-Gunn, 1992; Post & Crowther, 1985); low peer popularity (Jacobsen, Lahey, & Strauss, 1983); a decline in academic grades (Ebata & Petersen, 1992; Schulenberg, Asp, & Petersen, 1984; Simmons & Blyth, 1987); stressful life events (e.g., family responsibilities, arguments with peers, exposure to violence; Wagner, Compas, & Howell, 1988); and limited supportive social relationships (Daniels & Moos, 1990). The plethora of risks associated with depression underscores its complexity, as well as the inherent challenges to professionals who strive to improve the lives of these youths.

The proposed trajectories in the development of depression are numerous. As with adults, depression among youths is likely to be a multidetermined process, potentially resulting from various combinations of genetic and familial factors, biological dysregulation, individual predispositions, environmental events, developmental changes, or the use of particular coping mechanisms. Regardless of the trajectory, at the point at which an individual suffers from depression, he or she forever stands at significantly greater risk for future mental health concerns. The negative outcomes associated with depression leave youths more vulnerable to a downward spiral most difficult to escape.

REVIEW AND CRITIQUE OF THE LITERATURE

Relatively few empirical studies (e.g., Brent, Poling, McKain, & Baugher, 1993; Kahn, Kehle, Jenson, & Clark, 1990; Reynolds & Coates, 1986) have examined the effectiveness of prevention efforts targeted directly at childhood and adolescent depression. Despite this paucity of research, the limited emerging evidence supports the effectiveness of prevention interventions aimed at the circumvention and reduction of depressive symptomatology among children and adolescents (Klerman, Weissman, Rounsaville, & Chevron, 1984; Lewinsohn, Clarke, Hops, & Andrews, 1990). Other studies discussed here also address stress-related prevention programs that may provide secondary benefits in reducing the incidence of depression.

Cognitive-behavioral prevention programs have demonstrated significant success in improving skills believed to buffer youths against the development of depressive symptoms. Broadly focused programs instill problem-solving skills and enhance social competence, qualities believed to protect youths from depressive mood and symptoms (Weissberg, Caplan, & Harwood, 1991). Similarly, several prevention programs successfully have assisted adolescents in coping with stressors associated with divorce (see Grych & Fincham, 1992, for a review), a risk factor frequently correlated with increased risk of child and adolescent depression. Indeed, such interventions have been designed to improve social competencies and life skills that aid adolescents in social, emotional, and intellectual development. Yet, despite the logical connection between these skills and the reduction of depression, few studies have included outcome measures of depressed mood, syndromes, or disorders.

Some limited evidence supports the use of primary prevention cognitive-behavioral group interventions directly aimed at the reduction and/or prevention of depression. In a review of such programs for use with adolescents, Kaslow and Thomson (1998) found one form of cognitive-behavioral coping skills training to demonstrate particular efficacy. This curriculum, the *Coping with Depression* course, developed by Lewinsohn, Clarke, Rhode, Hops, and Seely (1996), originally was designed for use with adults. Subsequently, Clarke et al. (1995) adapted this prevention program for use in a school-based setting for children at risk for depression based on pre-existing parental depression. Adolescents aged 14 to 18 were randomly assigned to intervention groups and wait list groups. The prevention program focused on experiential learning, conflict resolution, reframing techniques, and coping-skills training. The results (Lewinsohn et al., 1996) suggested that the adolescents who participated in the course had lower rates of self-reported depression, more adaptive and positive cognitions, and increased activity levels when compared with the wait-list controls.

A cognitive-behavioral model of prevention designed by Zubernis, Cassidy, Gillham, Reivich, and Jaycox (1999), evaluated the efficacy of the depression prevention program with children in the fifth and sixth grades. This school-based program focused on enhancing children's cognitive and social problem solving skills. The study demonstrated efficacy in preventing depressive symptomatology among these children; however, the results diminished over time for children of divorced parents. Another school-based program, designed by Shochet et al., (2001), evaluated the effectiveness of a depression prevention program for adolescents. The study targeted 260 ninth grade students who were first assessed for levels of depressive symptom and hopelessness and then randomly assigned to three groups. The first group of students participated in a curriculum-based resiliency building program. The second group not only participated in the resiliency building program, but also involved parents in a three-session parent program. The third group served as a comparison group.

Findings suggested significantly lower levels of depressive symptomatology and hopelessness for those students involved in the resiliency programs (groups 1 and 2) as compared with the control group (group 3). In addition, students reported satisfaction with the program and evidenced a low (5.8%) attrition rate.

Another area of primary prevention approaches among older adolescents and adults involves media-based or other school-based interventions. Jason and Burrows (1986) designed a school-based transition training program for high school seniors aimed at improving cognitive restructuring, coping strategies, rational beliefs, and feelings of self-efficacy for diverse types of transitions. All of these factors, as discussed above, are particularly relevant to buffering depression among youth. The program produced increased self-efficacy and decreases in irrational beliefs among participating students. These findings are suggestive of the potential usefulness of such programs in decreasing depression rates. In another project, Jason, Curran, Goodman, and Smith (1989) combined daily television broadcasts with accompanying manuals for stress management among community members. The program's focus was to encourage and assist individuals in the identification of life stressors, available support, and the development of coping strategies useful in dealing with stress. The program resulted in the acquisition of new coping strategies and significant improvements on adjustment measures among community members. Another study, the San Francisco Mood Survey Project, (Munoz, Glish, Soo-Hoo, & Robertson, 1982), involved a 2-week television prevention program aimed at the adaptation of social learning and cognitive-behavioral treatment approaches aimed at reducing depression. The findings suggested that mood level was significantly improved among a symptomatic group that observed the program compared with individuals with similar levels of symptoms who did not watch the programming. Although these programs were targeted primarily at adults, programs such as these may well demonstrate even greater effectiveness among youths. Because the media reaches a large proportion of youths (e.g., 70% of all adolescents between the ages of 12 and 17 spend more than 3 hours daily in front of the television [Nielsen, 1987]), properly designed and implemented, media prevention efforts hold great promise in reaching the largest portions of youths and producing the greatest impact.

Primary prevention programs such as these may particularly benefit children and adolescents who possess or have been exposed to known risk factors or extraordinary environmental factors potentially contributing to the development of depressive disorders (Petersen & Crockett, 1985). For example, adolescents whose parents are clinically depressed stand at greater risk for the development of depressive disorders. Similarly, youths growing up in lower socioeconomic neighborhoods are exposed to multiple stressors, such as exposure to violence and limited resources, leaving them significantly more vulnerable to depression (Jonen, 1999). Researchers are only beginning to develop prevention efforts aimed at such populations (Robinson, 2000).

Given the likely trajectory of future depressive episodes subsequent to child-hood or adolescent onset of depression, secondary prevention programs tar-geting youths with depressive symptomatology at subclinical levels of depressed mood will ideally reduce the development of major depressive disorders. One such secondary prevention model producing promising results, the Depression Preventive Program (DPP), was implemented by Gillham, Revich, Jaycox, and Seligman (1995). The program, incorporating both cognitive and social prob-lem-solving techniques, demonstrated a significant decrease in depressive symp-toms with an even greater improvement in depressive symptoms over a 2-year follow-up period compared with a control group. Another study, by Jaycox, Reivich, Gillham, and Seligman (1994) tested the preliminary efficacy of a sec-ondary prevention program targeting depressive symptoms among at-risk youths and comorbid difficulties of depression, including conduct problems, low aca-demic achievement, low social competence, and poor peer relations. Not only was depressive symptomatology significantly reduced, but classroom behavior also improved compared with controls at posttest. At a 6-month posttest, these results continued to increase, with the greatest gains evidenced in youths origi-nally identified as being most at risk at the onset of the project.

The coordination of prevention programs aimed at large groups of youths and programs targeting high-risk groups offers the most efficient and com-plementary form of intervention (Compas, 2000). Mounting evidence indi-cates the need for interventions at multiple levels that address cognitive processes, coping skills, and strategies dealing with interpersonal difficulties. These themes ultimately support hypotheses suggesting that improved self-efficacy among youths will buffer them from future depressive episodes. The initial groundwork for these skills would be established in preventive inter-ventions delivered at the population level (Petersen, Schulenberg, Abramowitz, Offer, & Jarcho, 1988), followed by enhancement of these skills for those indi-viduals exhibiting some symptomatology (Beardslee, 1990). Finally, for those youths experiencing depressive disorders despite primary and secondary inter-vention efforts, individual therapeutic options combined with psychopharma-cology would be necessary (Lewinsohn etal., 1990). Only through such integrated efforts will adequate safety nets be established for youths at all ages and stages of vulnerability for depression.

CASE EXAMPLE

Recognizing the need for the prevention of depression among high-risk youths, the present authors' work has focused on providing services for inner-city, African-American adolescents. Toward this aim, our research team adapted and implemented *The Adolescent Coping With Stress Course* (Clarke & Lewinsohn, 1995) among inner-city adolescents attending a school-based health center (SBHC). Such youth face the chronic social and environmental stressors predominant in the lives of inner-city, low-income, African-American adolescents, leaving them particularly vulnerable to depression, among other disorders. Originally intended for use with White, middle-class adolescents, Clarke and Lewinsohn's (1995) program is an empirically based 15-session course grounded in a cognitive-behavioral model. The course leader is provided with explicit instructions for carrying out the course, and each student is provided a course workbook. Participants engage in discourse around issues of stress and are encouraged to practice a variety of coping techniques during and outside of sessions. This program is designed for students identified as at-risk for depression, based on such familial factors as having a parent with a diagnosis of depression.

Community Entry

The research team involved this project included the authors and a group of clinical-psychology graduate students. Entry into the participating pilot public high-school was facilitated by prior collaborative working relationships on previous research projects within the school and a painstakingly earned track record with school staff and administration. These well-nurtured working relationships and previously successful research endeavors fostered a sense of trust and confidence by school personnel in the research team that proved enormously beneficial in implementing the program. A SBHC nurse practitioner served as a liaison between the research team and the school's administration. This liaison embraced the program and shared a common vision regarding the program's goals and long-term potential benefits. A shared vision such as this among all members of a community-based research project provides an essential foundation for its implementation and success.

Goal Identification and Program Design

The project's conceptual philosophy focused on understanding the unique aspects of inner-city African-American students, aspects that might leave them more vulnerable to depression and less likely to benefit from traditional approaches. From the onset, a commitment to collaboration was critical to the development and survival of this school- and community-based intervention. Collaborative and horizontal relationships encourage engagement and program bonding; program developers from outside the system often provide guidance at the onset for the program's development, but the program is owned by the many who ultimately share in its construction. This collaborative spirit helps to ensure that the needs and goals of those served are truly met, as they too contribute to goal identification and program design. Collaboration clarifies that the working relationship is one of sharing, parity, and respect.

Through this collaborative and participatory process, two major goals were identified. First, the program aimed to provide a preventive intervention for those youth who were at risk for depression based on their challenging life experiences. Second, the research team aspired to gain a greater understanding of the experiences and needs of inner-city African-American adolescents, knowledge that could be used to design more efficacious future interventions containing a more culturally sensitive and relevant curriculum.

Implementation

Project implementation primarily consisted of introducing the depression curriculum described above with 15 inner-city, African-American students identified by SBHC staff as being at risk for depression. This pilot project largely adhered to Clarke and Levinsohn's (1995) original format and content; however, after completion of the 15-session curriculum, students were asked to participate in focus groups to capture their general reaction to the program and the applicability of the course to their own issues and lives.

The students' focus group responses underscored the need for preventive interventions among adolescents, particularly programs developed with respect for the cultural realities facing them. All participating students endorsed the utility of the coping strategies acquired as a result of their participation in the program. They also reported the program's applicability to their everyday lives and interactions, as well as a reduced level of stress secondary to the use of these skills. Furthermore, each student commented that he or she would continue attending the group if it could be made permanently available. Despite their positive reactions, many of the students were candid in sharing their preference for programming that included "Black slang" and examples more congruent with their typical interactions and life circumstances. They also commented on their desire to see more African-American images such as cartoons and artwork. Additionally, they recommended the inclusion of more salient scenarios reflecting their everyday experiences, such as pressure to have sex, exposure to violence, and the death of close friends and family members. The school staff also provided positive feedback on the program; however, they also concurred that a more culturally sensitive model would be more beneficial for students. Thus, they agreed to work with the research team on future projects to develop such a curriculum.

Pilot projects such as these emphasize not only the need for prevention programs aimed at youths but also elucidate the need to develop intervention models specific to the needs of particular groups of individuals. Undoubtedly, youth faced with the challenges of individuals living in inner-city neighborhoods stand at increased risk for depression; however, without options reflecting their personal and collective experiences, the effects of such efforts will be less than optimal.

FUTURE DIRECTIONS

The emergence of depression during childhood or adolescence has crucial implications for later mental health. The age of onset for depression has been found to predict later mental health outcomes, with earlier onset predicting poorer future outcomes such as more frequent and severe depressive episodes (Kovacs et al., 1984). Of particular concern is mounting evidence (e.g., Klein et al., 1997) that untreated depressive symptoms leave youths at risk for continued limited social, educational, and professional opportunities. Moreover, given the likely progression of depressive symptomatology to serious depressive disorders, the threat of suicide becomes a serious reality for adolescents and young adults, representing the third leading cause of death during mid-adolescence (Centers for Disease Control and Prevention [CDC], 1999; Hoyert, 1999). Preventive interventions offer the potential for the avoidance and reduction of these negative outcomes and the potentially catastrophic events associated with depression.

One issue relevant to the development of programs aimed at the prevention of depression is the poor consensus evidenced among mental health providers with respect to their support of treatment or prevention (Albee, 1982, 1990). Battle lines have been drawn based largely on professional proponents of treatment versus prevention modalities. The harsh realities of depression underscore the untenable nature of such battles and highlight the urgent need for a broad, unified effort to provide a continuum of services that can reach all youths. This broad approach must recognize that no single approach adequately addresses the complexity and suffering of so many children and adolescents.

Other issues require attention in future attempts to impact depression. The multidetermined nature of depression must be considered, with programs grounded in the multiple pathways by which depression develops, and the varied personal and social factors that place youths at risk. Research aimed at understanding programs directed at factors other than depression must evaluated to understand their potential secondary impact on depressive symptomatology. Furthermore, multilevel interventions that involve families, schools, communities, and the media would appear to hold considerable potential for preventing depression.

The need for cultural sensitivity in the design of preventive interventions is becoming increasingly apparent (Bernal, 1999). Many individuals belonging to ethnic minority groups, many of whom are at increased risk for depression, believe that mental health services are intended only for White, European-Americans (United States Public Health Services, 2000). Therefore, our obligation, as mental health professionals, to design and deliver interventions responsive to the needs of all individuals, becomes even more salient in view of the limitations of current intervention approaches for use with ethnic minorities.

Another important future research direction involves the implementation of studies focusing not only on efficacy (i.e., the success of interventions when conducted by research teams or with staff trained by the research staff) but also on effectiveness studies (i.e., the success of a program using community personnel). Frequently, researchers enjoy promising results when examining the efficacy of their programs and then find that effectiveness studies yield poorer results. Not surprisingly, a strong focus on efficacy studies has resulted in a rigid concern for experimental factors without regard for the generalizability of programs. As Clarke et al. (1995) observed, if interventions are proven to be both efficacious and effective, they will undoubtedly lead to better outcomes and improved mental health services.

Also important is the implementation and utilization of longitudinal research in the area of adolescent depression. Conducting such research that spans infancy, childhood, and adolescence may offer invaluable insights into the epidemiological factors and trajectory of depression across the life course, shedding light on the multidetermined nature of this disorder and its accompanying features. Specifically, prevention efforts need to demonstrate a strong commitment to longitudinal prevention research that incorporates longer-term follow-up. This knowledge could then be utilized in the design and implementation of subsequent programs.

Depression and its concomitant adversities represent some of the most prevalent and detrimental risks facing our youth. If mental health professionals fail to recognize the potential benefit of preventive interventions, or delay in the implementation of such programs, we inadvertently increase the likelihood of youths facing a lifetime of depressive symptoms and its related difficulties. A broader approach to the prevention of depression is needed to integrate all available resources and mobilize society to participate in this commitment. Only through a concerted and comprehensive effort will we create the optimal environment in which youths can develop, mature, and transition successfully into adulthood.

REFERENCES

Akiskal, H. S. (1983). Dysthymic disorder: Psychopathology of proposed chronic depressive subtypes. *American Journal of Psychiatry, 140*, 11–20.

Albee, G. W. (1982). Preventing psychopathology and promoting human potential. *American Psychologist, 37*, 1043–1050.

Albee, G. W. (1990). The futility of psychotherapy. *Journal of Mind and Behavior, 11*, 369–384.

Allgood-Merten, B., Lewinsohn, P. A., & Hops, H. (1990). Sex differences and adolescent depression. *Journal of Abnormal Psychology, 99*, 55–63.

Anderson, J. C., & McGee, R. (1994). Comorbidity of depression in children and adolescents. In W. M. Reynolds & H. F. Johnson (Eds.), *Handbook of depression in children and adolescents* (pp. 581–601). New York: Plenum.

Anderson, J. C., Williams, S. C., McGee, R., & Silva, P. A. (1987). DSM-III disorders in preadolescent children: Prevalence in a large sample from the general population. *Archives of General Psychiatry, 44*, 69–76.

Angold, A., & Costello, E. J. (1993). Depressive comorbidity in children and adolescents: Empirical, theoretical, and methodological issues. *American Journal of Psychiatry, 150*, 1779–1791.

Asamarov, J. R., & Horton, A. A. (1990). Coping and stress in families of child psychiatric inpatients: Parents of children with depressive and schizophrenia spectrum disorders. *Child Psychiatry and Human Development, 21*, 145–157.

Attie, I., & Brooks-Gunn, J. (1992). Development issues in the study of eating problems and disorders. In J. H. Crowther, S. E. Hobfoll, M. A. P. Stephens, & D. L. Tennenbaum (Eds.), *The etiology of bulimia: The individual and familial context* (pp. 35–50). Washington, DC: Hemisphere.

Attie, I., Brooks-Gunn, J., & Petersen, A. C. (1990). A developmental perspective on eating disorders and eating problems. In M. Lewis & S. Miller (Eds.), *Handbook of developmental psychopathology* (pp. 409–420). New York: Plenum.

Baldwin, D. R., Harris, S. M., & Chambliss, L. N. (1997). Stress and illness in adolescence: Issues of race and gender. *Adolescence, 32*, 839–853.

Beardslee, W. R. (1990). Development of a clinician-based preventive intervention for families with affective disorders. *Journal of Preventive Psychiatry and Allied Disciplines, 4*, 39–61.

Beardslee, W., Keller, M., Lavori, P., Staley, J., & Sacks. (1993). The impact of parental affective disorder on depression in offspring: A longitudinal follow-up in a non-referred sample. *Journal of the American Academy of Child & Adolescent Psychiatry, 32*, 723–730.

Birmaher, B., Ryan, N. D., Williamson, D. E., Brent, D. A., Kaufman, J., Dahl, R. E., Perel, J., & Nelson, B. (1996). Childhood and adolescent depression: A review of the past 10 years. Part I. *Journal of the American Academy of Child and Adolescent Psychiatry, 35,* 1427–1439.

Brent, D. A., Poling, K., McKain, B., & Baugher, N. (1993). A psychoeducational program for families of affectively ill children and adolescents. *Journal of the American Academy of Child and Adolescent Psychiatry, 32,* 770–774.

Block, J. H., Block, J., & Gjerde, P. F. (1986). The personality of children prior to divorce: A prospective study. *Child Development, 57,* 827–840.

Burge, D., & Hammen, C. (1991). Maternal communication: Predictors of outcome at follow-up in a sample of children at high and low risk for depression. *Journal of Abnormal Psychology, 100,* 174–180.

Cantwell, D. (1992). Clinical phenomenology and nosology. *Child and Adolescent Psychiatric Clinics of North America, 1,* 1–11.

Centers for Disease Control and Prevention (1999). *Suicide deaths and rates per 100,000.* Available: http://www.cdc.gov/ncipc/ data/us9794/suic.htm

Cherlin, A. J., Furstenberg, F. F., Chase-Lansdale, P. L., & Kiernan, K. E. (1991). Longitudinal studies of effects of divorce on children in Great Britain and the United States. *Science, 252,* 1386–1389.

Clarke, G., Hawkins, W., Murphy, M., Sheeber, L. B., Lewinsohn, P. M., & Seeley, J. R. (1995). Targeted prevention of unipolar depressive disorder in an at-risk sample of high school adolescents: A randomized trial of a group cognitive intervention. *Journal of the American Academy of Child and Adolescent Psychiatry, 34,* 312–321.

Clarke, G., & Lewinsohn, P.M. (1995). *The adolescent coping with stress course.* Unpublished manuscript. Available: http://www.kpchr.org/ACWD/ ACWD.html#NewACWD.html

Compas, B. E., & Oppedisano, G. (2000). Mixed anxiety/depression in childhood and adolescence. In A. J. Sameroff & M. Lewis (Eds.), *Handbook of developmental psychopathology* (2nd ed., pp. 531–548). New York: Kluwer Academic/Plenum.

Daniels, D., & Moos, R. H. (1990). Assessing life stressors and social resources among adolescents: Applications to depressed youth. *Journal of Adolescent Research, 5,* 268–289.

Digdon, N., & Gotlib, I. H. (1985). Developmental considerations in the study of childhood depression. *Developmental Reviews, 5,* 162–199.

Downey, G., & Coyne, J. C. (1990). Children of depressed parents: An integrative review. *Psychological Bulletin, 108,* 50–76.

Ebata, A. T., & Petersen, A. C. (1992). *Pattern of adjustment during early adolescence: Gender differences in depression and achievement.*

Ebata, A. T., Petersen, A. C., & Conger, J. J. (1990). The development of psychopathology in adolescence. In J. E. Rolf & A. S. Masten (Eds.), *Risk and protective factors in the development of psychopathology* (pp. 308–333). New York: Cambridge University Press.

Fava, G. A., Grandi, S., Zielezny, M., & Canestrari, R. (1994). Cognitive behavioral treatment of residual symptoms in primary major depressive disorder. *American Journal of Psychiatry, 151,* 1295–1299.

Fava, G.A., Rafanelli, C., Grandi, S., Conti, S., & Belluardo, P. (1998). Prevention of recurrent depression with cognitive behavioral therapy: Preliminary findings. *Archives of General Psychiatry, 55,* 816–820.

Finch, A. J., Lipovsky, J. A., & Casat, C. D. (1989). Anxiety and depression in children and adolescents: Negative affectivity or separate constructs? In P. C. Kendall & D. Watson (Eds.), *Anxiety and depression: Distinctive and overlapping features* (pp. 171–202). San Diego, CA: Academic Press.

Fleming, J. E., & Offord, D. R. (1990). Epidemiology of childhood depressive disorders. A critical review. *Journal of the American Academy of Child and Adolescent Psychiatry, 29,* 571–580.

Garrison, C. Z., Jackson, K. L., Marsteller, F., & McKeown, R. (1990). A longitudinal study of depressive symptomatology in young adolescents. *Journal of the American Academy of Child & Adolescent Psychiatry, 29,* 581–585.

Garrison, C. Z., Waller, J. L., Cuffee, S. P., McKeown, R. E., Addy, C. L., & Jackson, K. L. (1997). Incidence of major depressive disorder and dysthymia in young adolescents. *Journal of the American Academy of Child and Adolescent Psychiatry, 36,* 458–465.

Ge, X., Conger, R. D., & Elder, G. H. (2001). Pubertal transition, stressful life events, and the emergence of gender differences in adolescent depressive symptoms. *Journal of Abnormal Psychology, 110,* 203–215.

Geller, B., Zimerman, B., Williams, M., Bolhofner, K., & Craney, J. L. (2001). Adult psychosocial outcome of prepubertal major depressive disorder. *Journal of the American Academy of Child & Adolescent Psychiatry, 40,* 673–677.

Gibbs, J. T., & Moskowitz-Sweet, G. (1991). Clinical and cultural issues in the treatment of biracial and bicultural adolescents. *Families in Society, 72,* 572–592.

Gillham, J. E., Revich, K. J., Jaycox, L. H., & Seligman, M. E. P. (1995). Prevention of depressive symptoms in school children: Two-year follow-up. *Psychological Science, 6,* 343–351.

Gould, M. S., Fisher, P., Parides, M., Flory, M., & Shaffer, D. (1996). Psychosocial risk factors of child and adolescent completed suicide. *Archives of General Psychiatry, 53,* 1155–1162.

Gove, W. R., & Tudor, J. F. (1973). Adult sex roles and mental illness. *American Journal of Sociology, 78,* 812–835.

Graber, J. A., & Petersen, A. C. (1991). Cognive changes at adolescence: Biological perspectives. In K. R. Gibson & A. C. Petersen (Eds.), *Brain maturation and cognitive development: Comparative cross-cultural perspectives* (pp. 253–279). Hawthorne, NY: Aldine de Gruyter.

Grych, J. H., & Fincham, F. D. (1992). Interventions for children of divorce: Toward greater integration of research and action. *Psychological Bulletin, 111,* 434–454.

Hammen, C. (1992). Cognitive, life stress, and interpersonal model of depression. *Development and Psychopathology, 4,* 189–206.

Hammen, C., & Compas, B. E. (1994). Unmasking unmasked depression in children and adolescents: The problem of comorbidity. *Clinical Psychology Review, 14,* 686–603.

Harrington, R., Fudge, H., Rutter, M., Pickles, A., & Hill, J. (1990). Adult outcomes of childhood and adolescent depression. I. Psychiatric status. *Archives of General Psychiatry, 47,* 465–473.

Harter, S. (1990). Causes, correlates and the functional role of global self-worth: A life-span perspective. In R. Sternberg & J. Kolligian (Eds.), *Competence considered* (pp. 68–97). New Haven, CT: Yale University Press.

Henry, D., Guerra, N., Huesmann, R., Tolan, P., VanAcker, R., & Eron, L. (1995). Stressful events and individual beliefs as correlates of economic disadvantage and aggression among urban children. *Journal of Consulting and Clinical Psychology, 63,* 518–528.

Hirschfeld, R., Keller, M., Panico, S., & Arons, B. (1997) The National Depressive and Manic-Depressive Association consensus statement on the undertreatment of depression. *Journal of the American Medical Association, 277,* 333–340.

Jacobsen, R., Lahey, B. B., & Strauss, C. C. (1983). Correlates of depressed mood in normal children. *Journal of Abnormal Child Psychology, 11,* 29–39.

Jason, L. A., & Burrows, B. A. (1986). Transition training for high school seniors. In R. A. Feldman & A. R. Stiffman (Eds.), *Advances in adolescent mental health: Vol. 1* (pp. 145–147). Greenwich, CT: JAI Press.

Jason, L. A., Curran, T., Goodman, D., & Smith, M. (1989). A media-based stress management intervention. *Journal of Community Psychology, 17,* 155–165.

Jaycox, L. H., Reivich, K. J., Gillham, J., & Seligman, M. E. P. (1994). Prevention of depressive symptoms in school children. *Behaviour Research and Therapy, 34,* 801–816.

Jonen, L. (1999). *Relationship between stress and depression among African-American adolescents.* Unpublished manuscript, DePaul University.

Kahn, J. S., Kehle, T. J., Jenson, W. R., & Clark, E. (1990). Comparison of cognitive-behavioral, relaxation, and self-modeling interventions for depression among middle-school students. *School Psychology Review, 19,* 196–211.

Kandel, D. B., & Davies, M. (1982). Epidemiology of depressive mood in adolescents. *Archives of General Psychiatry, 39,* 1205–1212.

Kashani, J. H., Carlson, G. A., Beck, N. C., Hoeper, E. W., Corcoran, C. M., McAllister, J. A., Fallahi, C., Rosenberg, T. K., & Reid, J. C. (1987). Depression, depressive symptoms, and depressed mood among a community sample of adolescents. *American Journal of Psychiatry, 144,* 931–934.

Kaslow, N. J., Rehm, L. P., & Siegel, A. W. (1984). Social-cognitive and cognitive correlates of depression in children. *Journal of Abnormal Child Psychology, 12,* 605–620.

Kaslow, N. J., & Thompson, M. P. (1998). Applying the criteria for empirically supported treatments to studies of psychosocial interventions for child and adolescent depression. *Journal of Clinical Child Psychology, 27,* 146–155.

Katon, W., Kleinman, A., & Rosen, G. (1982). Depression and somatization: A review. Part 1. *American Journal of Medicine, 72,* 127–135.

Katzev, A. R., Warner, R. L., & Acock, A. C. (1994). Girls or boys? Relationship of child gender to marital instability. *Journal of Marriage and the Family, 56,* 89–100.

Keating, D. (1990). Adolescent thinking. In S. S. Feldman & G. R. Elliott (Eds.), *At the threshold: The developing adolescent* (pp. 54–89). Cambridge, MA: Harvard University Press.

Keller, M. B., Lavori, P. W., Beardslee, W. R., & Wunder, J. (1991). Depression in children and adolescents: New data on "undertreatment" and a literature review on the efficacy of available treatments. *Journal of Affective Disorders, 21,* 163–171.

Kendler, K. (1985). Is seeking treatment for depression predicted by a history of depression in relatives? Implications for family studies of affective disorder. *Psychological Medicine, 25,* 807–814.

Kendler, K. S., Heath, A., Martin, N. G., & Eaves, L. J. (1986). Symptoms of anxiety and depression in a volunteer twin population. *Archives of General Psychiatry, 43,* 213–221.

Kessler, R. C., Avenevoli, S., & Merikangas, K. R. (2001). Mood disorders in children and adolescents: An epidemiologic perspective. *Biological Psychiatry, 49,* 1002–1014.

Klein, D. N., Lewinsohn, P. M., & Seeley, J. R. (1997). Psychosocial characteristics of adolescents with a past history of dysthymic disorder: Comparison with adolescents with past histories of major depressive and non-affective disorders, and never mentally ill controls. *Journal of Affective Disorders, 42,* 127–135.

Klerman, G. L., Weissman, M. M., Rounsaville, B. J., & Chevron, E. S. (1984). *Interpersonal psychotherapy of depression.* New York; Basic Books.

Kovacs, M. (1989). Affective disorder in children and adolescents. *American Psychologist, 44,* 209–215.

Kovacs, M. (1990). Comorbid anxiety disorders in childhood-onset depressions. In J. D. Maser & C. R. Cloniger (Eds.), *Comorbidity of mood and anxiety disorders* (pp. 272–281). Washington, DC: American Psychiatric Press.

Kovacs, M., Akiskal, H. S., Gatsonis, C., & Parrone, P. L. (1994). Childhood-onset dysthymic disorder: Clinical features and prospective naturalistic outcome. *Archives of General Psychiatry, 51*, 365–374.

Kovacs, M., Devlin, B., Pollock, M., Richards, C., & Mukerji, P. (1997). A controlled family history study of childhood-onset depressive disorder. *Archives of General Psychiatry, 54*, 613–623.

Kovacs, M., Feinberg, T. L., Crouse-Novak, M. A., Paulauskas, S. L., Pollack, M., & Finkelstein, R. (1984). Depressive disorders in childhood: 2. A longitudinal study of the risk for a subsequent major depression. *Archives of General Psychiatry, 41*, 643–649.

Lee, C. M., & Gotlib, I. H. (1991). Adjustment of children of depressed mothers: A 10-month follow-up. *Journal of Abnormal Psychology, 100*, 473–477.

Lewinsohn, P. M., Clarke, G. N., Rhode, P., Hops, H., & Seely, J. (1996). A course in coping: A cognitive-behavioral approach to the treatment of adolescent depression. In D. Hibbs & P. S. Jensen (Eds.), *Psychosocial treatments for child and adolescent disorders: Empirically based strategies for clinical practice* (pp. 109–135). Washington, DC: American Psychological Association.

Lewinsohn, P. M., Clarke, G. N., Hops, H., & Andrews, J. (1990). Cognitive-behavioral treatment for depressed adolescents. *Behavior Therapy, 21*, 385–401.

Lewinsohn, P. M., Clarke, G. N., Seeley, J. R., & Rohde, P. (1994). Major depression in community adolescents: Age at onset, episode duration, and time to recurrence. *Journal of the American Academy of Child and Adolescent Psychiatry, 33*, 809–818.

Lewinsohn, P., Hops, H., Roberts, R., Seeley, J., & Andrews, J. (1993). Adolescent psychopathology: I. Prevalence and incidence of depression and other DSM-III-R disorders in high school students. *Journal of Abnormal Psychology, 102*, 133–144.

Lewinsohn, P. M., Rohde, P., Klein, D. N., & Seeley, J. R. (1999). Natural course of adolescent major depressive disorder: I. Continuity into young adulthood. *Journal of the American Academy of Child and Adolescent Psychiatry, 38*, 56–63.

Lewinsohn, P. M., Steinmetz, J. L., Larson, D. W., & Franklin, J. (1981). Depression-related cognitions: Antecedent or consequence? *Journal of Abnormal Psychology, 90*, 213–219.

Linehan, M. M., Heard, H. L., & Armstrong, H. E. (1993). Naturalistic follow-up of a behavioral treatment for chronically parasuicidal borderline patients. *Archives of General Psychiatry, 50*, 971–974.

Munoz, R. F., Glish, M., Soo-Hoo, T., & Robertson, H. (1982). The San Francisco Mood Survey Project: Preliminary work toward the prevention of depression. *American Journal of Community Psychology, 10*, 317–329.

Nolen-Hoeksema, S. (1987). Sex differences in unipolar depression: Evidence and theory. *Psychological Bulletin, 101*, 259–282.

Nolen-Hoeksema, S., & Girgus, J. S. (1994). The emergence of gender differences in depression during adolescence. *Psychological Bulletin, 115*, 424–443.

Nolen-Hoeksema, S., Girgus, J. S., & Seligman, M. E. P. (1986). Learned helplessness in children: A longitudinal study of depression, achievement, and explanatory style. *Journal of Personality and Social Psychology, 51*, 435–442.

Nolen-Hoeksema, S., Girgus, J. S., & Seligman, M. E. P. (1991). Sex differences in depression and explanatory style in children. *Journal of Youth and Adolescence, 20*, 233–246.

Nolen-Hoeksema, S., Girgus, J. S., & Seligman, M. E. P. (1992). Predictors and consequences of childhood depressive symptoms: A 5-year longitudinal study. *Journal of Abnormal Psychology, 101*, 405–422.

Petersen, A. C., & Crockett, L. (1985). Pubertal timing and grade effects on adjustment. *Journal of Youth and Adolescence, 14*, 101–106.

Petersen, A. C., Kennedy, R. E., & Sullivan, P. (1991). Coping with adolescence. In M. E. Colten & S. Gore (Eds.), *Adolescent stress: Causes and consequences* (pp. 93–110). New York: Aldine de Gruyter.

Petersen, A. C., Sarigiani, P. A., & Kennedy, R. E. (1991). Adolescent depression: Why more girls? *Journal of Youth and Adolescence, 20*, 247–271.

Petersen, A. C., Schulenberg, J. E., Abramowitz, R. H., Offer, D., & Jarcho, H. D. (1984). A Self-Image Questionnaire for Young Adolescents (SIQYA): Reliability and validity studies. *Journal of Youth and Adolescence, 13*, 93–111.

Post, G., & Crowther, J. H. (1985). Variables that discriminate bulimic from nonbulimic adolescent females. *Journal of Youth and Adolescence, 14*, 85–98.

Puig-Antich, J., Goetz, D., Davies, M., Kaplan, T., Davies, S., Ostrow, L., Asnis, L., Twomey, J., Iyengar, S., & Ryan, N. (1989). A controlled family history study of prepubertal major depressive disorder. *Archives of General Psychiatry, 46*, 406–418.

Rao, U., Hammen, C., & Daley, S. E. (1999). Continuity of depression during the transition to adulthood: A 5-year longitudinal study of young women. *Journal of the American Academy of Child & Adolescent Psychiatry, 38*, 908–915.

Radloff, L. S. (1977). The CES-D scale: A self-report depression scale for research in the general population. *Applied Psychological Measurement, 1*, 385–401.

Renouf, A. G., & Harter, S. (1990). Low self-worth and anger as components of the depressive experience in young adolescents. *Development and Psychopathology, 2*, 293–310.

Reynolds, W. M., & Coates, K. L. (1986). A comparison of cognitive-behavioral therapy and relaxation training for the treatment of depression in adolescents. *Journal of Consulting and Clinical Psychology, 54*, 653–660.

Rivinus, T. M., Biederman, J., Herzog, D., Kemper, K., Harper, G., Harmatz, G., & Houseworth, S. (1984). Anorexia nervosa and affective disorders: A controlled family history study. *American Journal of Psychiatry, 14*, 1414–1418.

Robins, L. N., & Regier, D. A. (1991). *Psychiatric disorders in America: The Epidemiologic Catchment Area Study.* New York: Free Press.

Robinson, W. L. (2000). Rates of depressive symptomatology among inner-city African-American adolescents. Unpublished raw data.

Rohde, P., Lewinsohn P., & Seeley J. (1991). Comorbidity of unipolar depression: II. Comorbidity with other mental disorders in adolescents and adults. *Journal of Abnormal Psychology, 100*, 214–222.

Rutter, M. (1986). The developmental psychopathology of depression: Issues and perspectives. In M. Rutter, C. E. Izard, & P. B. Read (Eds.), *Depression in young people: Developmental and clinical perspectives* (pp. 3–32). New York: Guilford.

Schulenberg, J. E., Asp, C. E., & Petersen, A. C. (1984). School from the young adolescent's perspective: A descriptive report. *Journal of Early Adolescence, 4*, 107–130

Shaffer, D., & Craft, L. (1999). Methods of adolescent suicide prevention. *Journal of Clinical Psychiatry, 60* (Suppl. 2), 70–74.

Shaffer, D., Fisher, P., Dulcan, M., Davies, M., Piacentini, J., Schwab-Stone, M., Lahey, B., Bourdon, K., Jensen, P., Bird, H., & Canino, G. R. D. (1996). The second version of the NIMH Diagnostic Interview Schedule for Children (DISC–2). *Journal of the American Academy of Child and Adolescent Psychiatry, 35*, 865–877.

Shaffer, D., Gould, M. S., Fisher, P., Trautment, P., Moreau, D., Kleinman, M., & Flory, M. (1996). Psychiatric diagnosis in child and adolescent suicide. *Archives of General Psychiatry, 53*, 339–348.

Simmons, R. G., & Blyth, D. A. (1987). *Moving into adolescence: The impact of pubertal change and school context.* Hawthorne, NY: Aldine de Gruyter.

Shochet, I. M., Dadds, M. R., Holland, D., Whitefield, K., Harnett, P. H., & Osgarby, S. M. (2001). The efficacy of a universal school-based program to prevent adolescent depression. *Journal of Clinical Child Psychology, 30*, 303–315.

Suomi, S. J. (1991). Adolescent depression and depressive symptoms: Insights from longitudinal studies with rhesus monkeys. *Journal of Youth and Adolescence, 20*, 273–287.

United States Public Health Services (2000). *Mental health: A report of the Surgeon General.* Washington, DC: Author.

Wagner, B. M., Compas, B. E., & Howell, D. C. (1988). Daily and major life events: A test of an integrative model of psychosocial stress. *American Journal of Community Psychology, 16,* 189–205.

Weissberg, R. P., Caplan, M. Z., & Harwood, R. L. (1991). Promoting competent young people in competence-enhancing environments: A systems-based perspective on primary prevention. *Journal of Consulting and Clinical Psychology, 59,* 830–841.

Weissman, M. M. (1990). Evidence for comorbidity of anxiety and depression: Family and genetic studies of children. In J. D. Maser & C. R. Cloninger (Eds.), *Comorbidity of mood and anxiety disorders* (pp. 349–365). Washington, DC: American Psychiatric Press.

Weissman, M. M., & Klerman, G. L. (1977). Sex differences and the epidemiology of depression. *Archives of General Psychiatry, 34,* 98–111.

Weissman, M. M., Wolk, S., Goldstein, R. B., Moreau, D., Adams, P., Greenwald, S., Klier, C. M., Ryan, N. D., Dahl, R. E., & Wickramaratne, P. (1999). Depressed adolescents grown up. *Journal of the American Medical Association, 281,* 1707–1713.

Wender, P. H., Kety, S. S., Rosenthal, D., & Schulsinger, F. (1986). Psychiatric disorders in the biological and adoptive families of adopted individuals with affective disorders. *Archives of General Psychiatry, 43,* 923–929.

Zubernis, L., Cassidy, K. W., Gillham, J. E., Reivich, K. J., & Jaycox, L. H. (1999). Prevention of depressive symptoms in preadolescent children of divorce. *Journal of Divorce & Remarriage, 30,* 11–36.

CHAPTER 9

Preventing Alcohol, Tobacco, and Other Substance Abuse

Caryn C. Blitz,
Michael W. Arthur, and
J. David Hawkins

DESCRIPTION OF THE PROBLEM

Considerable research has been conducted over the past 20 years concerning the etiology and prevention of drug abuse. This research has increased our understanding of the antecedents of drug use among children and adolescents, the onset and developmental progression of drug use and abuse, and the role and relative importance of specific etiologic factors (Clayton, 1993; Gerstein & Green, 1993; Hawkins, Catalano, & Miller, 1992). It also has provided a firm foundation for the development and testing of a variety of interventions to prevent drug abuse. Interventions that target empirically validated predictors of drug abuse have demonstrated their efficacy in preventing drug abuse and related health and behavior problems (Durlak, 1998; Hawkins, Arthur, & Catalano, 1995).

Despite these advances, there is a gap between what research suggests should be done to prevent substance abuse and the approaches being used in communities (Kaftarian & Wandersman, 2000). The aims of this chapter are: (a) to summarize what is known about current trends in substance use and abuse by adolescents in the United States, (b) to summarize major findings from substance abuse prevention research, and (c) to describe an innovative approach that empowers communities to implement science-based prevention practices and policies.

Prevalence of Substance Use and Abuse

Data from two national surveys (Johnston, O'Malley, & Bachman, 1996, 2000; Substance Abuse and Mental Health Services Administration [SAMHSA], 1998, 2000) provide evidence that the prevalence of drug use among American adolescents peaked in the late 1970s, declined considerably during the 1980s, and then increased during the 1990s before leveling off in recent years. Monitoring the Future (MTF; Johnston, O'Malley, & Bachman, 2000) is a survey of a nationally representative sample of high school seniors conducted annually since 1975 by researchers at the University of Michigan. Since 1991, the MTF survey also has included representative samples of eighth- and tenth-grade students. The MTF survey documented substantial increases from 1992 to 1997 in the percentage of students reporting use of alcohol, tobacco, marijuana, and, to a lesser degree, other illicit drugs. The National Household Survey on Drug Abuse, a survey of a nationally representative sample of U.S. household members age 12 and over (SAMHSA, 1998; 2000), showed similar decreases in rates of drug use during the 1980s and similar increases between 1992 and 1997. Although rates for most substances have leveled off or begun to decrease slightly during the last several years, significant increases have continued in prevalence rates for the "club drug" Ecstasy, anabolic-androgenic steroids, and heroin (Johnston, O'Malley, & Bachman, 2000; SAMHSA, 2000). Within these general trends at the national level, the data reveal considerable variation in both levels of use and types of substances used most frequently across demographic groups and geographic regions of the country (Johnston, O'Malley, & Bachman, 2000; National Institute of Justice, 2000; SAMHSA, 2000; 2001).

Rates of self-reported drug use in samples of homeless and runaway youths have been found to be two to seven times higher than in public school samples (Kipke, O'Connor, Palmer, & MacKenzie, 1995; Unger, Kipke, Simon, Montgomery, & Johnson, 1997). A study of street youths in Hollywood (Kipke, O'Connor, Palmer, & MacKenzie, 1995), which included homeless youths as well as youths involved in the "street economy" of prostitution, drug-dealing, and selling stolen goods, found that substance use exceeded that of an in-school comparison group by twofold for marijuana use, over fourfold for stimulants, and over tenfold for cocaine. These data suggest that there are different types of adolescent drug users in this country. Prevention policies and practices must address these variations in patterns of use and include efforts to address the needs of youth populations at greatest risk for substance abuse.

Data on the epidemiology of substance use among adolescents also indicate that alcohol and tobacco are substances of particular relevance for prevention. Most important, they are the drugs most widely used in the United States. In the most recent MTF survey, approximately 80% of American high-school seniors reported having used alcohol at least once during their lifetime, and more than 70% reported having used alcohol in the past year (Johnston, O'Malley, & Bachman, 2000). About one-third reported having consumed five or more drinks in a row in a 2-hour period within the 2 weeks preceding the survey. Lifetime prevalence of tobacco use among high-school seniors is just over 60%, with 30% reporting use in the past 30 days and just over 11% reporting smoking half a pack or more per day. According to the American Lung Association (2000) over 400,000 Americans die of tobacco-related causes each year at a cost of $97.2 billion in health-care costs and lost productivity. In 1992, over 100,000 Americans died of alcohol-related causes, whereas 25,000 died from the abuse of illegal drugs at costs of $31.3 billion and $14.6 billion, respectively (Harwood, Fountain, & Livermore, 1998). From the public health perspective, tobacco and alcohol abuse clearly require preventive attention.

Moreover, longitudinal studies have revealed a fairly predictable pattern of stages of drug use (Hawkins, Hill, Guo, Battin-Pearson, & Collins, in press; Kandel, Yamaguchi, & Chen, 1992). In the United States, initiation of tobacco use often precedes initiation of alcohol use. In turn, alcohol use virtually always precedes initiation of marijuana use, which almost always precedes initiation of use of cocaine and other "hard" drugs. For these reasons, tobacco, alcohol, and marijuana have been referred to as "gateway" drugs. Onset of use of these "gateway" drugs in early adolescence is an important predictor of subsequent drug abuse (Kandel, 1982; Robins & Przybeck, 1985). These findings have influenced many prevention scientists and practitioners to concentrate on delaying the initiation of alcohol, tobacco, and marijuana use rather than on preventing the use of a specific category of "hard" drug.

Prevention Science and Substance Abuse Prevention

The emerging discipline of prevention science provides a general model that integrates epidemiological data on the prevalence of substance use and abuse among adolescents with information on the etiology of drug abuse and information on effective prevention strategies derived from controlled intervention trials (Coie et al., 1993; Kellam, Koretz, & Moscicki, 1999; Kellam & Rebok, 1992). Research has identified a variety of risk factors for adolescent substance abuse that exist within multiple ecological domains, including the individual, peer group, family, school, and community (for reviews of research on risk factors, see Dryfoos, 1990; Durlak, 1998; Hawkins et al., 1995; Hawkins, Catalano, & Miller, 1992; Mrazek & Haggerty, 1994) Studies also have identified protective factors that appear to buffer against or mitigate the negative effects of risk exposure (Garmezy, 1985; Hawkins, Catalano, & Miller, 1992; Luthar, 1991; Rutter, 1985; Werner & Smith, 1992). Specific risk and protective factors stabilize as predictors of substance abuse at different points in human development. If risk and protective factors are addressed at the developmental point at which they begin to predict later substance abuse, it is more likely that prevention efforts will be effective. Although risk factors are individually associated with an increased likelihood of substance abuse, studies also have shown that the prevalence and frequency of drug use is substantially higher among adolescents exposed to multiple risk factors (Bry, McKeon, & Pandina, 1982; Newcomb & Felix Ortiz, 1992; Pollard, Hawkins, & Arthur, 1999). This suggests that interventions to prevent drug abuse should focus on reducing multiple risk factors in individual, peer, family, school, and community environments. Findings from tests of preventive interventions also support a focus on predictors of substance abuse (Durlak, 1998). What follows is a summary of promising prevention approaches that have demonstrated both short- and long-term effects on substance use.

REVIEW AND CRITIQUE OF THE LITERATURE

School-Based Programs

School-based prevention programs have flourished since the 1970s. Early efforts took the form of alcohol, tobacco, and drug education curricula that sought to provide students with information about drugs and the negative effects of drug use and abuse. Other early efforts focused on the affective development of students via approaches designed to increase self-esteem, self-awareness, and acceptance, and to improve interpersonal relationships (Swisher, 1979). Evaluation of informational approaches (e.g., Schaps, Bartolo, Moskowitz, Palley, & Churgin, 1981) demonstrated some impact on drug knowledge and antidrug attitudes but consistently failed to demonstrate an impact on substance use and intentions to use. Although some studies produced evidence that affective education approaches had an impact on one or more correlates of drug use, they did not demonstrate a measurable impact on drug use behavior (Kearney & Hines, 1980; Kim, 1988).

In the 1980s, a paradigm shift occurred that moved prevention researchers toward more rigorous, theory-based interventions that focused on the development of skills for social problem solving and for resisting social influences to use drugs (Hawkins, Catalano, & Miller, 1992; Tobler et al., 2000). Some studies (e.g., Ellickson & Bell, 1990) focused almost exclusively on cigarette smoking, while other studies examined the effects of social influence curricula on the use of multiple substances. Unfortunately, methodological issues and challenges weakened evaluations of many of these interventions (Flay, 1985; Gerstein & Green, 1993). When rigorous evaluations of these school-based prevention programs were mounted, evidence of their effectiveness was usually weak (Tobler, 1994; Tobler et al., 2000).

Although there are some notable exceptions (Perry & Kelder, 1992; Sussman, Dent, Stacy, & Sun, 1993), most studies (Bell, Ellickson, & Harrison, 1993; Ellickson, Bell, & McGuigan, 1993; Flay et al., 1989) examining the social influence approach observed that its effects eroded after 1 or 2 years. Recent results from the Hutchinson Smoking Prevention Project, perhaps the most rigorous randomized controlled trial of a school-based social influences smoking prevention program for youth, revealed no difference in smoking prevalence for students in the control and experimental conditions, as assessed at grade 12 (10 years of intervention) and 2 years after high school (Peterson, Kealey, Mann, Marek, & Sarason, 2000).

In contrast, approaches that combine key elements of the problem-specific social influences model (Evans et al., 1978) and the broader competence enhancement approach (Botvin, Baker, Dusenbury, Botvin, & Diaz, 1995) appear to be more effective. A distinguishing feature of the competence enhancement approach is that resistance skills are taught within the context of a broader program designed to enhance generic personal and social skills (Botvin et al., 1995). Observed reductions in smoking and in alcohol and marijuana use have ranged from 30% to 75% for these approaches after the initial intervention (Donaldson, Graham, & Hansen, 1994; Perry, Kelder, & Komro, 1993). Moreover, longer-term follow-up studies (Botvin et al., 1995) of interventions that combined the social influence and competence-enhancement approaches also have demonstrated long-term prevention effects up to 6 years. Thus, although most school-based interventions have shown little evidence of long-term effects on drug use, the combined social competence-social influences strategy has produced sustained effects.

Family Interventions

The literature on family interventions (Ge, Best, Conger, & Simons, 1996; Hawkins, Catalano, & Miller, 1992; Kumpfer, Olds, Alexander, Zucker, &

Gary, 1998) shows that most strategies target risk and protective factors for youth substance abuse specific to the family context as well as interactions between the family and other contexts that may involve or have an impact on the child. Current evidence suggests that certain forms of family therapy and family skills training interventions are the most effective in reducing risk factors and increasing protective factors, as well as preventing substance abuse. An important factor that characterizes effective family-focused interventions is that, similar to school-based interventions, they concentrate on skill development rather than on simply informing parents about effective parenting practices.

Family therapy interventions are used with families in which preteens or adolescents are already manifesting behavior problems. Research (SAMHSA, 1998) has demonstrated that family therapy improves family communication, family control imbalances, and family relationships. Several specific family therapy programs have been identified as exemplary programs because of their effectiveness in reducing delinquency and drug use in preteens and adolescents (Kumpfer et al., 1998). These programs include Functional Family Therapy (FFT; Alexander & Parsons, 1982), Structural Family Therapy (SFT; Szapocznik, Scopetta, & King, 1978), and Multisystemic Therapy (MST; Henggeler, Mihalic, Rone, Thomas, & Timmons-Mitchell, 1998).

Family skills training approaches are frequently targeted at high-risk children and families. These youth are targeted because they exhibit characteristics, or are in circumstances, that are empirically associated with substance abuse. These interventions often include a combination of behavioral parenting skills training, children's social skills training, and behavioral family therapy or role-playing with special coaching by the trainers (Kumpfer & Alvarado, 1995). According to an outcome analysis conducted by Kumpfer (1996), family skills training appears to affect the largest number of measured family and youth risk and protective factors. Family skills training programs that have demonstrated positive effects on substance use include the Focus on Families (FOF) program (Catalano, Haggerty, Gainey, & Hoppe, 1997), the Preparing for the Drug-Free Years (PDFY) curriculum (Spoth, Redmond, Haggerty, & Ward, 1995), the Strengthening Families Program (SFP; Kumpfer, Molgaard, & Spoth, 1996), and the Iowa Strengthening Families Program (ISFP; Molgaard & Kumpfer, 1994). For example, at 4 years postintervention, results for the PDFY and the ISFP showed evidence of delayed initiation and lower levels of progressed use for alcohol, tobacco, and marijuana (Spoth, Redmond, & Shin, in press). Relative reductions in new user rates for marijuana were as high as 55.7% and 36.6% for IFSP and PDFY, respectively; relative reductions in past-month alcohol use were 30.0% and 40.6% for IFSP and PDFY, respectively (Spoth et al., in press).

Environmental Interventions

Researchers concerned with the health consequences of alcohol and tobacco use have investigated the effects of laws and regulatory mechanisms for reducing consumption of those substances that can be legally possessed and used by adults (for a review, see Pentz, 2000). In the last few years, attention has been focused specifically on the issue of illegal sales of cigarettes to minors (e.g., Forster et al., 1998; Jason, Biglan, & Katz, 1998; Rigotti et al., 1997). A number of studies (Forster & Wolfson, 1998) have shown that enforcing tobacco age-of-sale laws results in merchants altering their practices and in reductions in illegal sales to minors. These practices have involved developing new ordinances regarding enforcement of youth access laws, tracking purchase attempts by minors, imposing fines on and suspending the tobacco licenses of merchants who violated age restrictions on tobacco sales, and imposing fines on minors for tobacco possession (Altman, Wheelis, McFarlane, Lee, & Fortmann, 1999; Forster et al., 1998; Jason, Berk, Schnopp Wyatt, & Talbot, 1999; Rigotti et al., 1997).

Research shows that reduction of minors' ability to buy tobacco has resulted in decreased cigarette smoking among youth, and that these effects have been maintained over time (DiFranza, Carlson, & Caisse, 1992; Forster et al., 1998; Jason et al., 1999; Jason, Ji, Anes, & Birkhead, 1991). The interventions that have demonstrated lasting effects on smoking prevalence have included laws with several common characteristics: (a) civil, as opposed to criminal, penalties that are imposed on both the store owner and the clerk, (b) progressively increasing fees that culminate in the suspension or revocation of the store owner's tobacco license, and (c) regular enforcement of the law, using minors in unannounced purchase attempts to monitor compliance (Jason, Biglan, & Katz, 1998). Other characteristics of effective interventions include fining minors for tobacco possession (Jason et al., 1999) and combining laws reducing youth access to tobacco with larger community interventions (Forster et al., 1998).

Comprehensive Interventions

Both epidemiological and etiological investigations have revealed substance abuse to be a health and behavior problem with multiple causal roots. A number of factors have been shown to predict higher probability of substance abuse in longitudinal prospective studies (Hawkins, Catalano, & Miller, 1992; Kandel, Simcha Fagan, & Davies, 1986; Newcomb, Maddahian, & Bentler,

1986). These findings suggest that the prevention of substance abuse ultimately requires a multiple component strategy with elements focused on different predictors thought to be causal. Four examples of multicomponent projects seeking to address multiple risk and protective factors across domains are highlighted below.

Seattle Social Development Project

The Seattle Social Development Project (SSDP; Hawkins, Catalano, Kosterman, Abbott, & Hill, 1999) examined the long-term effects of an intervention combining teacher training, parent education, and social competence training for children during the elementary grades. The design was a nonrandomized controlled trial with follow-up 6 years postintervention. The participants included 76% of the fifth-grade students enrolled in participating schools, of which 93% were followed up and interviewed at age 18 years. The full intervention was provided in grades 1 through 6 and consisted of 5 days of in-service training for teachers each intervention year, developmentally appropriate parenting classes offered to parents when children were in grades 1 through 3, 5, and 6, and developmentally adjusted social competence training for children in grades 1 and 6. A late intervention, provided in grades 5 and 6 only, paralleled the full intervention at these grades.

Hawkins et al. (1999) found that students in the full intervention group reported greater commitment and attachment to school, better academic achievement, and less school misbehavior than control students. Moreover, fewer students receiving the full intervention, compared with the control condition, reported heavy drinking, violent delinquent acts, sexual intercourse, multiple sex partners, and pregnancy or causing pregnancy by age 18 years. Late intervention in grades 5 and 6 did not significantly affect health and behavior problems in adolescence beyond school misbehavior.

Midwestern Prevention Project

The Midwestern Prevention Project (MPP) was a comprehensive community-based drug abuse prevention program which consisted of five program components (school, parent, community organization, mass media, and health policy) introduced in sequence over a 5-year period (Pentz, Mihalic, & Grotpeter, 1997). The goal of the program was to decrease the rates of onset and prevalence of drug use in young adolescents (ages 10–15) and to decrease drug use among parents and other residents in two large communities. The components focused on promoting adolescent drug use resistance and counteraction skills, parent prevention practices and parent support of adolescent prevention practices, and dissemination and support of no-drug-use social norms and expectations in the community. MPP was tested in two major Midwestern metropolitan areas: (a) Kansas City, Kansas and Kansas City, Missouri, with a quasi-experimental design and (b) Indianapolis and Marion County, Indiana, with an experimental design.

The MPP demonstrated net reductions of up to 40% in daily smoking, similar reductions in marijuana use, and smaller reductions in alcohol use among students in the intervention schools, which were maintained up to grade 12 (Pentz, Mihalic, & Grotpeter, 1997). By the end of the fourth year in Kansas City (9th/10th grade), cocaine and crack use were significantly less prevalent in intervention schools, and by early adulthood (2 years postintervention), program youth also demonstrated reductions in the need for drug abuse treatment. The MPP also decreased parent alcohol and marijuana use, increased positive parent-child communications about drug use prevention, and facilitated development of prevention programs, activities, and services among community leaders (Pentz et al., 1997). Policy changes associated with MPP included institutionalization of the school program, establishment of youth drug abuse treatment beds, and cooperation from vendors to refuse tobacco and alcohol sales to minors (Pentz et al., 1997).

Project SixTeen

The objective of Project SixTeen was to evaluate a comprehensive communitywide program to prevent adolescent tobacco use (Biglan, Ary, Koehn, & Levings, 1996). Eight matched pairs of small Oregon communities were randomly assigned to receive a school-based program alone or a school-based program plus a community program. Effects were assessed through five annual surveys of students in grades 7 and 9 (age 12–15). The community program included: (a) media advocacy, (b) youth antitobacco activities, (c) family communications about tobacco use, and (d) reduction of youth access to tobacco. The school-based program was administered by trained classroom teachers and consisted of both social influence and life skills training, including peer-led discussions and skills practice.

The results indicated that the community program had significant effects on the prevalence of weekly cigarette use at time 2 and time 5, and the effect approached significance at time 4 (Biglan, Ary, Smolkowski, Duncan, & Black,

2000). The intervention affected the prevalence of smokeless tobacco among ninth-grade boys at time 2. There were also significant effects on the incidence of alcohol use among ninth graders and marijuana use for all students (Biglan et al., 2000).

Project Northland

Project Northland was a randomized community trial initially implemented in 24 school districts and communities in northeastern Minnesota, with goals of delaying onset and reducing adolescent alcohol use using communitywide, multiyear, multiple-component interventions (Perry et al., 1993; Perry et al., 1996). The study targeted all students ($n = 2,352$) enrolled in 24 public school districts who were in the sixth grade and who were present in subsequent follow-up years (1991–1998). The early-adolescent phase of Project Northland consisted of parent involvement/education programs, behavioral curricula, peer participation, and community task force activities (Perry et al., 1993; Wagenaar & Perry, 1994). Phase II of Project Northland, targeting 11th- and 12th-grade students, used five major strategies: (a) direct action community organizing methods to encourage citizens to reduce underage access to alcohol, (b) youth development involving high school students in youth action teams, (c) print media to support community organizing and youth action initiatives and communicate healthy norms about underage drinking, (d) parent education and involvement, and (e) a classroom-based curriculum for 11th-grade students. In both phases of Project Northland, the intervention components were designed to be complementary and developmentally appropriate.

At the end of Phase I (eighth grade) there was a 20% reduction in past-month drinking and a 30% reduction in past-week drinking for intervention students (Perry, Williams, Veblen Mortenson, Toomey, Komro, Anstine et al., 1996). By the end of the 10th grade, after 2 years without a substantive intervention program, there were no significant differences between the intervention and reference groups. By the end of the 11th grade, after 1 year of Phase II intervention activities, students in the intervention group were drinking less, but this was not statistically significant. However, among baseline nonusers (the two-thirds of the sample who had not started drinking until the sixth grade or later), the difference between groups in past-week use of alcohol use was marginally significant ($p < .07$), suggesting some impact from the 11th-grade intervention among these students (Perry et al., 2000). The results from the analysis of the 12th-grade surveys of students, parents, police, community leaders, school leaders, and merchants, as well as alcohol purchase attempts by young buyers, have not yet been reported.

Bridging the Gap Between Research and Practice

These studies of comprehensive interventions have added to the expanding knowledge base in prevention science. Other studies have begun to examine the effects of combining specific program components in various domains—individual, family, school, peer, and community—in an effort to elucidate which combinations of interventions have the largest effects on substance use and related problem behaviors. Such research has demonstrated that combining school-based programs with mass media campaigns and programs aimed at parents and community leaders has a greater impact on substance use than mass media or community organizing alone (Johnson et al., 1990; Pentz et al., 1989); that social influence programs combined with life skills training and parent interventions (written materials, homework assignments, and workshops) have a greater impact on substance use than either one of those programs alone (Scheier & Botvin, 1998); and that community mobilization and public awareness campaigns can increase the effectiveness of interventions to reduce youth access to tobacco in decreasing smoking prevalence (Forster et al., 1998).

Given all this information, why are we still faced with the widespread belief that prevention doesn't work? Numerous factors contribute to the gap between prevention research and prevention practice (Kaftarian & Wandersman, 2000; Morrissey et al., 1997). First, communities often lack the funding, research expertise, and implementation support necessary to carry out the planning, implementation, and evaluation of evidence-based interventions. Second, many prevention providers are unfamiliar with science-based prevention practices and instead rely on strategies with which they are familiar. Third, prevention planning decisions are often influenced more by community concerns and impressions rather than objective needs assessment data that could inform planning, monitoring, and evaluation efforts. What follows is a description of a community prevention approach designed to address some of these issues and to reduce the gap between research and practice.

CASE STUDY: THE COMMUNITIES THAT CARE(r) PREVENTION OPERATING SYSTEM

Studies of comprehensive community prevention initiatives suggest that implementation of science-based prevention activities can be promoted through training and technical assistance in needs assessment and strategic prevention planning (Arthur, Ayers, Graham, & Hawkins, in press; Arthur, Hawkins, &

Catalano, 2000; Greenberg, Osgood, Babinskik, & Anderson, 1999). For example, the Communities That Care (CTC) training and technical assistance package is a strategy for changing the way that communities approach and conduct prevention (Hawkins, Catalano, & Associates, 1992; Hawkins, Catalano, & Miller, 1992). The strategy provides (a) a framework of risk- and protection-focused prevention to orient community prevention action and (b) the tools for assessment and strategic planning needed to implement and institutionalize science-based prevention (Developmental Research and Programs, 1997, 2000a). It empowers communities to approach prevention analytically, and it leaves in place tools that communities can use to monitor and inform their progress in reducing risks, enhancing protection, and preventing health and behavior problems (Hawkins, 1999).

The CTC intervention consists of five phases designed to mobilize community leaders and a community prevention board to plan and implement a strategic set of research-based interventions designed to reduce specific risk factors and promote protective factors in the community (Developmental Research and Programs, 2000b). Phase I, *Community Board Mobilization*, begins the process with a Community Readiness Assessment focused on assessing attitudinal and organizational characteristics of community members, leaders, and organizations that influence the mobilization process (Arthur et al., 1996; National Institute on Drug Abuse, 1997). The readiness assessment informs the development of strategies and timelines to complete the subsequent phases of the intervention. Key issues that are addressed during this phase include defining the community, identifying individuals who will commit to leading the process, specifying the health and behavior issues to be addressed and the level of agreement among community members about the importance of these issues, promoting collaboration among service providers, and assessing community norms and the fit of the CTC approach with existing community initiatives and values.

Phase II, *Introduce and Involve*, begins with a workshop to orient key community leaders (i.e., mayor, police chief, school superintendent, and business and media leaders) to risk- and protection-focused prevention and community mobilization processes. Key community leaders are essential to the CTC approach because they have the status, position, authority, and control of resources to ensure that the programs and policies developed through the CTC planning process are fully implemented and institutionalized (Finnegan, Bracht, & Viswanath, 1989). The leaders nominate about 30 community members to constitute the community prevention board. The community prevention board includes the opinion shapers and grassroots leaders in the community, as well as those who are involved in delivering prevention programs and services to children, families, and the community. The key leaders make a commitment to actively support the project and maintain its visibility within the community, while the community prevention board is the main mechanism for carrying out the planning and implementation activities of the project.

To complete Phase II, the members of the community prevention board attend a two-day *community board orientation* workshop, which provides an overview of the CTC intervention and information on risk factors, the social development strategy, and strategies for developing and maintaining effective board organization and structure. Important issues in implementing Phase II include developing a clear, common vision for the community's prevention efforts, obtaining the commitment of the key leaders to support the process, defining the roles and responsibilities of the key leaders and those of the community prevention board, and recruiting and establishing an effective community prevention board.

In Phase III, *Develop a Data-Based Profile*, community prevention board members participate in a training workshop which describes how to conduct an assessment of risk and protective factors affecting youth in the community. The workshop provides methods for collecting, analyzing, and reporting survey and archival measures of research-based risk and protective factors for adolescent problem behaviors. These data are used to develop community profiles of risk and protective factors to assist the prevention board members in identifying the most prevalent risk factors and assessing the levels of protective factors in the community (see, for example, Figs. 9.1 and 9.2). This information empowers communities to prioritize specific risk and protective factors for preventive attention as well as to select specific areas or subpopulations within the community for concerted attention. It also provides baseline data for ongoing assessment of the community's progress in changing levels of the specific factors targeted by their strategic prevention plans.

Following the collection and profiling of the community's risk and protective factor data, community prevention board members attend a workshop on resource assessment. The resource assessment training provides methods and tools for surveying the community's existing prevention resources that address the risk and protective factors prioritized from the community profiles. The focus of this assessment is on identifying gaps in existing resources that could be mobilized or better utilized to address the prioritized factors. Key issues during the third phase include identifying and mobilizing the technical resources needed to collect, analyze, and interpret the community's data on risk, protection, and resources; obtaining broad community input and consensus on priority risk and protective factors and populations toward which prevention actions will be directed; and gathering complete and accurate information on existing prevention resources.

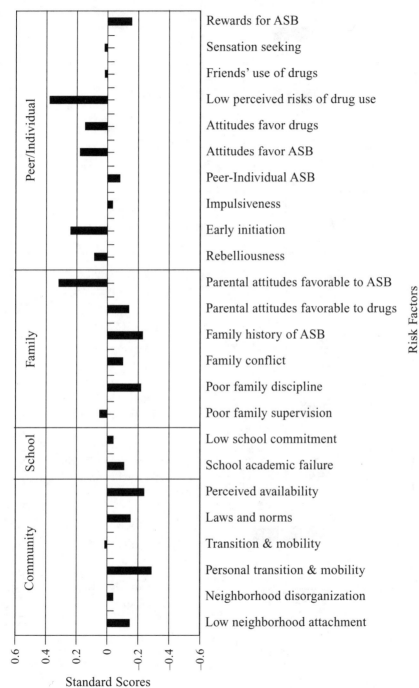

Figures 9.1 Community risk profile. (eighth Grade Student Survey)

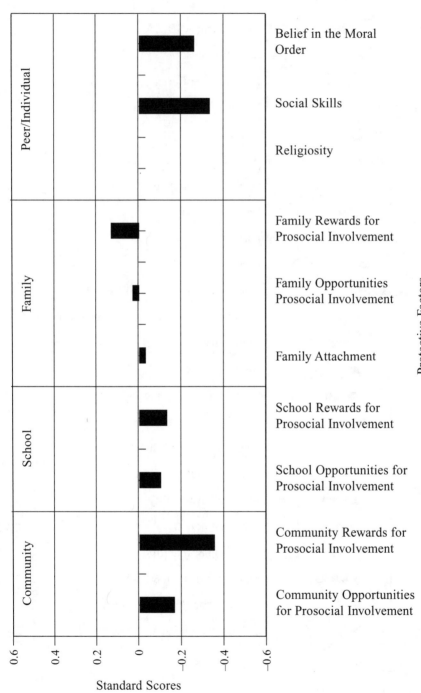

Figures 9.2 Community protection profile. (eighth Grade Student Survey)

Phase IV of the CTC process focuses on developing a comprehensive, communitywide prevention plan. Community board members attend a 2-day *effective prevention strategies* training event covering strategic action planning and the selection of interventions shown to be effective in well-designed evaluation studies. Board members learn about specific program elements in sessions with expert consultants describing each intervention and allowing for direct questioning by board members.

The community prevention board then develops a comprehensive substance abuse prevention plan for the community. The plan describes the prevention strategies that will be implemented to address each prioritized risk and protective factor, includes work plans to implement these new strategies, and specifies measurable objectives for each strategy. The plan also specifies how the new interventions will be coordinated with existing programs and resources. The community prevention board completes the action plan by specifying how it will monitor implementation quality and provide feedback to community prevention providers to support continuous quality improvement (Wandersman et al. 1998).

Phase V of the CTC intervention focuses on implementation and evaluation of the community's comprehensive prevention plan. Follow-up training and ongoing technical assistance is provided to develop the capacity within the community to implement the selected interventions effectively, including removing barriers to implementation, marshalling resources, and developing procedures to monitor the implementation of each element (Chavis, Florin, & Felix, 1992; Florin, Mitchell, & Stevenson, 1993). The community board also acts to change community norms, policies, and practices regarding substance use and related problem behaviors. Local media are used to: (a) educate community members about risk and protective factors for substance use and other problem behaviors, (b) communicate clear norms and enforcement policies regarding substance use in the community, (c) generate public support for regulatory measures, and (d) motivate community members to take part in efforts to reduce risk factors and promote protective processes in the community. Key issues during the implementation phase include developing the resources and capacity to implement the selected interventions with sufficient scope and fidelity to impact targeted risk and protective factors, reaching the populations in greatest need of the interventions, and addressing turnover and transitions in key leader and community board membership.

In summary, *Communities That Care* focuses community resources where risk exposure is high and protection is low, addresses prioritized predictors with preventive interventions shown to be effective at impacting those predictors, and facilitates the creation of a strategic plan for implementing and monitoring the selected strategies. By intervening at the systems level to reduce risk and enhance protective influences, Communities That Care attempts to change the community context for youth development, thereby promoting positive youth development and preventing substance use and related problems.

FUTURE DIRECTIONS

Advances in the science of prevention over the past 30 years have provided a substantial base of knowledge for the design of effective substance abuse prevention efforts. The technology exists to support communities in assessing the need for prevention services, prioritizing specific targets for intervention, selecting intervention strategies with demonstrated efficacy, and monitoring the impact of these services. Despite the promise of science-based approaches to the prevention of substance use, several important questions remain unanswered. Most important, factors that influence the implementation and effectiveness of prevention services delivered in community settings must be better understood. Interventions that have demonstrated efficacy in controlled research studies often fail to replicate their effectiveness when implemented on a large scale using existing services systems (Goodman, 2000). Implementing an efficacious intervention model on a large scale necessitates balancing fidelity to the core elements of the intervention model with adaptation to the varying contexts within which the intervention is delivered (Weissberg, 1990). In order to do this, more information is needed about the core elements of effective prevention models and about processes of adoption and adaptation in community contexts.

Another area for further research involves prevention services systems. For example, determining how much and what types of prevention training and technical assistance are necessary in order to support strategic, science-based, systems-level planning and continuous quality improvement of the community's prevention services system is an important question for prevention services research. Although evidence is mounting that multicomponent interventions can produce greater long-term impact than single-focused interventions, little is known about the characteristics of effective prevention service delivery systems. Further research is needed to understand community readiness, community resources, and other community characteristics that may influence the viability and implementation quality of systems-level interventions.

Finally, rapidly emerging developments in information technology are creating new possibilities in the efficient collection, analysis, and distribution of data and information that can be applied to strategic planning and the transfer of prevention technologies to communities. On-line training, technical assistance, and strategic planning tools can facilitate the dissemination and diffusion of effective preventive interventions. Technology will dramatically alter the way substance abuse preventive interventions are conceived and delivered in the 21st century.

ACKNOWLEDGMENT

This research has been partially supported by the National Institute on Drug Abuse, Grant #R43 DA10132-01A1 and Grant #R01 DA10768, and by the Center for Substance Abuse Prevention, Contract #277-93-1014.

REFERENCES

Alexander, J. F., & Parsons, B. V. (1982). *Functional family therapy: Principles and procedures*. Carmel, CA: Brooks/Cole.

Altman, D. G., Wheelis, A. Y., McFarlane, M., Lee, H. R., & Fortmann, S. P. (1999). The relationship between tobacco access and use among adolescents: A four-community study. *Social Science and Medicine, 48*, 759–775.

American Lung Association (2000). *American Lung Association fact sheet: Smoking*. Available: http://www.lungusa.org/tobacco/smoking_factsheet99.html

Arthur, M. W., Ayers, C. D., Graham, K. A., & Hawkins, J. D. (in press). Mobilizing communities to reduce risks for drug abuse: A comparison of two strategies. In W. J. Bukoski & Z. Sloboda (Eds.), *Handbook of drug abuse theory, science and practice*. New York: Plenum.

Arthur, M. W., Brewer, D., Graham, K. A., Shavel, D., Hawkins, J. D., & Hansen, C. (1996). *Assessing state and community readiness for prevention*. Rockville, MD: Center for Substance Abuse Prevention, National Center for the Advancement of Prevention.

Arthur, M. W., Hawkins, J. D., & Catalano, R. F. (2000). *Translating prevention research into action: Impact of community leader training on implementation of risk and protection-focused prevention*. Paper presented at the annual meeting of the Society for Prevention Research, Montréal, Quebec, Canada.

Bell, R. M., Ellickson, P. L., & Harrison, E. R. (1993). Do drug prevention effects persist into high school? How Project ALERT did with ninth graders. *Preventive Medicine, 22*, 463–483.

Biglan, A., Ary, D. V., Koehn, V., & Levings, D. (1996). Mobilizing positive enforcement in communities to reduce youth access to tobacco. *American Journal of Community Psychology, 24*, 625–638.

Biglan, A., Ary, D. V., Smolkowski, K., Duncan, T., & Black, C. (2000). A randomized controlled trial of a community intervention to prevent adolescent tobacco use. *Tobacco Control, 9*, 24–32.

Botvin, G. J., Baker, E., Dusenbury, L., Botvin, E. M., & Diaz, T. (1995). Long-term follow-up results of a randomized drug abuse prevention trial in a white middle-class population. *Journal of the American Medical Association, 273*, 1106–1112.

Bry, B. H., McKeon, P., & Pandina, R. J. (1982). Extent of drug use as a function of number of risk factors. *Journal of Abnormal Psychology, 91*, 273–279.

Catalano, R. F., Haggerty, K. P., Gainey, R. R., & Hoppe, M. J. (1997). Reducing parental risk factors for children's substance misuse: Preliminary outcomes with opiate-addicted parents. *Substance Use and Misuse, 32*, 699–721.

Chavis, D. M., Florin, P., & Felix, M. (1992). Nurturing grassroots initiatives for community development: The role of enabling systems. In T. Mizrahi & J. Morrison (Eds.), *Community organization and social administration: Advances, trends, and emerging principles*. Binghamton, NY: Haworth.

Clayton, R. R. (1993). *Basic/etiology research: Drug use and its progression to drug abuse and drug dependence*. Unpublished manuscript. University of Kentucky, Lexington, Center for Prevention Research.

Coie, J. D., Watt, N. F., West, S. G., Hawkins, J. D., Asarnow, J. R., Markman, H. J., Ramey, S. L., Shure, M. B., & Long, B. (1993). The science of prevention: A conceptual framework and some directions for a national research program. *American Psychologist, 48*, 1013–1022.

Developmental Research and Programs (1997). *Communities That Care—A comprehensive prevention program*. Seattle, WA: Author.

Developmental Research and Programs (2000a). *Communities That Care—A comprehensive prevention program*. Seattle, WA: Author.

Developmental Research and Programs (2000b). *Communities That Care— Information Packet*. Seattle, WA: Author.

DiFranza, J. R., Carlson, R., & Caisse, R. (1992). Reducing youth access to tobacco. *Tobacco Control, 1*, 58.

Donaldson, S. I., Graham, J. W., & Hansen, W. B. (1994). Testing the generalizability of intervening mechanism theories: Understanding the effects of adolescent drug use prevention interventions. *Journal of Behavioral Medicine, 17*, 195–216.

Dryfoos, J. G. (1990). *Adolescents at risk: Prevalence and prevention*. New York: Oxford University Press.

Durlak, J. A. (1998). Common risk and protective factors in successful prevention programs. *American Journal of Orthopsychiatry, 68*, 512–520.

Ellickson, P. L., & Bell, R. M. (1990). Drug prevention in junior high: A multi-site longitudinal test. *Science, 247*, 1299–1305.

Ellickson, P. L., Bell, R. M., & McGuigan, K. (1993). Preventing adolescent drug use: Long-term results of a junior high program. *American Journal of Public Health, 83*, 856–861.

Evans, R. I., Rozelle, R. M., Mittlemark, M. B., Hanson, W. B., Bane, A. L., & Havis, J. (1978). Deterring the onset of smoking in children: Knowledge of immediate physiological effects and coping with peer pressure, media pressure, and parent modeling. *Journal of Applied Social Psychology, 8*, 126–135.

Finnegan, J. R., Bracht, N., & Viswanath, K. (1989). Community power and leadership analysis in lifestyle campaigns. In C. T. Salmon (Ed.), *Information campaigns: Managing the process of social change* (pp. 54–84). Newbury Park, CA: Sage.

Flay, B. R. (1985). Psychosocial approaches to smoking prevention: A review of findings. *Health Psychology, 5*, 449–488.

Flay, B. R., Koepke, D., Thomson, S. J., Santi, S., Best, J. A., & Brown, K. S. (1989). Six-year follow-up of the first Waterloo School Smoking Prevention Trial. *American Journal of Public Health, 79*, 1371–1376.

Florin, P., Mitchell, R., & Stevenson, J. (1993). Identifying training and technical assistance needs in community coalitions: A developmental approach. *Health Education Research, 8*, 417–432.

Forster, J. L., Murray, D. M., Wolfson, M., Blaine, T. M., Wagenaar, A. C., & Hennrikus, D. J. (1998). The effects of community policies to reduce youth access to tobacco. *American Journal of Public Health, 88*, 1193–1198.

Forster, J. L., & Wolfson, M. (1998). Youth access to tobacco: Policies and politics. *Annual Review of Public Health, 19*, 203–235.

Garmezy, N. (1985). Stress-resistant children: The search for protective factors. *Journal of Child Psychology and Psychiatry, 4*(Suppl.), 213–233.

Ge, X., Best, K. M., Conger, R. D., & Simons, R. L. (1996). Parenting behaviors and the occurrence and co-occurrence of adolescent depressive symptoms and conduct problems. *Developmental Psychology, 32*, 717–731.

Gerstein, D. R., & Green, L. W. (Eds.). (1993). *Preventing drug abuse: What do we know?* Washington, DC: National Academy Press.

Goodman, R. M. (2000). Bridging the gap in effective program implementation: From concept to application. *Journal of Community Psychology, 28*, 309–321.

Greenberg, M. T., Osgood, D. W., Babinskik, L., & Anderson, A. (1999). *Developing community readiness for prevention: Initial evaluation of the Pennsylvania Communities That Care Initiative.* Paper presented at the annual meeting of the Society for Prevention Research, New Orleans, Louisiana.

Harwood, H. J., Fountain, D., & Livermore, G. (1998). Economic costs of alcohol abuse and alcoholism. In M. Galanter (Ed.), *Recent development in alcoholism: Vol. 14. The consequences of alcoholism: Medical, neuropsychiatric, economic, cross-cultural* (pp. 307–330). New York: Plenum.

Hawkins, J. D. (1999). Preventing crime and violence through Communities That Care. *European Journal on Criminal Policy and Research, 7,* 443–448.

Hawkins, J. D., Arthur, M. W., & Catalano, R. F. (1995). Preventing substance abuse. In M. Tonry & D. Farrington (Eds.), *Crime and justice: Vol. 19. Building a safer society: Strategic approaches to crime prevention* (pp. 343–427). Chicago: University of Chicago Press.

Hawkins, J. D., Catalano, R. F., & Associates. (1992). *Communities That Care: Action for drug abuse prevention.* San Francisco, CA: Jossey-Bass.

Hawkins, J. D., Catalano, R. F., Kosterman, R., Abbott, R., & Hill, K. G. (1999). Preventing adolescent health-risk behaviors by strengthening protection during childhood. *Archives of Pediatrics and Adolescent Medicine, 153,* 226–234.

Hawkins, J. D., Catalano, R. F., & Miller, J. Y. (1992). Risk and protective factors for alcohol and other drug problems in adolescence and early adulthood: Implications for substance abuse prevention. *Psychological Bulletin, 112,* 64–105.

Hawkins, J. D., Hill, K. G., Guo, J., Battin-Pearson, S. R., & Collins, L. M. (in press). Substance use norms and transitions in substance use: Implications for the gateway hypothesis. In D. Kandel (Ed.), *Examining the gateway hypothesis: Stages and pathways of drug involvement.* New York: Cambridge University Press.

Henggeler, S. W., Mihalic, S. F., Rone, L., Thomas, C., & Timmons-Mitchell, J. (1998). Multisystemic therapy. In D. S. Elliott (Series Ed.), *Blueprints for violence prevention* (Book 6). Boulder, CO: University of Colorado, Center for the Study and Prevention of Violence, Institute of Behavioral Science.

Jason, L. A., Berk, M., Schnopp Wyatt, D. L., & Talbot, B. (1999). Effects of enforcement of youth access laws on smoking prevalence. *American Journal of Community Psychology, 27,* 143–160.

Jason. L. A., Biglan, A., & Katz, R. (1998). Implications of the tobacco settlement for the prevention of teenage smoking. *Children's services: Social policy, research, and practice, 1,* 2.

Jason, L. A., Ji, P. Y., Anes, M. D., & Birkhead, S. H. (1991). Active enforcement of cigarette control laws in the prevention of cigarette sales to minors. *Journal of the American Medical Association, 266,* 3159–3161.

Johnson, C. A., Pentz, M. A., Weber, M. D., Dwyer, J. H., Baer, N. A., MacKinnon, D. P., Hansen, W. B., & Flay, B. R. (1990). Relative effectiveness of comprehensive community programming for drug abuse prevention with high-risk and low-risk adolescents. *Journal of Consulting and Clinical Psychology, 58,* 447–456.

Johnston, L. D., O'Malley, P. M., & Bachman, J. G. (1996). *National survey results on drug use from the Monitoring the Future study: Vol. 1. Secondary school students* (NIH Pub. No. 97-4139). Rockville, MD: National Institute on Drug Abuse.

Johnston, L. D., O'Malley, P. M., & Bachman, J. G. (2000). *The Monitoring the Future national survey results on adolescent drug use: Overview of key findings, 1999* (NIH Publication No. 00-4690). Rockville, MD: National Institute on Drug Abuse.

Kaftarian, S. J., & Wandersman, A. (2000). Bridging the gap between research and practice in community-based substance abuse prevention. *Journal of Community Psychology, 28,* 237–240.

Kandel, D. B. (1982). Epidemiological and psychosocial perspectives on adolescent drug use. *Journal of the American Academy of Clinical Psychiatry, 21,* 328–347.

Kandel, D. B., Simcha Fagan, O., & Davies, M. (1986). Risk factors for delinquency and illicit drug use from adolescence to young adulthood. *Journal of Drug Issues, 16,* 67–90.

Kandel, D. B., Yamaguchi, K., & Chen, K. (1992). Stages of progression in drug involvement from adolescence to adulthood: Further evidence for the gateway theory. *Journal of Studies on Alcohol, 53,* 447–457.

Kearney, A. L., & Hines, M. H. (1980). Evaluation of the effectiveness of a drug prevention education program. *Journal of Drug Education, 10,* 127–134.

Kellam, S. G., Koretz, D., & Moscicki, E. K. (1999). Core elements of developmental epidemiologically based prevention research. *American Journal of Community Psychology, 27,* 463–482.

Kellam, S. G., & Rebok, G. W. (1992). Building developmental and etiological theory through epidemiologically based preventive intervention trials. In J. McCord & R. E. Tremblay (Eds.), *Preventing antisocial behavior: Interventions from birth through adolescence* (pp. 162–195). New York: Guilford.

Kim, S. (1988). A short- and long-term evaluation of "Here's looking at you" II. *Journal of Drug Education, 18,* 235–242.

Kipke, M. D., Montgomery, S. B., Simon, T. R., & Iverson, E. F. (1997). "Substance abuse" disorders among runaway and homeless youth. *Substance Use and Misuse, 32,* 969–986.

Kipke, M. D., O'Connor, S., Palmer, R., & MacKenzie, R. G. (1995). Street youth in Los Angeles: Profile of a group at high risk for human immunodeficiency virus infection. *Archives of Pediatrics and Adolescent Medicine, 149,* 513–519.

Kumpfer, K. L. (1996, January). *Principles of effective family-focused parent programs.* Paper presented at the NIDA Family Intervention Research Symposium, Gaithersburg, Maryland.

Kumpfer, K. L., & Alvarado, R. (1995). Strengthening families to prevent drug use in multi-ethnic youth. In G. Botvin, S. Schinke, & M. Orlandi (Eds.), *Drug abuse prevention with multi-ethnic youth* (pp. 253–292). Newbury Park, CA: Sage.

Kumpfer, K. L., Molgaard, V., & Spoth, R. (1996). The Strengthening Families Program of the prevention of delinquency and drug use. In R. D. Peter & R. J. McMahon (Eds.), *Preventing childhood disorders, substance abuse, and delinquency* (pp. 241–267). Thousand Oaks, CA: Sage.

Kumpfer, K. L., Olds, D. L., Alexander, J. F., Zucker, R. A., & Gary, L. E. (1998). Family etiology of youth problems. In R. S. Ahsery, E. B. Robertson, & K. L. Kumpfer (Eds.), *Drug abuse prevention through family intervention for families of aggressive boys: A replication study* (NIDA Research Monograph No. 177, pp. 42–77). Washington, DC: U.S. Government Printing Office.

Luthar, S. S. (1991). Vulnerability and resilience: A study of high-risk adolescents. *Child Development, 62,* 600–616.

Molgaard, V., & Kumpfer, K. L. (1994). *Strengthening Family Program II.* Ames, IA: Iowa State University, Social and Behavioral Research Center for Rural Health.

Morrissey, E., Wandersman, A., Seybolt, D., Nation, M., Crusto, C., & Davino, K. (1997). Toward a framework for bridging the gap between science and practice in prevention: A focus on evaluator and practitioner perspectives. *Evaluation and Program Planning, 20,* 367–377.

Mrazek, P. J., & Haggerty, R. J. (1994). *Reducing risks for mental disorders: Frontiers for prevention intervention research.* Washington, DC: National Academy Press.

National Institute on Drug Abuse (1997). *Community readiness for drug abuse prevention: Issues, tips and tools.* Rockville, MD: U.S. Dept. of Health & Human Services, National Institutes of Health.

National Institute of Justice (2000). *1999 annual report on drug use among adult and juvenile arrestees.* Washington, DC: U.S. Department of Justice, Office of Justice Programs.

Newcomb, M. D., & Felix Ortiz, M. (1992). Multiple protective and risk factors for drug use and abuse: Cross-sectional and prospective findings. *Journal of Personality and Social Psychology, 63,* 280–296.

Newcomb, M. D., Maddahian, E., & Bentler, P. M. (1986). Risk factors for drug use among adolescents: Concurrent and longitudinal analyses. *American Journal of Public Health, 76,* 525–530.

Pentz, M. A. (2000). Institutionalizing community-based prevention through policy change. *Journal of Community Psychology, 28,* 257–270.

Pentz, M. A., MacKinnon, D. P., Flay, B. R., Hansen, W. B., Johnson, C. A., & Dwyer, J. H. (1989). Primary prevention of chronic diseases in adolescence: Effects of the Midwestern Prevention Project on tobacco use. *American Journal of Epidemiology, 130*, 713–724.

Pentz, M. A., Mihalic, S. F., & Grotpeter, J. K. (1997). The Midwestern Prevention Project. In D. S. Elliott (Series Ed.), *Blueprints for violence prevention* (Book 1). Boulder, CO: University of Colorado, Center for the Study and Prevention of Violence, Institute of Behavioral Science.

Perry, C. L., & Kelder, S. H. (1992). Models for effective prevention. *Journal of Adolescent Health, 13*, 355–363.

Perry, C. L., Kelder, S. H., & Komro, K. (1993). *The social world of adolescents: Family, peers, schools, and culture.* Washington, DC: Carnegie Council on Adolescents, Carnegie Corporation.

Perry, C. L., Williams, C. L., Forster, J. L., Wolfson, M., Wagenaar, A. C., Finnegan, J. R., McGovern, P. G., Veblen-Mortenson, S., Komro, K. A., & Anstine, P. S. (1993). Background, conceptualization and design of a community-wide research program on adolescent alcohol use: Project Northland. *Health Education Research, 8*, 125–136.

Perry, C. L., Williams, C. L., Komro, K. A., Veblen-Mortenson, S., Forster, J. L., Bernstein-Lachter, R., Pratt, L. K., Dudovitz, B., Munson, K. A., Farbakhsh, K., Finnegan, J., & McGovern, P. (2000). Project Northland high school interventions: Community action to reduce adolescent alcohol use. *Health Education and Behavior, 27*, 29–49.

Perry, C. L., Williams, C. L., Veblen Mortenson, S., Toomey, T. L., Komro, K. A., Anstine, P. S., McGovern, P. G., Finnegan, J. R., Forster, J. L., Wagenaar, A. C., & Wolfson, M. (1996). Project Northland: Outcomes of a communitywide alcohol use prevention program during early adolescence. *American Journal of Public Health, 86*, 956–965.

Peterson, A. V., Kealey, K. A., Mann, S. L., Marek, P. M., & Sarason, I. G. (2000). Hutchinson Smoking Prevention Project: Long-term randomized trial in school-based tobacco use prevention—results on smoking. *Journal of the National Cancer Institute, 92*, 1979–1991.

Pollard, J. A., Hawkins, J. D., & Arthur, M. W. (1999). Risk and protection: Are both necessary to understand diverse behavioral outcomes in adolescence? *Social Work Research, 23*, 145–158.

Rigotti, N. A., DiFranza, J. R., Chang, Y. C., Tisdale, T., Kemp, B., & Singer, D. E. (1997). The effect of enforcing tobacco-sales laws on adolescents' access to tobacco and smoking behavior. *New England Journal of Medicine, 337*, 1044–1051.

Robins, L. N., & Przybeck, T. R. (1985). Age of onset of drug use as a factor in drug use and other disorders. In C. L. Jones & R. J. Battjes (Eds.), *Etiology of drug abuse: Implications for prevention* (NIDA Research Monograph No. 56, pp. 178–192). Washington, DC: U.S. Government Printing Office.

Rutter, M. (1985). Resilience in the face of adversity: Protective factors and resistance to psychiatric disorder. *British Journal of Psychiatry, 147,* 598–611.

Schaps, E., Bartolo, R. D., Moskowitz, J., Palley, C. S., & Churgin, S. (1981). A review of 127 drug abuse prevention program evaluations. *Journal of Drug Issues, 11,* 17–43.

Scheier, L. M., & Botvin, G. J. (1998). Relations of social skills, personal competence, and adolescent alcohol use: A developmental exploratory study. *Journal of Early Adolescence, 18,* 77–114.

Spoth, R. L., Redmond, C., Haggerty, K., & Ward, T. (1995). A controlled parenting skills outcome study examining individual difference and attendance effects. *Journal of Marriage and the Family, 57,* 449–464.

Spoth, R. L., Redmond, C., & Shin, C. (2001). Randomized trial of brief family interventions for general populations: Adolescent substance use outcomes four years following baseline. *Journal of Consulting and Clinical Psychology, 69,* 627–642.

Substance Abuse and Mental Health Services Administration (1998). *Family-centered approaches: Prevention Enhancement Protocols Systems (PEPS).* Washington, DC: U.S. Government Printing Office.

Substance Abuse and Mental Health Services Administration (2000). *Summary of findings from the 1999 National Household Survey on Drug Abuse.* Rockville, MD: Author.

Substance Abuse and Mental Health Services Administration (2001). *Mid-year 2000 preliminary emergency department data from the Drug Abuse Warning Network.* Washington, DC: U.S. Department of Health and Human Services, Public Health Service.

Sussman, S., Dent, C. W., Stacy, A. W., & Sun, P. (1993). Project Towards No Tobacco Use: 1-year behavior outcomes. *American Journal of Public Health, 83,* 1245–1250.

Swisher, J. D. (1979). Prevention issues. In R. I. Dupont, A. Goldstein, & J. O'Donnell (Eds.), *Handbook on drug abuse* (pp. 49–62). Washington, DC: National Institute on Drug Abuse.

Szapocznik, J., Scopetta, M. A., & King, O. E. (1978). Theory and practice in matching treatment to the special characteristics and problems of Cuban immigrants. *Journal of Community Psychology, 6,* 112–122.

Tobler, N. S. (1994). Meta-analytical issues for prevention intervention research. In L. Seitz & L. Collins (Eds.), *Advances in data analysis for prevention intervention research* (NIDA Research Monograph No. 142, pp. 342–403). Washington, DC: U.S. Government Printing Office.

Tobler, N. S., Roona, M. R., Ochshorn, P., Marshall, D. G., Streke, A. V., & Stackpole, K. M. (2000). School-based adolescent drug prevention programs: 1998 meta-analysis. *Journal of Primary Prevention, 20,* 275–336.

Unger, J. B., Kipke, M. D., Simon, T. R., Montgomery, S., & Johnson, C. J. (1997). Homeless youths and young adults in Los Angeles: Prevalence of mental health problems and the relationship between mental health and substance abuse disorders. *American Journal of Community Psychology, 25,* 371–394.

Wagenaar, A. C., & Perry, C. L. (1994). Community strategies for the reduction of youth drinking: Theory and application. *Journal of Research on Adolescence, 4,* 319–345.

Wandersman, A., Morrissey, E., Davino, K., Seybolt, D., Crusto, C., Nation, M., Goodman, R., & Imm, P. (1998). Comprehensive quality programming and accountability: Eight essential strategies for implementing successful prevention programs. *Journal of Primary Prevention, 19,* 3–30.

Weissberg, R. P. (1990). Fidelity and adaptation: Combining the best of both perspectives. In P. Tolan, C. Keys, F. Chertok, & L. Jason (Eds.), *Researching community psychology: Issues of theory and methods* (pp. 186–189). Washington, DC: American Psychological Association.

Werner, E. E., & Smith, R. S. (1992). *Overcoming the odds: High-risk children from birth to adulthood.* Ithaca, NY: Cornell University Press.

PART III

Problems in Adulthood

CHAPTER 10

Preventing HIV and AIDS

Eric G. Benotsch and
Seth C. Kalichman

When first recognized, AIDS quickly became known as a global health crisis that would eventually affect everyone. However, over time AIDS has blended into the social fabric and has become removed from the consciousness of daily life for those who have not been affected directly. What were once outcries for public awareness and outrage over unresponsive public health officials have been replaced with AIDS complacency and apathy. The three decades since the first cases of AIDS were diagnosed have seen more than a million persons infected in North America and hundreds of thousands die (UNAIDS/WHO, 2000). We also have witnessed remarkable progress in the treatment of HIV infection, where combinations of potent medications can stall HIV disease processes and delay the onset of AIDS. There is no cure for HIV-AIDS, and a preventive vaccine remains a distant hope. Therefore, stemming the HIV epidemic can be achieved only through the practice of preventive behaviors by persons at risk for HIV infection.

This chapter reviews recent advances in prevention interventions aimed at reducing high-risk sexual behavior among groups at greatest risk for HIV infection. After a brief overview of the problem, we describe a conceptual model that provides a useful heuristic for understanding the mechanisms of HIV prevention interventions. We then summarize the approaches taken by theory-based HIV risk-reduction interventions delivered to individuals, groups, and communities. To provide greater detail on effective intervention strategies, we present a case example of an HIV risk-reduction intervention delivered to men at risk for HIV and other sexually transmitted diseases. We conclude with a discussion of future directions for HIV prevention.

DESCRIPTION OF THE PROBLEM

The best epidemiological evidence suggests that the first AIDS cases occurred in sub-Saharan Africa in the latter part of the 20th century, with the first recognized cases of AIDS diagnosed in 1981. At first believed to be a disease of young gay men and persons who share needles to inject drugs, we now understand AIDS to affect every group of persons on every continent. The World Health Organization (UNAIDS/WHO, 2000) estimates that more than 36 million people worldwide are infected with HIV, and more than 21 million people are known to have died of AIDS-related conditions. In many areas of the world, heterosexual contact remains the primary route of HIV transmission. However, HIV epidemics vary across populations and geographical regions. In the United States, for example, 47% of AIDS cases have occurred in men who have had sex with men, 31% of cases have occurred in persons who have injected drugs, and 10% of individuals diagnosed with AIDS have reported heterosexual contacts as their sole risk factor (Centers for Disease Control, 2000).

The vast majority of HIV infections are entirely preventable through behavioral change. HIV is a complex virus that is capable of evading immunological responses and preventive vaccines. Without a preventive vaccine in the foreseeable future, behavioral interventions to reduce the risk of HIV transmission offer our greatest hope for stemming the spread of HIV. Fortunately, progress in HIV prevention research demonstrates the effectiveness of theory-based behavioral interventions to reduce HIV transmission.

REVIEW AND CRITIQUE OF THE LITERATURE

Information-Motivation-Behavioral Skills (IMB) Model: A Heuristic for Understanding HIV Prevention Strategies

A number of theoretical models are available for understanding risky sexual behavior and structuring HIV prevention programs. The Information-Motivation-Behavioral skills (IMB) model, developed by Fisher and Fisher (1992), provides a valuable conceptual framework for understanding the correlates of HIV preventive behavior and offers guidance for the development of HIV primary prevention interventions. As its name implies, the IMB model focuses on the associations among the informational, motivational, and behavioral components of HIV preventive behavior.

According to the IMB model, individuals will engage in sustained HIV preventive behavior to the extent that they are informed, motivated, and have acquired the necessary behavioral skills. The IMB model specifies a set of causal relationships among the three interactive elements (see Fig. 10.1). Accurate information concerning HIV preventive behavior is a necessary prerequisite to engaging in risk reduction. Effective information includes not only accurate HIV preventive messages (e.g., "condom use can reduce HIV risk"), but also the absence of misinformation (e.g., "sex with a monogamous partner is always safe"). Motivation to engage in HIV preventive behavior is an additional prerequisite for behavioral risk reduction. According to the IMB model, motivation to reduce risk can be enhanced by increasing perceived vulnerability to HIV, other internal factors such as self-esteem and perceived control, and external motivating factors such as social approval for engaging in HIV preventive acts. The model holds that behavioral skills related to preventive acts are a final common pathway for information to result in AIDS preventive behavior change. The IMB model assumes that information and motivation activate behavioral skills to ultimately engage risk-reduction behaviors. The model also posits that information or motivation alone can have a direct effect on certain preventive behaviors. In the IMB model, behavioral skills become increasingly important when preventive actions require complex abilities, such as convincing a sex partner to use a condom. The IMB model also recognizes that risk behaviors occur within a social context that can impede or facilitate efforts to reduce risk.

The IMB model has been shown to predict specific risk-reduction practices across several at-risk populations (see Kalichman, 1998 for a review). The greatest strength of the IMB model is its direct articulation in HIV preventive interventions. Increases in information can be achieved through a variety of educational strategies, including the use of videotapes, didactic presentations, brochures, group discussions, and interactive games. Motivation is enhanced by changing attitudes and increasing the perceived personal relevance of AIDS. Recently, techniques adapted from motivational interviewing and motivational enhancement therapy developed by Miller, Zweben, DiClemente, and Rychtarik (1992) have been incorporated into AIDS preventive interventions to bolster the motivational component of HIV risk-reduction counseling (e.g., Belcher et al., 1998; Carey, Maisto, Kalichman, Forsyth, Wright, & Johnson, 1997; Kalichman, Cherry, & Brown-Sperling, 1999). Risk-reduction behavioral skills-building strategies have been the cornerstone of IMB model interventions. Skills building focuses on managing environmental cues for risk, personal correlates of risk, condom use, and sexual communication skills for negotiating safer sex. Finally, IMB model interventions integrate intervention activities into a meaningful and personally relevant context that is tailored and targeted to specific at-risk populations. The IMB intervention components have been successfully implemented in individual face-to-face counseling interventions, small-group workshop-style interventions, and risk-reduction strategies targeted to entire communities.

208

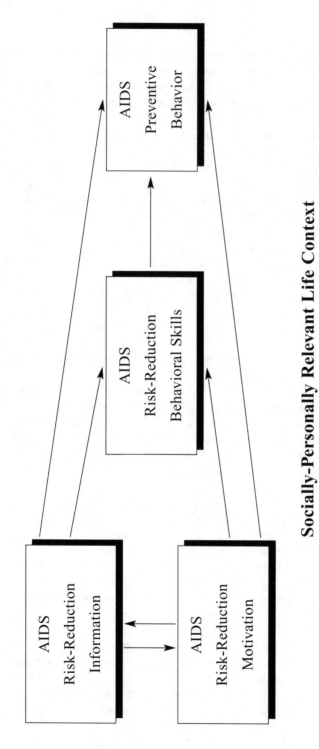

Socially-Personally Relevant Life Context

Figure 10.1 The Information-Motivation-Behavioral (IMB) skills model (Fisher & Fisher, 1992).

HIV Prevention Delivered to Individuals

A considerable body of research has evaluated the effectiveness of face-to-face interventions delivered to populations at risk for HIV infection. Individual-level interventions can resemble traditional public health education and counseling approaches, often encompassing a single encounter within a clinic setting. Alternately, individual-level interventions can consist of multiple sessions conducted over an extended period of time, such as in prevention case management and mental health care models. Most individual-level interventions have been structured around services for HIV antibody testing. Guidelines for HIV counseling and testing have been set forth by the Centers for Disease Control and Prevention (CDC) with the intent of incorporating counseling into the practices of facilities receiving public funds to provide HIV antibody testing services. When individuals appear for HIV testing at a public health clinic, they typically receive both pretest counseling and a posttest debriefing. Pretest counseling sessions are conducted immediately prior to blood collection, are typically brief in nature, and are focused on informed consent for the test. Pretest counseling may include a comprehensive personal assessment of sexual and drug use behaviors geared toward increasing awareness of actual risk and assuming responsibility for one's own behavior (Gerber et al., 1993). Ideally, posttest counseling incorporates at least some components of the IMB model, including providing information about HIV risk behaviors, furnishing the patient with individualized feedback on the risk of past behaviors, and helping the client develop a personalized risk-reduction plan that incorporates the use of relevant safer sex behavioral skills. Unfortunately, the ideal posttest counseling strategies are not the standard of practice. Rather, brief educational messages are the most common form of posttest counseling.

Research investigating the effectiveness of HIV counseling and testing as a risk reduction strategy has yielded mixed results. The effects of HIV counseling and testing have been examined in both naturalistic studies and in randomized field trials. Ross (1988) compared Australian men who received either counseling or testing, or both, and found that the combination resulted in greater risk reduction than either counseling or testing alone. Other studies also have suggested that the combination of counseling and HIV testing is more effective than counseling alone in reducing risk behaviors in men and women attending U.S. health clinics (Wenger, Linn, Epstein, & Shapiro, 1991), and in reducing risk behaviors in college students (Wenger et al., 1992). Research with other populations has not, however, consistently yielded positive findings. Caslyn, Saxon, Freeman, and Whitaker (1992) evaluated the effectiveness of HIV counseling and testing in reducing risk behaviors in injection-drug users and failed to find sustained behavioral changes. Similar negative findings have been reported for women attending public health clinics (Ickovics, Morrill, Beren, Walsh, & Rodin, 1994).

Weinhardt, Carey, Johnson, and Bickham (1999) completed a meta-analysis of 27 controlled studies investigating the effects of HIV counseling and testing on sexual risk behavior. This empirical review concluded that persons who test HIV positive are likely to reduce their unprotected intercourse and increase their use of condoms, but that counseling and testing does not result in sustained behavior change in people who test HIV negative. Thus, traditional, brief counseling and testing may be an effective prevention strategy for persons who test HIV positive, but does not appear to be effective for persons who test HIV negative.

As a result of the mixed evidence for behavioral effects of standard HIV counseling and testing, the CDC designed a large, multisite study of an enhanced HIV counseling intervention for use with HIV testing. Project RESPECT is the largest trial of an HIV risk-reduction intervention directed toward individual clients seen in one-on-one counseling services (Kamb et al., 1998). Participants in Project RESPECT were recruited from sexually transmitted disease (STD) clinics in five U.S. cities. The study randomly assigned, 5758 HIV negative men and women to receive one of three types of HIV counseling: (a) standard care control—one pretest and one posttest counseling session consisting of standard HIV information and education, (b) prevention counseling—one educational pretest counseling session and one posttest session of HIV risk-reduction counseling that included not only information but also techniques to increase participant risk perception, and (c) enhanced counseling—one educational pretest session and three posttest sessions of enhanced counseling that included risk-reduction information, exercises aimed at challenging risk-promoting beliefs, attitudes, and behavioral intentions, and behavioral skills-training activities. Results over a 12-month follow-up period showed that the enhanced counseling condition resulted in the greatest increases in condom use for both men and women (Kamb et al., 1998). However, participants in the two-session risk-reduction prevention counseling and the four-session enhanced counseling conditions both showed changes in HIV-risk behaviors and reduced rates of STDs compared with the standard care health education condition. These findings suggest that more intensive counseling delivered in a single post-test counseling session that includes all three of the components of the IMB model in conjunction with HIV testing can lead to reductions in HIV-risk behaviors.

In a smaller study that directly tested a brief counseling intervention derived from the IMB model, Belcher et aj. (1998) showed that a single two-hour risk-reduction counseling intervention effectively reduced high-risk sexual practices among women at risk for HIV and other STDs. Women recruited from an inner-city neighborhood in Atlanta were screened for high-risk behavior and randomly assigned to one of two conditions: (a) 2-hour HIV risk-reduction counseling based on the IMB model or (b) a 2-hour matched contact HIV information education session. The HIV risk-reduction counseling was based on Fisher and Fisher's (1992) IMB model. This intervention included the provision of personalized risk behavior feedback, individualized counseling around the personalized feedback, HIV risk and risk-reduction information, counseling to place personal risk behavior feedback in the context of risk information, communication skills training and behavioral rehearsal for negotiating safer sex and condom use with male partners, problem-solving situations in which partners are resistant to using condoms, managing risk situations including risk for violence and other negative repercussions of initiating condom use, and instruction in the correct use of male and female condoms. Women in the comparison intervention were exposed to information about HIV and STDs without the motivational and skills-building counseling components.

Outcome analyses showed that women in Belcher et al.'s (1998) HIV risk-reduction counseling intervention condition demonstrated significantly less unprotected vaginal intercourse and significantly greater condom use than women in the comparison condition. This study demonstrated significant effects of a 2-hour single session HIV risk-reduction counseling intervention. Using Cohen's (1988) d as a standardized index of effect size, the researchers found that the 2-hour counseling intervention demonstrated effects comparable to those found in interventions of much greater duration, participant burden, and expense.

HIV Prevention Delivered to Small Groups

In contrast to the relatively small number of HIV prevention trials undertaken at the one-on-one individual level, a much larger number of randomized, controlled trials have been conducted using small-group interventions. These rigorously conducted studies have demonstrated the effectiveness of small-group HIV risk-reduction interventions with diverse at-risk populations, including gay and bisexual men (Kelly, St. Lawrence, Hood, & Brasfield, 1989; Peterson et al., 1996; Roffman et al., 1998), women living in inner-cities (Carey et al., 1997; DiClemente & Wingood, 1995; Kalichman, Rompa, & Coley, 1996; Kelly et al., 1994), adolescents (Jemmott, Jemmott, & Fong, 1992; Rotheram-Borus, Koopman, Haignere, & Davies, 1991; St. Lawrence, Brasfield, Jefferson, Alleyne, & Shirley, 1995), inner-city health clinic patients (NIMH Multisite HIV Prevention Trial Group, 1998), homeless persons (Susser et al., 1995), persons with chronic mental illness (Kalichman, Sikkema, Kelly,

& Bulto, 1995), and military recruits in countries with high HIV incidence (Celentano et al., 2000).

Small-group interventions are typically intensive, involving several hours of face-to-face contact, and seek to facilitate interaction among participants. Despite the considerable diversity of populations with which small-group HIV prevention interventions have been studied, most published interventions have many common elements. In particular, group interventions emphasize collective experiences and encourage members to learn vicariously from each other. These interventions typically include information designed to dispel myths about HIV transmission and to increase participant knowledge about HIV prevention steps. Small-group interventions also have included components designed to enhance motivation for engaging in safer behaviors. In addition, an important component of most small-group interventions has been building behavioral skills necessary to implement risk-reduction plans. Key behavioral skills that have been incorporated into small-group interventions include identifying risky situations, developing strategies for coping with high-risk situations, direct training and performance rehearsal of proper condom use, sexual communication skills emphasizing talking to sexual partners about condom use, and assertiveness training to refuse unsafe sex. Special attention also is placed on tailoring small-group interventions to meet the unique needs and fit the social context of targeted populations.

The NIMH Multisite HIV Prevention Trial (1998) is the largest controlled small group intervention trial designed to test an HIV risk-reduction intervention. This investigation was conducted in STD clinics and inner-city health service settings in seven locations in six U.S. states. Overall, more than 3,700 persons deemed to be at risk for HIV and other STDs were included in the study and randomized to either a single-session AIDS education control group, or a seven-session small-group HIV risk-reduction intervention intended to produce changes in participant knowledge, motivation, and behavioral skills. The HIV prevention intervention employed information provision, group discussion, attitude change activities, communication skills training, and goal setting for behavioral changes between sessions. At 1-year follow-up, participants assigned to the HIV risk-reduction condition were more likely to consistently use condoms or to abstain from penetrative sexual activity. Using data from participants' clinic charts, it also was determined that participants in the HIV risk-reduction intervention were significantly less likely to experience a new STD during the follow-up period, relative to participants in the education-only control condition.

A considerable body of research has suggested that small-group interventions of the type described here are effective in reducing HIV risk behaviors in populations at high risk for HIV, including empirical reviews and meta-analyses (Kalichman & Hospers, 1997; Kalichman, Carey, & Johnson, 1997). Considering the intervention literature as a whole, several independent scientific review panels have concluded that small-group HIV risk-reduction interventions result in clinically significant changes in HIV risk behavior. The United States Office of Technology Assessment (1995), for example, concluded "Interventions developed through in-depth preliminary work with the target population that consist of small group programs that are interactive and include skills development, have been among the most successful at reducing risky sexual and drug-related behaviors" (p. 2). A strength of small-group interventions is the availability of manualized, intervention packages that embody IMB components tailored to the socially and personally relevant contexts of several at-risk populations.

There are, however, many challenges to implementing small-group interventions in community settings. Among the most significant limitations facing many small-group interventions are challenges to recruiting participants and high dropout rates. Research (Hoff et al., 1997) suggests that persons at highest risk for HIV infection are the least likely to attend intensive, community-based prevention programs. Small-group intervention studies with inner-city women have experienced significant rates of participant dropout, ranging from 38% (Kalichman, Carey, & Johnson, 1996) to 50% (Kelly et al., 1994). These high rates of attrition have occurred even in studies that provided participants with transportation, child care, and cash incentives for attendance. Participants' reluctance to attend groups and attrition from group interventions may be exacerbated by scheduling peoples' attendance at a given group session at a time when they have competing issues, such as unemployment, health care, housing, substance abuse, or coping with violent crime. Another potential source of attrition may be the reluctance of some persons to take part in potentially stigmatizing discussions of sexual behavior and drug use, particularly within the context of a peer group. Thus, there has been a movement toward delivering interventions to individuals in one-on-one counseling sessions or, alternately, toward intervention models that target entire communities.

HIV Prevention Delivered to Communities

Community-level interventions go beyond the face-to-face contact used in individual and small-group interventions to influence entire geographic regions and communities. These interventions seek to reduce the prevalence of HIV risk behaviors in a population or targeted segment of a population by bringing about community-wide changes in perceived social norms, risk awareness, attitudes, and perceived self-efficacy for behavior change. Community-level interventions can take many forms, including media campaigns, community outreach, and social influence models. Media-based interventions typically distribute brief prevention messages that deliver a simple bit of information or attract attention to shift attitudes or motivate change. Media-based interventions, therefore, are rarely capable of including all elements of the IMB model.

Outreach interventions occur in the natural environment, targeting the intervention to people who otherwise may not be exposed to HIV prevention messages. Outreach interventions do not impose a formal structure on their target populations. Rather, outreach occurs on the client's terms. Described as applied ethnography, outreach relies on unobtrusive infiltration of closed communities and participant-observer strategies for establishing trusting relationships with difficult-to-reach populations (Broadhead & Fox, 1990; Kotarba, 1990). The central feature of outreach interventions is the face-to-face contact between outreach workers and their contacts. In this sense, outreach is an individualistic intervention. However, because outreach interventions penetrate communities to achieve community-level change, outreach is conceptualized at the community level. Nevertheless, the face-to-face encounter is the mechanism of action in outreach interventions.

Outreach provides information and prevention materials such as condoms and bleach to at-risk persons in their natural environments. In most cases, populations that are otherwise hard to reach are identified and engaged by community health outreach workers. Outreach workers are trained to enter communities of known risk and become a trusted part of the environment (Watters & Guydish, 1994), without preaching, proselytizing, or judging their clients' behavior. Rather, outreach workers secure trusting relationships within the community and offer themselves as AIDS information and education resources. In using these strategies, outreach workers safely and effectively enter social systems to alter the course of the AIDS epidemic by becoming instruments of behavioral change. Therefore, in outreach programs the outreach worker implements elements of the IMB model within the context of encounters with at-risk persons in the natural environment.

The CDC AIDS Community Demonstration Projects Research Group (1999) undertook a large-scale trial of a community-level HIV prevention intervention in five U.S. cities. This project targeted a variety of different groups in each city, including intravenous drug users and their sexual partners, commercial sex workers, nongay-identified men who have sex with men, and high-risk youth. The intervention combined an outreach program with a media campaign. The outreach program utilized the use of "role model stories" that described how persons similar to the members of the target populations were changing their HIV risk behavior. The complementary media campaign presented similar role model stories in community newsletters and pamphlets. In addition, the outreach workers distributed condoms and bleaching kits. The results showed increased condom use with main and nonmain partners and increased carrying of condoms.

The most complete articulation of the IMB model in community level interventions has occurred in social influence interventions (Kelly et al. 1991; Kelly, St. Lawrence, Stevenson, & Hauth, 1992). Social influence interventions employ principles derived from diffusion of innovation theory (Rogers, 1983), which postulates that new behavioral trends in a social group can be initiated when popular, respected members of that group adopt and advocate for such changes. Social influence interventions identify key members of targeted groups and solicit them to participate as behavior change agents in their communities. Kelly et al. (1991, 1992) found that community-level social influence interventions produced significant changes in behavior and changed norms toward greater acceptance of safer sex practices. This intervention model consisted of three separate steps: (a) identification and recruitment of respected members ("popular opinion leaders") of the gay communities in three small southeastern U.S. cities, (b) training of popular opinion leaders to become risk-reduction behavioral change agents, and (c) dissemination of risk-reduction messages by popular opinion leaders to friends and other members of their social networks. Popular opinion leaders implemented the intervention by conversing with friends about risk reduction. These frequent conversational messages delivered by persons who were already known and respected by others in their social group constituted the intervention's active component.

Kelly et al. (1992) reported significant changes in each of three cities following implementation of the social influence intervention. The percentage of men in each city who reported engaging in unprotected receptive anal intercourse dropped significantly after the intervention. Similar changes were noted for insertive anal intercourse and total number of sex partners. In addition, social norms in each city changed to allow greater acceptance of safer sexual behavior. Kelly et al. (1997) replicated this intervention in gay bars in four small cities across four regions of the United States. The same intervention methods were used, but the replication utilized a randomized experimental design with four matched control cities. At 12-month follow-up, men in the intervention cities reported lower rates of unprotected anal intercourse. In addition, condom use during intercourse increased from 45% at baseline to 66% at follow-up in intervention cities, with no similar changes in control cities. Supplemental analyses indicated that men who came to the gay bar, which served as the intervention venue, more frequently showed greater reductions in risk behaviors, suggesting that changes were moderated by exposure to opinion leaders delivering the interventions.

Other research with gay and bisexual men has evaluated community-level HIV prevention interventions that incorporated elements of the popular opinion leader model but included additional components. Kegeles, Hays, and Coates (1996) reported on the effects of a program for young men that combined HIV prevention outreach by a group of popular opinion leaders with an HIV prevention media campaign and small-group risk-reduction sessions. The results again showed significant reductions in unprotected anal intercourse from baseline to post-intervention. This intervention study is important because it demonstrated the positive effects of a social influence model delivered to gay and bisexual men in a larger city (i.e., San Francisco) with a higher HIV prevalence rate than the cities where Kelly et al. (1991, 1997) intervened.

Community-level social influence interventions also have been shown to be effective in promoting HIV risk-reduction activities in women of lower socioeconomic status. Sikkema et al. (2000) implemented a social influence model in nine low-income, inner-city housing developments in five U.S. cities. Nine demographically matched housing units in the same cities served as controls. Control sites were provided with safer sex brochures and a coupon that could be redeemed for ten male condoms. The intervention condition included, besides these same materials, training women regarded as popular opinion leaders in risk reduction and encouraging these women to form "Women's Health Councils" and to recruit female friends to participate in risk-reduction workshops. The intervention also included assisting the Women's Health Councils to carry out community events designed to promote HIV risk reduction. Twelve-month follow-up results showed that the proportion of women reporting unprotected intercourse in the previous 2 months declined from 50% at baseline to 38% at follow-up, and the percentage of condom use during intercourse increased from 30% to 47%. For women who reported participating in at least one community event, increases in condom use were even more substantial. In addition, requests for condoms from the project staff were nearly twice as high for women living in the intervention housing developments compared with the control housing developments.

Taken as a whole, the literature supports the effectiveness of community-level interventions in promoting HIV risk-reduction behavior across diverse populations. A considerable strength of intervening at the community level is the ability of such programs to reach individuals who are unmotivated to attend facility-based programs or unable to invest the time and effort to complete an individual-level or small-group intervention.

CASE EXAMPLE

This case example describes a small-group intervention for inner-city African-American men based on the IMB model with enhanced motivational components, using techniques described by Miller, Zweben, DiClemente, and Rychtarik (1992) as adapted for HIV prevention (Carey et al., 1997). The educational, motivational, and skills-building components of the intervention relied on videotapes for implementation in an effort to increase the transportability of the intervention to community service agencies and health clinics. The intervention itself was delivered by community-based prevention service providers to further test its feasibility for technology transfer. Finally, the study used an experimental effectiveness trial design to test the effects of the intervention against a contact-matched alternative HIV prevention intervention that represented the community standard of care for HIV prevention education. The results of the intervention trial were reported by Kalichman, Cherry, and Brown-Sperling (1999).

The participants were 133 African-American men recruited from a county STD clinic. Because the intervention was tailored for heterosexual relations, men who reported only male sex partners in the three months prior to the baseline assessment ($n = 16$) were excluded. The participants were an average of 33 years old ($SD = 9.0$), and reported an average of 11.7 years of formal education ($SD = 1.9$). Ninety percent reported annual incomes under $20,000. The sample demonstrated risk for HIV infection and other STDs. Eighty-two percent of the men had been treated for an STD, 71% had exchanged sex for money or drugs, and 16% had both male and female sex partners in the previous three months. Substance use was also common: 85% of the sample had used alcohol, and more than 70% had used at least one other street drug in the previous three months.

Group sessions consisted of six to ten participants, led by one male and one female community-based service provider who served as group facilitators. The intervention required 6 hours of contact time, delivered in two 3-hour blocks. Both sessions were delivered in the same week; either Monday-Wednesday or Tuesday-Thursday. The participants were provided with snacks and lunch and received condoms after each group session.

Session 1: Information and Motivational Enhancement

The group facilitators introduced the intervention by explaining that the project was designed to inform people about AIDS and ways that they could protect themselves and others from the deadly virus that causes AIDS. They were told that the program had three main goals: (a) to educate people about AIDS and how it was affecting their community, (b) to bring groups of men together to share information and experiences about AIDS, and (c) to help people learn new ways to protect themselves and others from AIDS. Following brief introductions where each man said a little about himself, the facilitators initiated the information component of the intervention. They started with a group discussion that was stimulated by questions posed to the group such as: "What information have you heard about AIDS?," "Where did you hear it?," "Who is at risk for AIDS?," "How does AIDS affect people?", and "What are the ways that persons can protect themselves from AIDS?" This discussion led to the viewing of a 25-minute educational videotape that showed a group of men asking questions about AIDS that were answered by a female AIDS educator. The group viewed the video and then discussed the issues raised in the tape.

The group then participated in an "AIDS Myths and Facts" activity that used flash cards to distinguish between accurate and inaccurate information about AIDS. The participants were encouraged to explain why they believed the statement was either a myth or fact, and group members who disagreed about whether the statement was a myth or fact were asked to explain why. This often generated a lively discussion. Group facilitators provided accurate answers and moved the group along. Also, as part of the session's information component, the group participated in an activity that required it to conceptualize risk behaviors on a continuum and agree on relative levels of risk for a variety of sexual behaviors. This activity led to a discussion of condoms and how they protect against HIV and other STDs. In addition, the group identified sex behavior options that reduce risks, including not having sex, having sex without intercourse, and using condoms during sex. Problem-solving skills to implement these strategies also were discussed. The group ended by watching another videotape that was edited from existing educational tapes, including a video featuring basketball star Magic Johnson and celebrity Arsenio Hall.

The group then watched a video that showed five men infected with HIV, representing different transmission modes and stages of HIV disease. The group viewed the tape and discussed its content. The group facilitators tried to connect each of the participants to the men in the tape by exploring how they felt watching the tape. The tape was used as a bridge to discussion about what people could do to reduce their risks for HIV and other STDs.

Group members were then given personalized feedback forms, modeled after procedures designed by Carey et al. (1997), that reported back to them their own risk and protective behaviors based on the baseline assessment. This information was provided in the form of a private feedback report that was not shared with the group. The facilitators walked the group through the feedback report and asked each man to consider his own personal risks and the goals that he might have for reducing risk. In thinking about their personal risks, the participants explored their own situations that they believed put them at risk. Using a group process and brainstorming technique, the facilitators had the group generate situational characteristics, or "triggers," associated with risky situations. The group then was instructed in a problem-solving technique that could be used to manage situational triggers. Problem solving included: identifying the sexually risky situation and its triggers, identifying the goal for that situation, brainstorming alternative courses of action, evaluating choices, acting on the best choice, and walking through each step to address sexual risk-producing situations.

Session 2: Risk Reduction and Communication Skills Building

The group reviewed information presented in the first session, revisited the discussion of risky situations, and discussed condoms in the context of risk-reduction strategies. The facilitators then led a discussion of the "pros and cons of condoms." After working through various attitudes about condoms brought up by group members, the facilitators initiated the condom skills-building component of the intervention. First, the group viewed a videotape, "It's All About Condoms," that demonstrated condom application. Next, the facilitators demonstrated correct condom use on a wooden penis model. Group members then practiced applying and removing condoms with facilitator guidance and feedback from other group members. In-session behavioral rehearsal was the key element of condom-use skills building. Although the technical aspects of correct condom use were important, this activity served to desensitize the men to using condoms, reduce condom anxiety, and promote a positive attitude toward condoms. The group session ended with a brief review of how to identify risky situations and problem-solving triggers, and how to devise a plan for practicing safer sex that could include condom use.

The facilitators then led a discussion of what constituted sexual communication, both verbal and nonverbal, and why it was important. Communication skills building requires in-session practice accomplished through role playing. However, asking heterosexually identified men to role-play sexual situations with each other is quite challenging. To create realistic and meaningful situations that men could use to generate safer sex communication messages, the group facilitators used scenes identified from popular films to set up role plays. All of the scenes were from PG and R-rated motion pictures with African-American men and women, including *Boyz in the Hood*, *Jason's Lyric*, and *Rage in Harlem*. (The use of these movie clips in group settings for the purpose of education and without profit is legal under fair-use statutes.) Following a brief introduction by the facilitators to set up the scenes, the movie clips (2–3 minutes each) were shown one at a time. Scenes were stopped at predetermined points, and the participants were asked what the man in the scene could say or do at that moment to create a safer sex experience.

The seven movie clips were played, and the participants practiced communication skills as well as trigger identification and problem-solving skills for each scene. Viewing the scenes presented in the movie clips, the participants identified triggers in the situation, generated safer sex options, and stated a line that the man could have said to initiate condom use. Each movie clip was played through once and then repeated for skills practice.

The end of the session was dedicated to reviewing all of the information, motivation, and behavioral skills building that occurred in the intervention. Each participant was encouraged to discuss what he thought was most and least useful about the intervention, and the participants were reinforced for having come to the group and for making an effort to change their behavior to reduce risks for HIV and other STDs.

FUTURE DIRECTIONS

The HIV-AIDS behavioral prevention research conducted over the past decades represents progress in basic and applied prevention sciences. There remain, however, unanswered questions and many important avenues for future research. Here we consider three areas that we believe are important for future research: the transfer of HIV prevention technologies from science to practice, the development of interventions that can be implemented by community service providers, and the implementation of interventions that target people who know they are HIV infected.

Studies are Needed to Examine the Barriers to HIV Prevention Technology Transfer

Despite the successful testing of several behavioral risk-reduction interventions for populations that are vulnerable to HIV, there is little evidence that science-based interventions make their way into community practice. Interventions that do not fit community needs and lack personal relevance to targeted individuals will be rejected by community service providers. Interventions run the greatest risk of being irrelevant when they are handed down to front-line practitioners by an authoritarian system. Including practitioners in the planning and development of an intervention fosters community relevance. Traditional models of technology transfer offer the least opportunity for such collaborations, and are therefore at greatest risk for delivering irrelevant interventions. Research is needed to formally evaluate the channels through which prevention information and innovations flow to community-based services.

Theory-Based Behavioral Interventions That Have Maximum Utility in Community and Public Health Settings Are Needed

Since 1985 several theory-based behavioral interventions for HIV risk-reduction have been developed and tested in clinical studies. Comprehensive literature reviews conducted by governmental panels and published in peer-reviewed journals consistently have shown that behavioral risk-reduction interventions that are grounded in behavioral change theories demonstrate significant reductions in unprotected sexual acts and increased use of condoms. Unfortunately, these interventions usually require individuals to attend multiple small group sessions delivered independently of other clinical or community services. Although group intervention models are clearly promising, they have proven difficult to transfer to community and public health services. Among the most significant limitations facing many interventions are challenges to recruiting participants and high dropout rates. Research (e.g., Hoff, Kegeles, Acree, Stall, Paul, Ekstrand, et al., 1997) suggests that persons at highest risk for HIV infection are the least likely to attend intensive community-based prevention programs. The gap between research showing the effectiveness of cognitive-behavioral interventions and the state of prevention practice can be bridged by structuring effective intervention components into a format that can be more feasibly implemented in service delivery settings. Therefore, effective behavioral prevention intervention models that can and will be implemented in community services are urgently needed.

HIV Prevention Interventions Are Needed That Target People Who Know They Are HIV Infected

Research suggests that as many as one-third of HIV seropositive men who have sex with men engage in unprotected anal intercourse, and the rate of risky sex among seropositive men may not be any less than that observed among seronegative men. Given the risks posed by even a single unprotected sex act with an HIV infected partner, interventions must offer maximum promise for establishing long-term risk reduction. In addition, in order to offer transferable and sustainable prevention technologies, interventions must be developed in collaboration with community members and existing service delivery systems. A review of the scientific literature suggests that there are a number of factors that are plausible correlates of continued risk behavior among seropositive persons. Studies of continued sexual-risk behavior in seropositive men have concentrated on frequencies of high- and low-risk sex acts as well as predictors of sexual risk practices. Identified risk correlates among seropositive men include relationship types, economic conditions, affective states, substance use, and behavioral disinhibition. In addition, self-disclosure of HIV serostatus is an important stressor for seropositive persons and has direct implications for their own and their partner's safety. These and other factors are potentially important in addressing the next generation of HIV prevention interventions—those designed for people who know they are HIV infected.

Our survey of the field suggests that considerable progress has been made in the behavioral science of HIV prevention. There is good evidence that theory-based prevention efforts reduce risk behavior, prevent new HIV infections, and save lives. Multiple intervention modalities have shown promise, including individual, face-to-face interventions, interventions implemented with small groups of people, and interventions targeted at entire communities. Although behavioral science has advanced tremendously since the early AIDS epidemic, more work remains to be done. Interventions that are practical and feasible for adoption by community-service agencies are especially needed. Continued refinement and increasing sophistication of intervention techniques coupled with increased attention to adaptability in community settings will help combat a disease that, despite 20 years of effort, continues unnecessarily to claim too many lives.

ACKNOWLEDGMENT

Preparation of this chapter was supported by National Institute of Mental Health (NIMH) Grant R01-MH61672 and Center Grant P30 MH52776. Correspondence should be addressed to Seth C. Kalichman, Center for AIDS Intervention Research (CAIR), Medical College of Wisconsin, 8701 Watertown Plank Road, Milwaukee, WI 53226, Phone (414) 456-7728, Fax (414) 287-4209, E-mail sethk@mcw.edu

REFERENCES

Belcher, L., Kalichman, S. C., Topping, M., Smith, S., Emshoff, J., Norris, F., & Nurss, J.A. (1998). Randomized trial of a brief HIV risk-reduction counseling intervention for women. *Journal of Consulting and Clinical Psychology, 66*, 856–861.

Broadhead, R. S., & Fox, K. J. (1990). Takin' it to the streets: AIDS outreach as ethnography. *Journal of Contemporary Ethnography, 19*, 322–348.

Carey, M. P., Maisto, S. A., Kalichman, S. C., Forsyth, A. D., Wright, E. M., & Johnson, B. T. (1997). Enhancing motivation to reduce risk of HIV infection for economically disadvantaged urban women. *Journal of Consulting and Clinical Psychology, 65,* 531–541.

Caslyn, D. A., Saxon, A., Freeman, G., & Whittaker, S. (1992). Ineffectiveness of AIDS education and HIV antibody testing in reducing high-risk behaviors among injection drug users. *American Journal of Public Health, 82,* 573–575.

Celentano, D. D., Bond, K. C., Lyles, C. M., Eivmtrakul, S., Go, V. F. L., Beyrer, C., Chainacong, C., Nelson, K. E., Khamboonrung, C., & Vaddhanaphuti, C. (2000). Prevention intervention to reduce sexually transmitted infections: A field trial in the Royal Thai Army. *Archives of Internal Medicine, 160,* 535–540.

Centers for Disease Control AIDS Community Demonstration Projects Research Group. (1999). Community-level HIV intervention in five cities: final outcome data from CDC AIDS community demonstration projects. *American Journal of public Health,* 89, 336–345.

Centers for Disease Control (2000). U.S. HIV and AIDS cases reported through June 2000. *Surveillance Report, 12.*

Cohen, J. (1987). *Statistical Power Analysis.* (2nd ed.). Hillsdale, NJ: Erlbaum.

DiClemente, R. J., & Wingood, G. M. (1995). A randomized controlled trial of an HIV sexual risk reduction intervention for young African American women. *Journal of the American Medical Association, 274,* 1271–1276.

Gerber, A. R., Valdiserri, R. O., Holtgrave, D. R., Jones, S., West, G. R., Hinman, A. R., & Curran, J. W. (1993). Preventive services guidelines for primary care clinicians caring for adults and adolescents infected with the Human Immunodeficiency Virus. *Archives of Family Medicine, 2,* 969–979.

Hoff, C. C., Kegeles, S., Acree, M., Stall, R., Paul, J., Ekstrand, M., & Coates, T. (1997). Looking for men in all the wrong places...: HIV prevention small group programs do not reach high risk gay men. *AIDS, 11,* 829–831.

Ickovics, J. R., Morril, A. C., Beren, S. E., Walsh, U., & Rodin, J. (1994). Limited effects of HIV counseling and testing for women: A prospective study of behavioral and psychological consequences. *Journal of the American Medical Association, 272,* 443–448.

Jemmott, J. B., Jemmott, L. S., & Fong, G. T. (1992). Reduction in HIV risk-associated sexual behavior among Black male adolescents: Effects of an AIDS prevention intervention. *American Journal of Public Health, 82,* 372–377.

Kalichman, S. C. (1998). *Preventing AIDS: Sourcebook for behavioral interventions.* Hillsdale, NJ: Erlbaum.

Kalichman, S. C., Carey, M. P., & Johnson, B. T. (1996). Prevention of sexually transmitted HIV infection: Meta-analytic review and critique of the theory-based intervention outcome literature. *Annals of Behavioral Medicine, 18*, 6–15.

Kalichman, S. C., Cherry, C., & Brown-Sperling, F. (1999). Effectiveness of a video-based motivational skills-building HIV risk-reduction intervention for inner-city African American men. *Journal of Consulting and Clinical Psychology, 67*, 959–966.

Kalichman, S. C., & Hospers, H. (1997). Efficacy of behavioral skills enhancement HIV risk-reduction interventions in community settings. *AIDS, 11 (Suppl A)*, S191–S199.

Kalichman, S. C., Rompa, D., & Coley, B. (1996). Experimental component analysis of a behavioral HIV/AIDS prevention intervention of inner-city women. *Journal of Consulting and Clinical Psychology, 64*, 687–693.

Kalichman, S. C., Sikkema, K. J., Kelly, J. A., & Bulto, M. (1995). Use of a brief behavioral skills intervention to prevent HIV infection among chronically mentally ill adults. *Psychiatric Services, 46*, 275–280.

Kamb, M. L., Fishbein, M., Douglas, J. M., Rhodes, F., Rogers, J., Bolan, G., Zenilman, J., Hoxworth, T., Malotte, K., Iatesta, M., Kent, C., Lentz, A., Graziano, S., Byers, R. H., Peterman, T. A., & Project RESPECT Study Group (1998). Efficacy of risk-reduction counseling to prevent human immunodeficiency virus and sexually transmitted diseases. *Journal of the American Medical Association, 280*, 1161–1167.

Kegeles, S. M., Hays, R. B., & Coates, T. J. (1996). The Mpowerment Project: A community-level HIV prevention intervention for young gay men. *American Journal of Public Health, 86*, 1129–1136.

Kelly, J. A., Murphy, D. A., Sikkema, K. J., McAuliffe, T., Roffman, R. A., Solomon, L. J., Winett, R. A., & Kalichman, S. C. (1997). Randomised, controlled, community-level HIV-prevention intervention for sexual-behaviour among homosexual men in U.S. cities. *Lancet* 350:1500–1505.

Kelly, J. A., Murphy, D. A., Washington, C. D., Wilson, T. A., Koob, J. J., Davis, D. R., Ledezma, G., & Davantes, B. (1994). The effects of HIV/AIDS intervention groups for high-risk women in urban clinics. *American Journal of Public Health, 84*, 1918–1922.

Kelly, J. A., St. Lawrence, J. S., Diaz, Y. E., Stevenson, L. Y., Hauth, A. C., Brasfield, T. L., Kalichman, S. C., Smith, J. E., & Andrew, M. E. (1991). HIV risk behavior reaction following intervention with key opinion leaders of a population: An experimental analysis. *American Journal of Public Health, 81*, 168–171.

Kelly, J. A., St. Lawrence, J. S., Hood, H. V., & Brasfield, T. L. (1989). Behavioral intervention to reduce AIDS risk activities. *Journal of Consulting and Clinical Psychology, 57*, 60–67.

Kelly, J. A., St. Lawrence, J. S., Stevenson, Y. L., & Hauth, A. C. (1992). Community AIDS/HIV risk reduction: The effects of endorsements by popular people in three cities. *American Journal of Public Health, 82*, 1483–1489.

Kotarba, J. A. (1990). Ethnography and AIDS: Returning to the streets. *Journal of Contemporary Ethnography, 19*, 259–270.

Miller, W. R., Zweben, A., DiClemente, C., & Rychtarik, R. (1992). *Motivational enhancement therapy manual* (DHHS Publication No. ADM 92–1894). Washington, DC: U.S. Government Printing Office.

National Institute of Mental Health Multisite HIV Prevention Trial Group (1998). The NIMH multisite HIV prevention trial: Reducing HIV sexual risk behavior. *Science, 280*, 1889–1894.

Office of Technology Assessment (1995). *The effectiveness of AIDS prevention efforts*, Washington, DC: American Psychological Association Office on AIDS.

Peterson, J. L., Coates, T. J., Catania, J., Hauck, W. W., Acree, M., Daigle, D., Hillard, B., Middleton, L., & Hearst, N. (1996). Evaluation of an HIV risk reduction intervention among African-American homosexual and bisexual men. *AIDS, 10*, 319–325.

Roffman, R. A., Picciano, J. F., Ryan, R., Beadnell, B., Fisher, D., Downey, L., & Kalichman, S. C. (1997). HIV prevention group counseling delivered by telephone: An efficacy trail with gay and bisexual men. *AIDS & Behavior, 1*, 137–154.

Rogers, E. M. (1983). *Diffusion of innovations*. New York: Free Press.

Ross, M. W. (1988). Attitudes toward condoms as AIDS prophylaxis in homosexual men: Dimensions and measurement. *Psychology and Health, 2*, 291–299.

Rotheram-Borus, M. J., Koopman, C., Haignere, C., & Davies, M. (1991). Reducing HIV sexual risk behaviors among runaway adolescents. *Journal of the American Medical Association, 266*, 1237–1241.

Sikkema, K. J., Kelly, J. A., Winett, R. A., Solomon, L. J., Cargill, V. A., Roffman, R. A., McAuliffe, T. L., Heckman, T. G., Anderson, E. A., Wagstaff, D. A., Norman, A. D., Perry, M. J., Crumble, D. A., & Mercer, M. B. (2000). Outcomes of a randomized community-level HIV prevention intervention for women living in 18 low-income housing developments. *American Journal of Public Health, 90*, 57–63.

St. Lawrence, J. S., Brasfield, T. L., Jefferson, K. W., Alleyene, E., & Shirley, A. (1995). Cognitive-behavioral intervention to reduce African American adolescents for HIV infection. *Journal of Consulting and Clinical Psychology, 63*, 221–237.

Susser, E., Valencia, E., Miller, M., Tsai, W. Y., Meyer-Bahlburg, H., & Conover, S. (1995). Sexual behavior of homeless mentally ill men at risk for HIV. *American Journal of Psychiatry, 152*, 583–587.

UNAIDS/WHO (2000). *AIDS epidemic update: December 2000*. Geneva: Author.

United States Office of Technology Assessment. (1995). The effectiveness of AIDS prevention efforts. (OTA Publication No. OTA-BP-H-172). Washington D.C.: Government Printing Office.

Watters, J. K., & Guydish, J. (1994). HIV AIDS prevention for drug users in natural settings. In R. S. Diclemente & J. L. Peterson (ed.), Preventing AIDS: Theories and Methods of Behavirol Intervention.

Weinhardt, L. S., Carey, M. P., Johnson, B. T., & Bickham, N. L. (1999). Effects of HIV counseling and testing on sexual risk behavior: A meta-analytic review of published research, 1985–1997. *American Journal of Public Health, 89,* 1397–1405.

Wenger, N. S., Greenberg, J. M., Hilborne, L. H., Kusseling, F., Mangotich, M., & Shapiro, M. F. (1992). Effect of HIV antibody testing and AIDS education on communication about HIV risk and sexual behavior. *Annals of Internal Medicine, 117,* 905–911.

Wenger, N. S., Linn, L., Epstein, M., & Shapiro, M. (1991). Reduction of high-risk sexual behavior among heterosexuals undergoing HIV antibody testing: A randomized clinical trial. *American Journal of Public Health, 81,* 1580–1585.

CHAPTER 11

Preventing Chronic Health Problems

Joel A. Minden and
Leonard A. Jason

DESCRIPTION OF THE PROBLEM

According to data gathered by the Centers for Disease Control and Prevention (CDC, 2000a), the four leading causes of death in this country are heart disease, cancer, stroke, and chronic lung disease. The CDC has estimated that chronic diseases such as these affect over 90 million Americans and account for 70% of deaths in the United States. In addition to the significant health consequences, chronic illness is a financial burden, with the medical expenses of individuals with chronic diseases accounting for more than 60% of the nation's medical care costs (Institute for the Future, 2000). Given the significance of chronic health problems in this country, it is appropriate that a chapter focusing on chronic health problems be included in this volume, broadening the types of preventive interventions reviewed in the editors' previous book on health promotion (Glenwick & Jason, 1993).

Although the problem of chronic medical illness is widespread, the development of such problems among Americans is not inevitable. By identifying risk factors and eliminating causal links, there is some potential for disease prevention. The difficulty lies in selecting from among the numerous predictors of chronic disease the factors that both influence disease development and are modifiable through intervention. For example, for the various forms of cancer, risk factors include family history, height, exposure to radiation, tobacco, aspirin, air and water pollutants, alcohol, age at first intercourse,

227

sexually transmitted diseases, sun exposure, and socioeconomic status (Golditz et al., 2000). Yet the extent to which these risk factors are causal and what constitutes suitable intervention targets varies considerably.

The CDC (2000b) estimated that "lifestyle behaviors alone contribute to 50% of an individual's health status," and McGinnis and Foege (1993) reported that smoking, poor diet, and lack of exercise are the three leading actual causes of death in the United States. Since an entire chapter in this book is devoted to tobacco, alcohol, and other substance abuse prevention, this chapter focuses exclusively on interventions targeting diet and exercise. There is a large body of research supporting the importance of diet and exercise in the prevention of chronic health problems. For example, in their review of epidemiologic data, the Centers for Disease Control and Prevention and the American College of Sports Medicine argued that a causal link between inactivity and chronic heart disease is clearly supported in the literature (Pate et al., 1995). Pate et al. (1995, p. 406) concluded that "(1) caloric expenditure and total time of physical activity are associated with reduced cardiovascular disease incidence and mortality; (2) there is a dose-response relationship for this association, (3) regular moderate physical activity provides substantial health benefits; and (4) intermittent bouts of physical activity, as short as 8–10 minutes, totaling 30 minutes or more on most days provide beneficial health and fitness effects." In addition to the role of lifestyle factors in the development of cardiovascular disease, the Food and Nutrition Science Alliance (FANSA, 1999) estimated that one-third of cancer cases can be attributed to poor diet and lack of exercise.

The likelihood of developing cancer or heart disease is dramatically reduced if one participates in regular aerobic exercise and consumes a diet that is high in fruits, vegetables, and whole grains and low in saturated fats and refined, processed food (CDC, 2000b). Furthermore, among those who have developed chronic health problems, lifestyle changes can result in a reduction of symptoms or disease elimination (CDC, 2000b). Nevertheless, despite the overwhelming and consistent evidence of the importance of eating habits and physical activity in the development of chronic disease, the significant impact of chronic health problems in this country suggests that Americans are neglecting to modify diet and exercise behaviors for their preventive benefits.

The fields of community psychology and public health have much to contribute to the prevention of chronic illness. This chapter reviews published innovative strategies for preventing chronic health problems through interventions targeting diet and exercise. Strategies were considered to be innovative if they were prevention focused, cost-effective, and directed toward groups in natural environments, rather than toward individuals in medical or other health settings. All studies reported behavioral outcome data, rather than changes in knowledge exclusively, and had been published in the previous 10 years. In addition to these global criteria, studies were categorized based on whether they had a youth-directed or media-based format.

REVIEW AND CRITIQUE OF THE LITERATURE

Youth-Directed Interventions

Results from the 1999 Youth Risk Behavior Survey (YRBS), a school-based assessment of high school students, indicated that 70% of youths surveyed ate fewer than five servings of fruits and vegetables on the previous day, 35% participated in vigorous physical activity on fewer than three of the previous seven days, and 70% did not attend physical education class daily (CDC, 2000c).

These data suggest that identifying risk factors and promoting changes in dietary and exercise behaviors among young people may make the onset of some chronic diseases less likely. Children and adolescents who adopt healthy behaviors are more likely to maintain those behaviors as adults. The relationship between young adult and future exercise behavior was demonstrated in a longitudinal study (Schnurr, Vaillant, & Vaillant, 1990) of Harvard University students that found that physical activity in young adulthood predicted adult exercise frequency, even among men in their 50s and 60s.

The Pawtucket Heart Health Program (PHHP) aimed to encourage community-wide involvement in a cardiovascular disease prevention program (Carleton et al., 1991). The Heart Healthy Cook-Off was a PHHP-sponsored program designed to influence adolescents' food preferences, knowledge about food, and food preparation skills. Junior high and high school students learned about the relationship between certain dietary risk factors and cardiovascular disease and then were given the chance to have their cholesterol measured and assessed. After assessment, counseling was offered to help students improve their eating behaviors. Students then participated in the Heart Healthy Cook-Off, a contest in which they designed and prepared meals that follow specific guidelines for fat and sodium content. Meals were judged for nutritional value and adherence to content guidelines. The top three students in each food category won prizes such as chef's hats, aprons, and T-shirts, and all participants received certificates of appreciation. Carleton et al. (1991) compared the cholesterol levels of students before and after participating in the Heart Healthy Cook-Off. Among those with elevated blood cholesterol levels prior to the beginning of the program, the mean blood cholesterol level decreased by 10.7% upon completion of the cook-off.

The San Diego Family Health Project (Atkins et al., 1990) is another program that attempted to improve cardiovascular health by encouraging risk-reducing dietary habits and physical activity. In this study, Mexican-American and White families of fifth- and sixth-grade students participated in the program. Families attended 12 weekly sessions followed by six maintenance sessions. The first 10 weekly sessions focused on self-monitoring, physical activity, and sodium and fat intake. Week 11 was a review session, and Week 12 was a potluck dinner where families brought heart healthy foods. The six maintenance sessions helped families deal with lifestyle problems associated with high-risk behavior. The results revealed that attendance at the program meetings was positively related to greater knowledge of health facts and to exercise behavior, and negatively related to blood pressure.

Citing national trends of low in-school activity as a rationale, the Sports, Play, and Active Recreation for Kids (SPARK) program (Sallis, McKenzie, Alcaraz, Kolody, Faucette, & Hovell, 1997) in Poway, California, was an effort to increase physical activity levels among fourth- and fifth-grade students at home and school. Seven elementary schools were targeted. In two schools, students participated in the SPARK curriculum led by a physical education specialist, in another two schools the same SPARK curriculum was presented by regular classroom teachers, and the final three schools received standard physical education instruction and served as comparison schools. Sessions were held for 30 minutes, three days each week. They aimed at increasing both health-related (e.g., aerobic exercise) and skill-related (e.g., basketball) activity levels through lessons that progressed in intensity and complexity. Once each week, students also developed self-management skills and set fitness goals in a 30-minute class. Initially, until students developed self-management skills, small prizes were awarded to those who met weekly goals. The results indicated that students participating in the SPARK curriculum received more physical education classes overall and spent more minutes engaged in exercise during physical education classes than those in the comparison schools. Regarding activity levels outside of school, however, there were no differences among the groups. Effects of the intervention on fitness outcomes were mixed. Girls in the specialist-led classes ran the mile one minute faster and were able to do more sit-ups than those in the comparison classes. There were no differences among the girls' groups on three other measures of fitness, and no differences among the boys' groups on all five fitness measures. The authors argued that perhaps the self-management techniques were difficult to learn or implement for the students and that high baseline levels of extracurricular sports or exercise involvement may have had an impact on the extent to which out-of-school activity levels could increase.

The Washington Heights-Inwood Healthy Heart Program focused in part on reducing saturated fat intake through the selection of reduced-fat milk (Wechsler, Basch, Zybert, & Shea, 1998). The study was developed as a response to the high rate of saturated fat intake, due to the consumption primarily of whole milk, among Latino children in the New York City area. Six largely Latino elementary schools in New York City participated, with three receiving an intervention bolstered by advertising techniques and entertaining education, and three control schools receiving no intervention. All schools gave children the choice of whole or reduced-fat milk. Children in the intervention schools participated in a session in the school auditorium, advertised for two weeks in posters placed throughout the schools. The session featured a cartoon character cow performing in costume and appearing on educational materials as a symbol promoting low-fat milk consumption. Students viewed a presentation given by the costumed performer, participated in low-fat milk taste tests, and competed in games and contests for prizes such as T-shirts and magnets. Comparisons of 5-day average milk selections immediately following the intervention revealed large increases in low-fat milk consumption for the intervention schools compared with the control schools, with these differences remaining during a 3- to 4-month follow-up period.

Gimme 5 was a multicomponent intervention aimed at increasing fruit, juice, and vegetable intake among fourth and fifth graders in 16 southeastern elementary schools (Baranowski, Davis, Resnicow, Baranowski, Doyle, Lin et al., 2000). Prior to the development of the intervention, focus groups were conducted with children, parents, and school personnel to identify barriers to children's fruit, vegetable, and juice consumption. The most frequently noted barriers were the lack of availability of these foods in the home; children's dislike of fruits, vegetables, and juices; and the absence of healthy food preparation skills. These barriers were important intervention targets. After being matched on demographic characteristics, eight schools received treatment, and eight served as control schools. Students in the treatment schools received 45- to 55-minute curricula, twice weekly, for 6 weeks. The pupils' primary teachers presented the material following a 1-day training session. Focus areas included skill building, such as asking for fruits and vegetables at home or at restaurants, food preparation techniques, tasting food in class, and setting goals to increase fruit and vegetable consumption. Prizes could be won for meeting goals. In addition to the school curriculum, newsletters and videos were sent home so parents could encourage dietary change and reinforce what the students learned in school. Finally, families were encouraged to attend evening workshops on produce selection, tasting, and preparation in local grocery stores. Following the intervention, students completed a food diary for one week. The results revealed significant group by time interactions in the expected direction. Those in the schools receiving treatment maintained a relatively consistent intake of fruits, juices, and vegetables, while consumption in the control groups declined over the study period. Although the effects were small, it should be noted that treatment fidelity was compromised because teachers in the study provided fewer than 50% of planned lessons.

The National Cancer Institute funded the 5-a-Day Power Plus program (Perry, Bishop, Taylor, Murray, Mays, Dudovitz et al., 1998) in an attempt to increase fruit and vegetable consumption among fourth- and fifth-grade students. The pupils in the program were attending 20 elementary schools in St. Paul, Minnesota. Of the 20 schools, ten were assigned to intervention conditions during the spring of the fourth-grade year and the autumn of the fifth-grade year. The other ten schools, matched to the original ten schools by demographic characteristics, served as the control schools. The classroom intervention consisted of twice weekly in-class sessions for eight weeks. The curriculum focused on comic book and adventure story characters. In addition, individual and team competitions with prizes were held, food preparation skills were developed, and students participated in taste testing. Parents participated in assignments and food preparation activities with the children at home. For each home activity, parents signed a card that would enter the child into a classroom drawing. The intervention also included food service components, such as increasing the visibility and variety of fruit and vegetable items. Finally, industry involvement was maintained by a local supplier of produce and other businesses that presented lectures to all students and provided food for the classroom activities and take home snacks. In the winter of the fifth-grade year, follow-up comparisons revealed that greater proportions of fruits and vegetables were consumed (a) during school lunch hours, (b) during the previous 24 hours, and (c) in general by students receiving the intervention than by those in the control settings.

Several program characteristics emerge consistently from this review of youth-directed diet and exercise programs. These components include health education, knowledge-building or activity-driven competitions with prizes or incentives, self-management skill development with goal setting, and advertising campaigns. Although these interventions are promising, the effect sizes were generally small. This may be due, in some instances, to low treatment fidelity. Another explanation may be that most of the aforementioned programs focused primarily on health education, physical education, food service programs, and other aspects of the school already directed toward diet and exercise. Wechsler, Devereaux, Davis, and Collins (2000) suggested additional, but often overlooked, school-related characteristics that may be important to consider as potential intervention components. For example, recess periods, intramural sports, and alternative foods (e.g., vending machines) deserve more exploration as plausible chronic disease prevention program elements.

Media-Based Programming

Both mass and minor media (e.g., mailings, computers) are ideal for conveying positive health promotion messages to communities (Jason, Crawford, &

Gruder, 1989). In addition to being cost-effective, media-based approaches allow for the portrayal of role models engaging in a target behavior, they bring community members and the media together, and they benefit the public reputations of both the media and the program's administrators (Jason, 1998).

The National Heart Foundation (NHF) of Australia initiated two mass-media campaigns in consecutive years to increase exercise behavior, specifically brisk walking (Owen, Bauman, Booth, Oldenburg, & Magnus, 1995). Using the slogans "Exercise: Make it part of your day" in the first year, and "Exercise: Take another step" in the following year, citizens were exposed to nationally delivered educational messages on radio and television and in newspapers and magazines. Celebrities and health experts publicly endorsed the campaign's messages, and advertisements featuring the slogans and other educational messages were made through posters, brochures, stickers, and clothing. Television coverage also was supported by messages presented in the scripts of two popular television shows. In addition, these national efforts were bolstered by community-level activities organized by NHF offices in each state. In each study year, the campaigns lasted four weeks. To evaluate changes in behavior and intent as well as recognition of media exposure, 2500 participants were interviewed in their homes 2 weeks before and 3 to 4 weeks following the media campaigns. During both study years, participants were more likely to report being exposed to exercise messages in the media following the campaigns. In the first study year, significant post-campaign increases in walking prevalence for participants greater than 40 years old was revealed, but these differences were not present in the second year. There was also a minor increase in intentions to exercise following the campaign in the first year, but there were no differences following the second campaign.

A mass media approach also was taken to encourage the consumption of reduced-fat milk in the 1% Or Less campaign in West Virginia (Reger, Wootan, & Booth-Butterfield, 1999). Residents of Wheeling were targeted by the media campaign, and residents of Parkersburg served as the control community, receiving no intervention. Both cities had populations of approximately 35,000, with each having a distinctive (i.e., not overlapping) media market. In Wheeling, over a 6-week period, approximately 400 advertisements were placed on television and radio and in newspapers. In addition, a public relations campaign, consisting of a press conference, press releases, and taste tests, was held to increase media coverage. Random telephone surveys were conducted, and supermarket milk sales data were collected. The surveys revealed that more than 80% of the interviewed residents in the intervention community had been exposed to 1% or less advertisements or news coverage. In Wheeling, low-fat milk sales increased from 29% 1 month before the intervention to 46% the month after the intervention, and remained at 42% 6 months after the intervention; no changes in milk sales were evident in Parkersburg. In addition, the telephone surveys revealed a significant change in the proportion of residents in the intervention community who switched from high- to low-fat milk, but no change in the control community.

The Health Education Board for Scotland sponsored a national media campaign to encourage physically inactive people to begin walking for exercise (Wimbush, MacGregor, & Fraser, 1998). Targeting 30- to 55-year-old sedentary men and women, a 40-second television commercial was presented in numerous markets across the country for 4 weeks in the autumn and 4 weeks in the spring. The ad showed a popular retired professional athlete endorsing walking as a form of exercise equal to more strenuous activities in its fitness-promoting effects. The television spot also included a phone number for a service called Fitline, which provided additional information about walking. Fitline callers were able to request a free packet of information about adopting an exercise program, the health benefits of walking, and finding walking groups in their area. In addition, local radio stations presented programs on walking that featured community residents. Among a random sample of adults, recognition of the television and radio ads and the Fitline service was approximately 70% greater following the interventions than in the months in which no media coverage was available. General population surveys did not reveal changes in exercise behavior. However, among those using the Fitline service, comparisons with baseline surveys prior to the first ad revealed that, at both ten weeks and one year following the baseline survey, approximately half of the callers had increased their levels of physical activity. Of those who reported engaging in more frequent exercise, 86% reported increases in walking.

In Victoria, Australia, the 2 Fruit 'n' 5 Veg Every Day program, coordinated by the Victorian Health Promotion Foundation, used mass media advertising to promote fruit and vegetable consumption (Dixon, Borland, Segan, Stafford, & Sindall, 1998). The name of the program served as the campaign slogan in an effort to increase public knowledge about the minimum number of fruit and vegetable servings one should consume each day. During the 4 years of the campaign, consumer-directed television commercials were aired for 3 weeks in each of the first 2 years and for 1 week in the 3rd year. The majority of televised commercials were intended to be entertaining and comedic, and all depicted the health benefits of eating fruits and vegetables. To a lesser extent, radio and newspaper advertisements were promoted as well. Prior to the public airing of the commercials, stakeholder awareness and involvement were targeted through a meeting in which media, health care professionals, food industry workers, and community leaders were invited. In addition, print materials, covering a range of topics, such as recipes, local campaign strategies, and health benefits of fruits and vegetables, were distributed to health professionals, food service workers, and food retailers. Telephone surveys with approximately 500 randomly sampled adults were conducted each year, beginning 2 to 3 weeks following the advertising campaign. From the 1st to 2nd years of the program, respondents' ratings of the number of servings of fruits and vegetables they believed they should eat, as well the actual number of servings they reported consuming, increased. As media coverage declined in the study's 3rd and 4th years, the mean ratings of beliefs and consumption remained stable.

The Coeur en Santé St-Henri program aimed to reduce cardiovascular risk factors among residents of a low-income community in Montreal, Canada, through direct mass mailings of newsletters and a behavior change kit (O'Laughlin, Paradis, & Meshefedjian, 1997). For a 2-year period, all households in St-Henri received approximately one newsletter each month in the mail. Newsletters included educational articles on nutrition, smoking, and exercise, healthful recipes, and announcements of upcoming community events related to cardiovascular health. The newsletters consisted of messages presented at a sixth-grade reading level, with large print, pictures, and puzzles to appeal to residents having a range of academic skills. In addition, during the second year of newsletter mailings, residents were sent a "Heartfelt Kit" which included a 16-page educational booklet focused on diet, exercise, smoking, and stress management. Instructions were given in the booklets for systematically modifying health-related behaviors. Comparisons were made between 345 households in St-Henri that had received the newsletters and kits and 227 households from a nearby neighborhood that did not receive the mailings. Of the intervention community respondents, 38.6% recalled receiving newsletters, 27.9% had read them, 21.7% reported receiving the Heartfelt Kit, 10.8% had read them, and 8.1% had followed some of the instructions in the kit. Of the participants who read the newsletter, 14.7% reported increasing their exercise behavior and 28.4% reported improving their eating habits. Of the participants who read the Heartfelt Kit, 43.2% claimed an increase in their exercise behavior, and 35.1% an improvement in their eating habits.

In response to high levels of nutritional night blindness among children in Bangladesh due to vitamin A deficiencies, Hussain, Aarø, and Kvåle (1997) implemented a media-based program to encourage the consumption of foods high in vitamin A. A northern Bangladesh community with a population greater than 2,700,000 received the intervention over a 3-year period. The intervention's goal was to increase public knowledge about the characteristics of nutritional blindness and dietary strategies for prevention. A total of 13 strategies were used to impart the message. Citizens were presented with intervention messages through (a) local community volunteers and health professionals, who facilitated educational discussions at neighborhood meetings and home visits, (b) educational presentations featuring folk music performances, short films, and lectures in schools and other community settings, and (c) programs and advertisements on radio, television, and posters. Approximately 2 months following the conclusion of the 3-year campaign, randomly sampled parents in more than two thousand households were interviewed to assess changes in knowledge and behavior. When asked to provide the sources from which they received the campaign message, respondents most frequently identified folk singers at local markets and villages, home visits from women volunteers, and the short films shown in the villages. However, the most frequent sources of exposure were not always related to dietary behavior. Consumption of leafy green vegetables among those reporting direct contact with local volunteers and health professionals was significantly greater than for those reporting no direct contact, and animal protein consumption was greater for those who reported exposure to mass media messages. Although the folk singers and short films were recognizable, those reporting exposure to these approaches did not report related dietary changes.

Overall, the results from mass media efforts to improve exercise and dietary behaviors appear to be mixed. The recall of messages is often quite high in media-based programming, frequently reaching 70% or greater (Marcus, Owen, Forsyth, Cavill, & Fridinger, 1998). However, the extent to which both knowledge and behavior increase appears to be much more limited. Although blanket promotion of health behaviors through radio, television, and print media were common among the interventions, lasting change was most evident when specific behaviors were targeted and when some degree of direct contact, in addition to media distribution, was initiated and maintained between the target population and program representatives, health care professionals, or volunteers and support group members. Although media-based approaches are a cost-effective means for communicating a message to a large target audience, behavioral change may depend on proximal social influences as well.

CASE STUDY

The following case study describes a media-based weight control program (Jason, Greiner, Naylor, Johnson, & Van Egeren, 1991) that owed much of its success to the inclusion of social support groups as an adjunct component. Following the study description we present considerations and actions that shaped the program's development and outline steps, based on the implementation experiences, for the successful development of future large-scale prevention programs.

Targeting obesity, this media-based weight-loss program in Chicago focused on increasing physical activity and improving the quality of both exercise and diet (Jason, Greiner, Naylor, Johnson, & Van Egeren, 1991). During 15 weeknight news broadcasts, presented over 3 weeks, a popular television reporter explained progressive approaches for changing exercise and diet, and also informed viewers about a free, self-help, Body Basics manual, available from local businesses. The estimated citizen exposure totals were 300,000 to 500,000 for the broadcasts and 100,000 for the manuals. Prior to the first broadcast, viewers were asked to volunteer for the evaluation and were retained for the study if they were overweight (defined as greater than 1.5 times their ideal weight). Of the 74 participants, half were requested to participate in a support group, obtain the manual, and view the broadcast. The remaining participants were exposed to the media components without the support group. Eligible participants were assisted by research assistants to locate support groups. For the support group members, pre- and postintervention comparisons revealed an average loss of nine pounds of body weight, reductions in caloric intake and dietary fat, and increases in protein and aerobic activity. For the media-only group members, pre- and post-intervention comparisons revealed a non-significant change in body weight, although group members reported significant reductions in caloric intake. At a 3-month follow-up assessment, support group members maintained their health behaviors, and media-only group members reported a significant decrease in weight that had not been evident at the first posttest. These delayed effects suggest that, although the media-only group members may not have received the degree of social reinforcement that support group members experienced, the long-term practice of obesity management ultimately resulted in the expected reductions in weight.

There are abundant opportunities to find local resources to develop and implement these types of large-scale preventive and health-promoting interventions. However, the success of this approach might depend on associating and working with networks of supportive media outlets, businesses, and grass-roots organizations. Prior to the launching of the program described here, one of its developers (Jason) had already, in the course of previous projects, established relationships with and gained access to a number of for-profit businesses and television stations. Success in these earlier projects facilitated entry into other television stations and organizations, and we were therefore able to launch our media-based weight loss program.

A key factor in our success was our patience and readiness to use a vast set of networks, each of which gained direct, tangible benefits from its participation. For a number of these interventions, the Chicago Lung Association and PruCare Health Maintenance Organization provided staff to develop the programs and funds to print the manuals in exchange for considerable media coverage. Approximately two hundred 15- and 30-second promotions aired prior to many of the interventions, and the primary sponsors were identified in each promotion. The distributors (e.g., True Value Hardware) also provided financial resources in exchange for publicity on television, association with a worthy public health effort, and potential customers coming to their stores to pick up manuals. Each of the sponsors also had its organization's name printed prominently on all of the self-help manuals and promotional materials. The television stations were able to be identified with a credible, community-based health promotion program, and the program helped to attract new viewers to their stations.

The media is an excellent way to alert thousands of community residents to health promotion initiatives. Once alerted to these programs, participants can pick up materials and resources that reinforce the concepts that were broadcast and that encourage opportunities for practice. Perhaps the most exciting possibilities lie in more interactive interventions. Groups can be assembled to watch the programs, or participants can be provided additional support by actually being put in contact with helpers, self-help groups, or other community agencies. Many of our efforts to alter addictive behaviors have been unsuccessful in producing long-term change. Perhaps by lowering barriers to participation in programs, and devising imaginative ways to enable participants to continue receiving support and encouragement following the media programs, sustained improvement can be engendered.

FUTURE DIRECTIONS

Although some innovative strategies for preventing chronic health problems through diet- and exercise-focused interventions were identified in this review, the future success of such programming will benefit from the exploration of service delivery in new and multiple settings, the use of technological aids, and the targeting of those lifestyle behaviors having the greatest positive impact on health.

As with school-based health promotion efforts, worksite interventions deserve further consideration because of their potential for peer support, accessibility, and cost-effectiveness. Recent reviews suggest that worksite interventions are promising with respect to eliciting short-term changes in dietary habits (Glanz, Sorensen, & Farmer, 1996) and improvements in physical activity and fitness (Shepard, 1996); however, considerable variability in measured outcomes in worksite research as well as frequent methodological flaws, such as a lack of randomization, the absence of control groups, and assessments of knowledge but not behavior change, preclude drawing strong conclusions about the effectiveness of worksite programming. Winett et al. (1999) argued that worksite programs may be less effective for eliciting change than are interventions set in smaller settings, such as rural churches, in which the likelihood for developing and maintaining social network support is greater.

In addition to exploring new settings, future diet and exercise programs also may improve outcomes by implementing context-specific components in a variety of settings, including schools, worksites, media, churches, and medical and psychological health care agencies. An ecological approach might increase the likelihood that patterns of roles, relations, and activities related to health behavior will maintain across settings and lead to lasting change. For example, a family-focused diet and physical activity program might target both schools and religious institutions. Educational strategies, social marketing techniques, and support groups could be employed as behavior change agents for both adults and their children, potentially increasing modeling, health behavior salience, and generalization to the home environment for all family members.

Regarding technological aids to health behavior change, recent research has revealed that computers and other novel devices may dramatically influence health behavioral change. In response to reports that eating snacks and drinking regularly accompany viewing television (Van den Bulck, 2000), that children who watch more television are less likely to participate in vigorous activity (Anderson, Crespo, Bartlett, Cheskin, & Pratt, 1998), and that reducing media use may prevent childhood obesity (Robinson, 1999), Jason and Johnson (1995) employed a device which required a child to ride a bicycle in exchange for TV viewing. This device attached to the wheel and corresponding wheel rim of a stationary bicycle and was programmed to require that the child ride the bicycle for 15 minutes to earn 30 minutes of television viewing time. Reductions in television viewing and in children's weight have been found using this approach (Jason & Brackshaw, 1999).

The utilization of computerized devices to generate individualized recommendations and prompts regarding health behavior also has yielded promising results and deserves further investigation. For example, the Nutrition for a Lifetime System, an interactive, computer-based intervention, was implemented with supermarket customers to track purchases and self-reported dietary habits (Winett et al., 1997). This information was used by the computer program to provide specific dietary recommendations and dispense coupons for produce, low-fat, and high-fiber foods over a ten-week period. Compared with control participants receiving purchase tracking but no computer prompts or coupons, individuals participating in the intervention made significant improvements from baseline in produce, and low-fat, and high-fiber food purchases, and consumption maintained at a 3-month follow-up. Similarly, Brug, Glanz, Van Assema, Kok, and Van Breukelen, (1998) used questionnaires assessing dietary habits to develop computer-tailored feedback and recommendations to reduce fat and increase fruit and vegetable intake. At a 4-week comparison to baseline, those receiving personalized feedback reported significant differences in the expected directions for all three outcomes, whereas those receiving general feedback reported no differences. In addition, longer-term effects (i.e., at 8 weeks) were evident when additional feedback was provided after 4 weeks. These results suggest that, given the promising effects of personalized computer programming on dietary habits, this line of research should continue and the effects of computer-tailored feedback on exercise behavior should be explored as well.

Our final recommendation for future research concerns the specific health behaviors targeted for change. Chronic health problem prevention programs that encourage participants to increase the frequency and amount of time spent engaging in physical activity, without specific messages related to type of exercise or intensity, may result in weak changes in fitness and poor program adherence (Winett, 1998). Similarly, programs that promote low-fat food consumption, but advocate the use of dairy products, meat, and processed grains and sugar, may result in low-fiber diets, associated with an increased risk for colon cancer (Cousens, 2000). In addition, recommendations to consume greater quantities of fruits and vegetables may lead to increases in pesticide consumption, if the importance of eating pesticide-free, organic produce is not indicated to program participants. Given the consistent evidence that pesticide consumption leads to a variety of chronic health problems, including various forms of cancer and cardiovascular disease (Cousens, 2000), there is some concern about the extent to which dietary health promotion programs inadvertently encourage, rather than prevent, chronic disease.

The exploration of alternative health practices is recommended. Often presented in the popular media, clinical research by Ornish (2001) supports an integrated approach to heart disease prevention and treatment through lifestyle change. Plant-based diets with limited amounts of processed foods and low-impact, yet aerobically intense, activities such as yogic postures (asana) and breathing exercises (pranayana) are emphasized. Meditation, visualization, and stress management techniques are additional program components meriting greater attention from researchers regarding potential physical and mental health benefits and improvements in program adherence. Controlled research comparing behavioral and health-related outcomes associated with traditional versus alternative health practices (e.g., Plakosh-Smith & Jason, 1986) should improve researchers' ability to identify the most efficacious health practices and potentially lead to the development of stronger effects in preventive interventions targeting chronic health problems.

REFERENCES

Anderson, R. E., Crespo, C. J., Bartlett, S. J., Cheskin, L. J., & Pratt, M. (1998). Relationship of physical activity and television watching with body weight and level of fatness among children: Results from the third national health and nutrition examination survey. *Journal of the American Medical Association, 279*, 938–942.

Atkins, C. J., Senn, K., Rupp, J., Kaplan, R. M., Patterson, T. L., Sallis, Jr., J. F., & Nader, P. R. (1990) Attendance at health promotion programs: Baseline predictors and program outcomes. *Health Education Quarterly, 17*, 417–428.

Baranowski, T., Davis, M., Resnicow, K., Baranowski, J., Doyle, C., Lin, L., Smith, M., & Wang, D. T. (2000). Gimme 5 fruit, juice, and vegetables for fun and health: Outcome evaluation. *Health Education and Behavior, 27*, 96–111.

Brug, J., Glanz, K., Van Assema, P., Kok, G., & Van Breukelen, G. J. P. (1998). The impact of computer-tailored feedback and iterative feedback on fat, fruit, and vegetable intake. *Health Education and Behavior, 25*, 517–531.

Carleton, R. A., Sennett, L., Gans, K. M., Levin, S., Lefebvre, R. C., & Lasater, T. M. (1991). The Pawtucket Heart Health Program: Influencing adolescent eating patterns. *Annals of the New York Academy of Sciences, 623*, 322–326.

Centers for Disease Control and Prevention, (2000a). *About chronic disease.* Available: *http://www.cdc.gov/nccdphp/about.htm*

Centers for Disease Control and Prevention, (2000b). *Physical activity and good nutrition. Essential elements for good health.* Available: *http://www.cdc.gov/nccdphp/dnpa/dnpaaag.htm*

Centers for Disease Control and Prevention, (2000c). *Youth risk behaviors.* 1999 YRBS Data. Available: *http://www.cdc.gov/nccdphp/youthris.htm*

Cousens, G. (2000). *Conscious eating.* Berkeley, CA: North Atlantic Books.

Dixon, H., Borland, R., Segan, C., Stafford, H., & Sindall, C. (1998). Public reaction to Victoria's "2 fruit 'n' 5 veg every day" campaign and reported consumption of fruit and vegetables. *Preventive Medicine, 27*, 572–582.

Food and Nutrition Science Alliance (1999). FANSA statement on diet and cancer prevention in the United States. Available: *www.faseb.org/ascn/fansa12-99.htm*

Glanz, K., Sorensen, G., & Farmer, A. (1996). The health impact of worksite nutrition and cholesterol intervention programs. *American Journal of Health Promotion, 10*, 453–470.

Glenwick, D. S., & Jason, L. A. (Eds.). (1993). *Promoting health and mental health in children, youth, and families.* New York: Springer Publishing.

Golditz, G. A., Atwood, K. A., Emmons, K., Monson, R. R., Willett, W. C., Trichopoulos, D., & Hunter, D. J. (2000). Harvard Report on Cancer Prevention. Volume 4. Harvard Cancer Risk Index. *Cancer Causes and Control, 11*, 477–488.

Hussain, A., Aarø, L. E., & Kvåle, G. (1997). Impact of a health education program to promote consumption of vitamin A-rich foods in Bangladesh. *Health Promotion International, 12*, 103–109.

Institute for the Future (2000). *Health and health care 2010: The forecast, the future*. Jossey-Bass, San Francisco, CA.

Jason, L. A. (1998). Tobacco, drug, and HIV preventive media interventions. *American Journal of Community Psychology, 26*, 145–187.

Jason, L. A., & Brackshaw, E. (1999). Case study: Reducing TV viewing and corresponding increases in physical activity and subsequent weight loss. *Journal of Behavior Therapy & Experimental Psychiatry, 30*, 145–151.

Jason, L. A., Crawford, I., & Gruder, C. L. (1989). Using a community model in media-based health promotion interventions. *Journal of Primary Prevention, 9*, 233–246.

Jason, L. A., Greiner, B. J., Naylor, K., Johnson, S. P., & Van Egeren, L. (1991). A large-scale, short-term, media-based weight loss program. *American Journal of Health Promotion, 5*, 432–437.

Jason, L. A., & Johnson, S. (1995). Reducing excessive television viewing while increasing physical activity. *Child & Family Behavior Therapy, 17*, 35–44.

Marcus, B. H., Owen, N., Forsyth, L. H., Cavill, N. A., & Fridinger, F. (1998). Physical activity interventions using mass media, print media, and information technology. *American Journal of Preventive Medicine, 15*, 362–378.

McGinnis, J. M., & Foege, W. H. (1993). Actual causes of death in the United States. *Journal of the American Medical Association, 270*, 2207–2212.

O'Laughlin, J., Paradis, G., & Meshefedjian, G. (1997). Evaluation of two strategies for heart health promotion by direct mail in a low-income urban community. *Preventive Medicine, 26*, 745–753.

Ornish, D. (2001). *Dr. Dean Ornish's program for reversing heart disease: The only system scientifically proven to reverse heart disease without drugs or surgery*. New York: Ballantine Books.

Owen, N., Bauman, A., Booth, M., Oldenburg, B., & Magnus, P. (1995). Serial mass-media campaigns to promote physical activity: Reinforcing or redundant? *American Journal of Public Health, 85*, 244–248.

Pate, R. R., Pratt, M., Blair, S. N., Haskell, W. L., Macera, C. A., Bouchard, C., Buchner, D., Ettinger, W., Heath, G. W., King, A. C. (1995). Physical activity and public health: A recommendation from the Centers for Disease Control and Prevention and the American College of Sports Medicine. *Journal of the American Medical Association, 273*, 402–407.

Perry, C. L., Bishop, D. B., Taylor, G., Murray, D. M., Mays, R. W., Dudovitz, B. S., Smyth, M., & Story, M. (1998). Changing fruit and vegetable consumption among children: The 5-a-Day Power Plus program in St. Paul, Minnesota. *American Journal of Public Health, 88*, 603–609.

Plakosh-Smith, T., & Jason, L. A. (1986). Use of time budgets in a preventive program. *Evaluation and the Health Professions, 9*, 53–61.

Reger, B., Wootan, M. G., & Booth-Butterfield, S. (1999). Using mass media to promote healthy eating: A community-based demonstration project. *Preventive Medicine, 29*, 414–421.

Robinson, T. N. (1999). Reducing children's television viewing to prevent obesity: A randomized controlled trial. *Journal of the American Medical Association, 282*, 1561–1567.

Sallis, J. F., McKenzie, T. L., Alcaraz, J. E., Kolody, B., Faucette, N., & Hovell, M. F. (1997). The effects of a 2-year physical education program (SPARK) on physical activity and fitness in elementary school students. *American Journal of Public Health, 87*, 1328–34.

Schnurr, P. P., Vaillant, C. O., & Vaillant, G. E. (1990). Predicting exercise in late midlife from young adult personality characteristics. *International Journal of Aging & Human Development, 30*, 153–160.

Shepard, R. J. (1996). Worksite fitness and exercise programs: A review of methodology and health impact. *American Journal of Health Promotion, 10*, 436–452.

Van den Bulck, J. (2000). Is television bad for your health? Behavior and body image of the adolescent "couch potato." *Journal of Youth & Adolescence, 29*, 273–288.

Wechsler, H., Basch, C. E., Zybert, P., & Shea, S. (1998). Promoting the selection of low-fat milk in elementary school cafeterias in an inner-city Latino community: Evaluation of an intervention. *American Journal of Public Health, 88*, 427–433.

Wechsler, H., Devereaux, R. S., Davis, M., & Collins, J. (2000). Using the school environment to promote physical activity and healthy eating. *Preventive Medicine, 31*, S121–S137.

Wimbush, E., MacGregor, A., & Fraser, E. (1998). Impacts of a national mass media campaign on walking in Scotland. *Health Promotion International, 13*, 45–53.

Winett, R. A. (1998). Developing more effective health behavior programs: Analyzing the epidemiological and biological bases for activity and exercise programs. *Applied & Preventive Psychology, 7*, 209–224.

Winett, R. A., Anderson, E. S., Bickley, P. G., Walberg-Rankin, J., Moore, J. F., Leahy, M., Harris, C. E., & Gerkin, R. E. (1997). Nutrition for a lifetime system: A multimedia system for altering food supermarket shoppers' purchases to meet nutritional guidelines. *Computers in Human Behavior, 13*, 371–392.

Winett, R. A., Anderson, E. S., Whiteley, J. A., Wojcik, J. R., Rovniak, L. S., Graves, K. D., Galper, D. I., & Winett, S. G. (1999). Church-based health behavior programs: Using social cognitive theory to formulate interventions for at-risk populations. *Applied & Preventive Psychology, 8*, 129–142.

CHAPTER 12

Preventing Marital Disorder

Peter Fraenkel and
Howard Markman

In this chapter, we describe the current state of theory, intervention, and research pertaining to the prevention of marital disorder. In the first section we review the state of marriage in the United States and abroad and the mental, physical, and social problems associated with marital distress and disruption (i.e., separation and divorce). These findings provide a powerful rationale for developing and disseminating preventive interventions. We also review the literature on the variables that distinguish distressed from satisfied couples, as well as those that predict marital distress and disruption from groups of (initially) happy premarital or newlywed couples. In the second section we describe the typical contents and range of formats of preventive interventions for couples, and review the empirical outcome literature on these interventions. In the third section, as a case example, we describe the development and contents of one such intervention, focusing on issues of program implementation and dissemination. In the fourth and final section we discuss future directions of preventive interventions for couples.

Before turning to the first section, a few notes on language are in order. The notion of prevention of marital *disorder* marks a territory that includes both the goal of preventing serious distress or disharmony in marriage, as well as the marital disruption or dissolution that often follows from such distress. In recent years, some in the broader profession of couple and family therapy and beyond have looked with some degree of suspiciousness and alarm at the growing field of preventive couple interventions when the activities of this field are cast as *divorce* prevention. Feminist family therapists, in particular (e.g., Laird, 1999), have raised concerns about the so-called "marriage movement" often associated with preventive programs, especially because some within the movement seek to tighten divorce laws and redirect federal funding from welfare programs (which largely support poor, single, or divorced women with children) to marriage education programs.

Our position is to cast the field as marital *distress, conflict*, or *discord* prevention rather than as divorce prevention per se. Not only does this language potentially allow groups of varying religious, political, and social policy persuasions regarding divorce to agree on the unquestionable goal of promoting couple wellness and reducing risk of serious conflict, but it also is, in fact, a more accurate description of the focus of preventive efforts. The reader of this book is no doubt familiar with the terms *primary, secondary*, and *tertiary* prevention (Glenwick & Jason, 1993). In the domain of couples, primary prevention refers to interventions targeting nondistressed, well-functioning couples to help them remain so, with the reasoning that currently high divorce rates suggest that all couples are at risk simply by virtue of being married. Secondary prevention refers to interventions targeting either groups of happy couples known to be particularly at risk, or couples beginning to show signs of distress. As in other areas of mental disorder for which prevention programs are developed, tertiary prevention comprises treatment of those couples already experiencing significant distress and/or considering separation or divorce.

Technically speaking, the sorts of interventions and formats (typically brief contact in a group setting) that characterize most preventive programs are not adequate to assist a couple in moving back from the brink of divorce. Indeed, assisting distressed couples when one or both partners are considering divorce may require a specialized form of marital therapy (which Fraenkel (1999) has entitled "last chance couple therapy") to work with the damage done to the couple's level of commitment and trust. Two theories of the path toward marital dissolution (Gottman, 1993; Stanley, 1995) locate thoughts of separation and divorce as several steps into this sequence, and some data (Notarius & Buongiorno, 1992) suggest that the average length of time couples experience distress prior to seeking marital therapy (not necessary with divorce yet in mind) is 6 years. Thus, true preventive efforts are better cast as *distress* or *conflict* prevention, terms that characterize much of what is meant by marital disorder. If effective, such efforts have the added benefit of assisting couples and children to avoid the extra pain often associated with divorce. However, to the extent that divorce is associated with negative sequelae for adults and children alike, it appears to be due, at least initially, to the high conflict that often precedes and accompanies divorce (Howes & Markman, 1984). Indeed, separation and/or divorce may be the best option when high conflict, especially accompanied by violence or abuse, seems unlikely to abate because of the unwillingness of one or both partners to engage in change efforts.

We also would like to note that although this chapter focuses exclusively on prevention of *marital* disorder, and thus on research with heterosexual, legally married, or engaged to be married couples, we believe that the basic preventive principles and practices described apply as well to other forms of long-term committed relationships, including common-law marriages and gay and lesbian committed relationships. Although there are a number of excellent studies and clinical writings on gay and lesbian relationships (Julien, Arellano, & Turgeon, 1997; Kurdek, 1998; Laird & Green, 1996), much more research is needed, which might in turn indicate important adaptations in the preventive practices best suited to promoting them.

DESCRIPTION OF THE PROBLEM

The State of Marriage

Although divorce prevalence statistics vary somewhat among studies, depending on time frame and other sampling issues, by all accounts, divorce has been an alarmingly frequent outcome of marriage for many years—alarming especially when one considers that this outcome is the last one newlyweds expect or intend as they confirm plans to share a life together. In 1970, the divorce rate for first marriages was 50% (Cherlin, 1981) and by the mid-1980s was found to be 67% (Martin & Bumpass, 1989). It is common for divorced persons to marry again, but the divorce rate for second marriages is estimated to be even higher than for first marriages (Brody, Neubaum, & Forehand, 1998; Cherlin, 1992), and, according to Glick (1984), up to 10% higher. More recent statistics suggest that beginning in the late 1980s (National Center for Health Statistics, 1996) up to the most current estimate published in the late 1990s (U.S. Bureau of the Census, 1998) there has been a steady decline in divorce rates. Even so, current findings indicate that between 40% (Norton & Miller, 1992) and 50% (Teachman, Tedrow, & Crowder, 2000) of couples will divorce. Although for many years the United States held the dubious distinction of world leader in divorce, international statistics indicate that divorce rates in many other countries are now quite high, including 42% in the United Kingdom, 35% in Australia, and 37% in Germany (Berger & Hannah, 1999). In addition, although even more couples may experience separation without divorce, separated couples are 75% more likely to divorce than to reconcile (Bloom, Hodges, Caldwell, Systra, & Cedrone, 1977).

Of course, most couples do not divorce within days of first experiencing conflict. Although a large percentage of marriages end within 2 years, and the average length of marriage is only six years (Olson & Defrain, 1997), the path to divorce typically involves many months or years of conflict. Thus, in any period sampled for divorce rates, a percentage of intact marriages that may or may not eventually end in divorce are experiencing significant levels of discord. Mace and Mace (1980) reported that approximately half of those who remain married do so unhappily, and others (O'Leary, Barling, Arias, & Rosenbaum, 1989; Straus & Gelles, 1990) have found that many marriages are characterized by high levels of discord, and even violence and abuse. Given the central role of marriage to an individual's overall life satisfaction (Glenn & Weaver, 1981), the finding of a significant decrement in marital quality since the mid-1970s (Glenn, 1991; Rogers & Amato, 1997) suggests the importance of efforts to stave off marital disorder.

Correlates and Sequelae of Marital Discord and Disruption

Marital discord and dissolution are typically highly stressful and are described by the majority of people seeking any form of therapy as the primary source of their malaise (Veroff, Kulka, & Douvan, 1981). Indeed, research increasingly has identified negative mental health correlates of marital discord and dissolution. We describe these conditions as correlated with, rather than caused by, marital disorder because, to date, most of the research has not clearly established a causal relation between these variables (Bradbury, Fincham, & Beach, 2000; Gotlib & McCabe, 1990). In addition, we must note that most of the research on the effects of marital disorder has not teased apart the impact of distress from the impact of divorce, nor for that matter has it usually simultaneously studied predictors of distress versus predictors of divorce (Karney & Bradbury, 1995; Rogge & Bradbury, 1999). Given that divorce is almost always preceded and accompanied by marital distress, it may be difficult if not impossible to definitively establish their separate impact. Even when certain sequelae only appear following divorce, these might also be due to the accumulated impact of marital distress rather than divorce per se.

From a systemic theoretical and interventive perspective that looks at problems from a circular or reciprocal causal framework rather than a linear unidirectional framework (Fraenkel, 1997), it may be just as important to note the correlation between marital discord and an individual mental health disorder as it would be to identify a clear causal pathway from discord to such a disorder. For instance, a number of researchers and clinicians (Gotlib & McCabe, 1990; Papp, 2000) have argued coherently for a systemic perspective on the relationship between marital discord and depression, noting that a discordant marriage may elicit and maintain depression in an individual partner, and, in contrast, a positive, supportive marriage may provide a powerful buffer or mediator against nonmarital causes of depression. From this perspective, preventive marital interventions lower whatever percentage of *risk* for depression can be attributed to marital conflict and strengthen *protective* factors attributable to a satisfying marriage. A similar perspective captures contemporary thinking about the relationship between marital discord or dissolution and physical health (Schmaling & Sher, 1997), as well as other negative correlates of marital problems, such as employment issues (Barling, 1990). Indeed, this conceptualization of preventive interventions as simultaneously decreasing risk and increasing protection represents the current paradigm in prevention science (Coie et al. 1993).

Keeping these points in mind, we can summarize the findings on the correlates of marital distress and divorce. Distress and divorce are related to an increased risk for psychopathology, including anxiety and depressive disorders, as well as substance and alcohol abuse (see extensive reviews by Bloom, Asher, & White, 1978; Gotlib & McCabe, 1990; Kelly & Fincham, 1999; and several chapters in Halford & Markman, 1997). In addition to its relation to a higher likelihood of psychopathology, marital dissolution (separation or divorce) is predictive of a higher risk of automobile accidents and resulting fatalities, a higher risk of suicide and homicide, a greater likelihood of physical illness and mortality from disease, and overall shorter lifespan (see reviews in Gottman, 1994a, 1999). The emerging literature (Burman & Margolin, 1992; Kiecolt-Glaser et al. 1993; Schmaling & Sher, 1997) documents the physical health risks of marital distress and divorce.

A large body of literature documents the impact of marital distress and divorce on the mental and physical health and the social adjustment of children (see reviews by Amato, 2000; Emery, 1982; Gottman, 1994a, 1999; Grych & Fincham, 1990; Jenkins, 2000; Luthar & Zigler, 1991). Many of the studies are cross-sectional and cannot establish a causal link between marital distress, divorce, and child problems. However, at least one longitudinal study assessed relationship quality before marriage and after the birth of the child and found a causal link between premarital relationship satisfaction, level of premarital and marital conflict and communication quality, and quality of mother-child attachment (Howes & Markman, 1984). As alluded to earlier, research (Amato, 2000; Emery, 1982; Gottman, 1999; Markman & Jones-Leonard, 1985) suggests that it is marital conflict or parental conflict during and following separation and divorce, rather than the separation or divorce per se, that has a negative impact on children.

In sum, there is much evidence linking marital distress and dissolution to all manner of mental and physical health problems for both adults and children. Aside from the enormous suffering entailed, the economic costs of marital strife for families and society as a whole due to health care needs, engagement of the legal system, and decreased work productivity is estimated to be in the billions of dollars yearly (Forthofer, Markman, Cox, Stanley, & Kessler, 1996). Preventive approaches to marital disorder, therefore, potentially could have enormous impact on the general well being of society.

Limitations of Marital Therapy

Another problem with marital disorder is that it is difficult to reverse. A number of studies and reviews (Gottman, 1999; Hahlweg & Markman, 1988; Jacobson & Addis, 1993) suggest that although marital therapy may result in statistically significant improvement as compared with no treatment, the majority of treated couples do not move from distressed to nondistressed status, and there is a high rate of relapse. Furthermore, although it is estimated that the majority of distressed couples do not seek treatment (Bradbury & Fincham, 1990; Kelly & Fincham, 1999), if they did, the need would far outstrip the availability of competent services.

What Goes Wrong in Distressed and Disrupted Marriages?

There are a number of excellent reviews of longitudinal studies on the variables that predict separation and divorce, as well as a growing number of studies that examine the interpersonal and intrapsychic (i.e., cognitive, emotional, physiological) processes that characterize distressed couples or those bound for future distress (Gottman, 1994a, 1999; Gottman & Levenson, 1999a, 1999b; Karney & Bradbury, 1995; Rogge & Bradbury, 1999). As the focus of this chapter is more on the nature of preventive interventions for couples than on a careful review and critique of these studies, we will summarize the main findings, particularly as they provide the basis for creation of interventions.

Karney and Bradbury (1995) reviewed 115 longitudinal studies, many of which had serious methodological flaws. Their review identified a few predictive variables that we would describe as stable attributes of persons, their backgrounds, or their contexts—those not readily amenable or impossible to prevent or change through short-term interventions. These include divorce of one's own parents, young age at marriage, poverty, and personality variables such as "neuroticism" (which is essentially the tendency to view life negatively). Other variables identified can be described as dynamic, in that they are more amenable to change or prevention through acquisition of skills and ideas (Stanley, Markman, St. Peters, & Leber, 1995).

Foremost among these dynamic variables are the quality and patterning of communication, including the types of affects expressed, particularly around discussing and solving problems. The paradigmatic research procedure generating these observational data involves the couple identifying the topic or domain (e.g., housework, childcare, time together, money, sex) about which they experience their greatest level of conflict and discussing the topic with an attempt to resolve it. These discussions are video- or audiotaped and later coded by independent observers using one of a number of available coding systems (Gottman & Notarius, 2000; Notarius & Markman, 1987). Indeed, in a recent review of predictors of divorce, Rogge and Bradbury (1999, p. 338) found that both behavioral observation and self-report studies with follow-up periods ranging from 2 to 12 years "reported rates of accuracy between 75% and 95%" in predicting dichotomous categories of either married versus separated/divorced, or satisfied versus unsatisfied, based largely on these variables. Thus, it is widely accepted that particular patterns of affect expression and communication characterize distressed versus nondistressed couples and powerfully predict marital outcomes.

A number of studies (DeMaris, 2000; Rogge & Bradbury, 1999) also have found incidents of physical violence and aggression to be strong predictors of marital dissolution. Such studies support the need for prevention programs to address the precursors to relational violence.

Although the language used to describe destructive communication behaviors varies somewhat across laboratories, there is general agreement as to the patterns that characterize the interactions of distressed couples more than satisfied couples and that are strong predictors of later problems in presently happy newlywed or engaged couples. Problem patterns include contempt, criticism, defensiveness, withdrawal, stonewalling (a particular style of withdrawal more common in men, in which the musculature of the face assumes a frozen, inexpressive state), negative escalation (described in different studies either as repetitive exchanges of negative affect, particularly those listed above, or as a powerfully negative response to a neutral or mildly negative comment), invalidation (putting down the thoughts, opinions, and efforts of the partner), and negative interpretations/mindreading (statements that assume negative intent on the part of the partner (Gottman, 1993, 1994a, 1994b, 1999; Gottman, Coan, Carrere, & Swanson, 1998; Markman, 1981; Markman, Floyd, Stanley, & Storaasli, 1988; Markman, Renick, Floyd, Stanley, & Clements 1993; Roberts, 2000). Importantly, Gottman and his colleagues found that expression of anger per se (without contempt or criticism) was not predictive of later marital difficulties (Gottman, 1993; Gottman, Coan, Carrere, & Swanson, 1998; Gottman & Krokoff, 1989), correcting a myth perpetuated by numerous professional and popular psychology books.

Gottman (1993, 1994a, 1999) has provided the most comprehensive theory of the "cascade" toward marital dissolution. The theory provides conceptual and empirical links among moment-to-moment marital interaction, perceptions/cognitions, and physiology. In brief, the theory suggests that marital interactions characterized by the above-described destructive behaviors result in the experience of physiological flooding and thoughts either of hurt and "righteous indignation" (accompanied by feelings of sadness, anger, contempt) or hurt and perceived attack (accompanied by internal whining, sense of "innocent victimhood," fear, and worry). In addition, hypervigilance to behavioral cues associated with flooding leads to interpretation of otherwise affectively ambiguous partner behavior as negative. Over time, these interpretations become codified into fixed attributions that cast the partner's behavior as selfish, characteristic of them in multiple contexts (globality), and stable (based on a trait rather than on current state or context) (see Fincham, Bradbury, & Scott, 1990, and Karney & Bradbury, 2000, for reviews of the impact of negative attributions on marriage). These attributions then guide perception of subsequent interactions and events through the process of confirmation bias, which in turn leads to more negative behavior and flooding.

In addition, Gottman has presented data supporting the notion that the critical issue is to achieve balance both within each subsystem involved in marital functioning (interactional behavior, cognition, physiology) and among these subsystems. In this model, balance is not necessarily achieved through equal occurrence of opposite behaviors. For instance, Gottman (1994a) found that a ratio of 5:1 for positive to negative behaviors predicted marital stability, whereas a ratio closer to 1:1 predicted marital disruption. In addition, as noted above, not all "negative" behaviors have the same interpersonal effects, and the expression of contempt or criticism, even if less frequent, can undo the relationship-strengthening impact of positive statements (Notarius & Markman, 1993).

REVIEW AND CRITIQUE OF THE LITERATURE

Efforts to strengthen couples so as to prevent serious levels of distress and divorce actually characterized many of the activities of the early marital counselors as far back as the 1930s (Gurman & Fraenkel, 2000). However, virtually none of these early efforts were based on empirical research, and in many cases not even on clear theory about processes related to preventing negative marital outcomes. The contemporary field of marital distress prevention began in the early 1970s when interventions began to be based on the research reviewed in the previous section, which involved careful empirical study of variables that distinguish distressed from happy couples and that predict distress and divorce. At around the same time, a number of more theoretically based approaches emerged. In this section, we describe the characteristic components of preventive interventions for couples and the range of theoretical premises, and we review the efficacy and effectiveness research on these interventions.

Components of Preventive Interventions and Range of Theoretical Premises

All programs designed to strengthen marriages are based on a philosophy of psychoeducation—the notion that ideas and skills believed to enrich marriages and/or protect them from destructive conflict can be directly taught to couples in a fairly brief period of time, mostly in a group setting, and that couples then can put these ideas and skills into practice without much ongoing assistance. Virtually all programs include information about communication and, usually, skills training; at least some attention to partners' beliefs about intimacy and marriage; and some focus and/or activities designed to increase the pleasurable aspects of relationship, such as fun, friendship, and sensuality. However, as a group the programs vary greatly in terms of theoretical premises about the nature of relationships, problems, and change, with all major theories of couple therapy represented (i.e., cognitive-behavioral, psychodynamic, intergenerational, experiential), as well as some more religious or cosmological belief systems.

Although some have suggested that only programs directly focused on decreasing marital risk factors and enhancing protective factors be considered true preventive approaches, as opposed to those that focus solely on enriching marriages (Kelly & Fincham, 1999), we view all of these programs as potentially preventive interventions. In our view, whether or not an intervention is preventive must be determined entirely by empirical, longitudinal study of its effectiveness in assisting happy couples or those just beginning to show signs of distress to remain stable and to maintain relatively high levels of quality years after the program, as compared with couples that did not participate in the program. Research demonstrating the positive impact of a program immediately post-intervention does not establish it as preventive. (For a meta-analysis of such studies concluding that enrichment programs are generally effective, see Giblin, Sprenkle, & Sheehan, 1985. However, see also critiques of this analysis in Bradbury & Fincham, 1990, and Kelly & Fincham, 1999.) Likewise, studies demonstrating the effectiveness of these interventions with distressed samples do not establish them as preventive, as these constitute treatment studies, whether or not they are conducted within the context of a program stated to be preventive (see DeMaria, 1998, and Durana, 1996, for examples of this confusion).

Our hope is that all programs interested in the prevention of marital distress and divorce will engage in the hard but exciting work of conducting randomized, long-term clinical trials as well as more naturalistic effectiveness studies with primary or secondary prevention samples. However, to date, only the Prevention and Relationship Enhancement Program (PREP) has been subjected to this sort of rigorous scrutiny (Kelly & Fincham, 1999). Thus, our review of efficacy and effectiveness research focuses on PREP.

Efficacy and Effectiveness of Preventive Interventions

The original efficacy study of PREP was reported by Markman et al. (1988) and by Markman et al. (1993). Nondistressed, premarital couples participating in a larger community study of predictors of marital quality and stability were matched in dyads or triads on the basis of variables found in previous research (Markman, 1981) to predict future satisfaction and stability (engaged versus planning marriage, relationship satisfaction, self-ratings of communication impact, confidence in getting married). One or two couples in each matched set were then randomly invited to participate in the intervention, while the other served in an untreated control group. Half of those invited into the intervention declined, so that there were three groups: intervention, decline control, and no-treatment control. With respect to relationship stability, at 1 1/2- and 3-year follow-up, intervention couples were significantly more likely than no-treatment control couples to be together (data were not presented in the 1988 article for decline control couples), and at 4- and 5-year follow-up, intervention couples were significantly more likely than either control group to be together. With regard to marital quality, as expected in a prevention study, there were no group differences immediately after intervention. However, at 1 1/2-, 3-, and 4-year follow-up, intervention couples showed higher relationship satisfaction than did control couples, and, for men, this difference continued at 5 years. In addition, at 3 years, intervention couples showed higher sexual satisfaction and lower problem intensity, as well as more positive self-ratings of communication impact.

Concerning interaction processes, at post intervention PREP couples demonstrated more positive and less negative communication, as determined by ratings of independent coders. This indicates that intervention couples learned and used the skills. At 4-year follow-up, intervention couples showed greater use of communication skill, greater positive affect, more problem-solving skill, and more support and validation than did control couples, and less denial, dominance, negative affect, conflict, and overall negative communication than did controls. Similar results distinguished the intervention from the decline control group. These differences did not appear at 5-year follow-up (except for greater use of communication skill by intervention men), possibly due to attrition of the least skilled control couples by that time or possibly due to a fading of the intervention impact. These behavioral findings suggest that couples can sustain improved communication and problem-solving skills for years following a relatively brief program, but that booster sessions might be critical to promote long-term use. Indeed, at the completion of the workshop many participants have asked for such sessions, anticipating the decline in their use or memory of the skills.

One other striking finding was that at 5-year follow-up, intervention couples were significantly less likely than control couples to report instances of physical violence. As well as further suggesting that PREP helps couples handle conflict more successfully, it may be that the intervention lowers the likelihood of some of the precursors to violence in some men, such as physiological flooding and withdrawal/stonewalling (Jacobson & Gottman, 1998).

Other studies have replicated PREP's effectiveness in decreasing relationship dissolution and maintaining relationship quality over time. For instance, a study (Hahlweg, Markman, Thurmaier, Engl, & Eckert, 1998) conducted in Germany compared couples who took PREP with those who engaged in the typical premarital training offered in their churches, as well as to those who took no premarital training. Five years later, PREP couples had significantly lower divorce rates and higher relationship satisfaction than either control group. However, the findings are limited because lack of random assignment to conditions meant that couples who chose PREP might have been systematically different from the other couples.

Several ongoing studies are attempting to replicate and extend these findings. For instance, Fraenkel and his colleagues are conducting a longitudinal study of the impact of PREP on partners' quality of life, stress, health, and health-related behavior. This study also is designed to examine the variables that enhance or impede implementation of program ideas and skills in couples' daily lives. In-depth interviews with intervention couples 1 and 2 years after the course found, among other things, that the majority of couples experienced it as useful but did not frequently use the skills exactly as taught. However, they believed the skills training and practice sessions to be essential in their becoming more attuned to the need to respect their partners' differing opinions and for resolving problems without resorting to destructive patterns (Fraenkel & Whittet, 1998).

One study has reported null findings on PREP's efficacy. Van Widenfelt, Hosman, Schaap, and Van Der Staak (1996) conducted a controlled study in Holland and found no benefits for intervention couples compared with controls immediately following the course, or 6 months later, or 2 years later. However, there were certain methodological problems with this study, includ-

ing reliance only on self-report measures, a sample that was already somewhat distressed, group differences in length of relationships, and differential
attrition.

CASE EXAMPLE

In this section we describe PREP's content and format in more depth, and discuss our efforts to disseminate the program. In doing so, we also address the
"barriers" (Bradbury & Fincham, 1990) and challenges facing efforts to promote primary and secondary preventive programs for couples.

Program Content

PREP focuses on teaching skills, ideas, and life practices designed to decrease
risk factors and to enhance protective factors. Content focused mostly on reducing risk factors includes (a) identifying and illustrating (with videotaped examples) common destructive communication patterns; (b) teaching a constructive
approach to expressing concerns or complaints, one that acts against the tendency to develop global, stable, and negative attributions by focusing instead
on specific partner behaviors and the emotional reactions these generate; (c)
teaching the speaker-listener technique, a form of structured, active listening,
as well as a problem-solving sequence; (d) discussing the negative impact of
unrecognized or undisclosed expectations about married life, which can result
in conflict as well as form the basis of negative attributions when the partner
violates these expectations; (e) raising awareness of potential conflict around
differences in religious and ethical values and practices, which many couples
seem to overlook until these concerns are raised by certain life events, such as
the birth of the first child; (f) presenting a model for identifying the hidden
issues or relationship themes, such as control, caring, respect and recognition,
commitment, trust, and acceptance, that often underlie repetitive, unresolved
issues or those that typically generate explosive reactions or avoidance; and
(g) encouraging partners to commit to enacting certain ground rules for handling conflict and maintaining positive aspects of the relationship.

Content focused mostly on increasing protective factors includes (a) lectures and suggested activities for increasing and maintaining time for fun,
friendship, and sensuality and (b) lectures on the two aspects of commitment
(dedication and constraint) and the importance of forgiveness, and suggestions
about how to strengthen these protective aspects of relationship. Figure 12.1

depicts the program's core components, with the sequence of conflict management skills shown in a flow chart and the protective activities arranged around the perimeter to represent how these can form a critical boundary around conflict and between the couple and the stressors that can impinge on their relationship.

Program Format

PREP combines group lectures delivered by one or two workshop leaders and individual skills practice sessions for each couple, facilitated by coaches or "consultants" trained and supervised by the workshop leader. The full PREP course is 15 hours long. The original schedule involved five meetings of 3 hours each. One of us (Fraenkel) found that busy New York City couples had difficulty attending each week, and created a format of 1 weekend day (8 hours) followed by two Thursday evenings of $3^{1}/_{2}$ hours each. This format resulted in virtually zero missed sessions (for both research and paying couples) over the past 6 years (approximately 24 workshops and roughly 120 couples). PREP has now adopted this format (1 weekend day plus 2 Thursday evenings) as the basic schedule. A weekend version has been used in Denver and in the German study described earlier. A 1-day workshop also has been implemented, and a special manual created for it. Shorter versions are possible as well (for example, an introductory "learning evening" or "half-day intensive"), with the understanding that reduced program content (and particularly, less in-session skills practice) may mean reduced long-term effectiveness.

Although the longitudinal findings from Germany suggest that couples can benefit as much from a weekend version as one that extends over a few weeks, no study has yet directly compared the two versions to determine which "dosage" is most effective. One important future direction for research is to determine the bare minimum of intervention necessary for couples to notably benefit in a sustained manner.

Professional Training

A key aspect of prevention program dissemination is training others to present the materials. Since 1990 PREP has offered a 3-day instructor training as a requirement to conduct the full 15-hour program and to train coaches to assist in workshops. Training in the 1-day workshop format is now available as well.

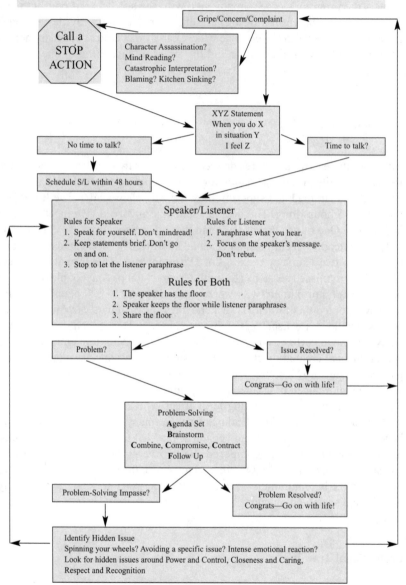

PREP AT A GLANCE

Gripe/Concern/Complaint

Call a STOP ACTION

Character Assassination?
Mind Reading?
Catastrophic Interpretation?
Blaming? Kitchen Sinking?

XYZ Statement
When you do X
in situation Y
I feel Z

No time to talk?

Time to talk?

Schedule S/L within 48 hours

Speaker/Listener

Rules for Speaker
1. Speak for yourself. Don't mindread!
2. Keep statements brief. Don't go on and on.
3. Stop to let the listener paraphrase

Rules for Listener
1. Paraphrase what you hear.
2. Focus on the speaker's message. Don't rebut.

Rules for Both
1. The speaker has the floor
2. Speaker keeps the floor while listener paraphrases
3. Share the floor

Problem?

Issue Resolved?

Congrats—Go on with life!

Problem-Solving
Agenda Set
Brainstorm
Combine, **C**ompromise, **C**ontract
Follow Up

Problem-Solving Impasse?

Problem Resolved?
Congrats—Go on with life!

Identify Hidden Issue
Spinning your wheels? Avoiding a specific issue? Intense emotional reaction?
Look for hidden issues around Power and Control, Closeness and Caring,
Respect and Recognition

Figure 12.1 Major components of the Prevention and Relationship Enhancement Program (PREP®).

© 1999 Peter Fraekel, Ph.D. & Amanda Salzhauer, MSW
PREP® at NYU Child Study Center (212) 263 8664

Initially we limited training to mental health professionals and pastoral counselors or those in graduate school in these professions. In recent years we have offered the training to selected paraprofessionals (such as clergy or senior persons in a church congregation, who generally provide the program in particular settings, such as in their religious communities. Training of professionals and paraprofessionals each presents particular challenges. Our experience is that experienced mental health professionals often have a difficult time staying within the role of coaching skills; on the other hand, paraprofessionals must become acquainted with fundamental rules about confidentiality and with how to respond sensitively to personal material.

As in the previous steps in developing PREP, we are attempting to answer questions about the relative strengths of professional versus paraprofessional trainers through empirical study. We (Stanley et al. 2001) currently are conducting a long-term effectiveness study comparing outcomes for couples in church and synagogue communities who were randomly assigned to receive either PREP presented in the usual academic setting by our workshop leaders, PREP presented by the community's own clergymen or clergywomen, or the usual premarital programs provided in that church. Initial pre/post findings supported the conclusion that paraprofessionals can deliver the program as well as mental health professionals. Data indicated no differences between the couples who received the program in the university setting and those who received it from their clergy, but a significant difference between PREP delivered in either context and the usual premarital program presented in the religious institution. These findings are extremely promising, as religious institutions provide a natural context for implementation of preventive interventions, given that over 75% of couples still marry in a church or synagogue and often already receive some sort of premarital information or counseling.

Materials

We find a variety of written and audiovisual materials critical to program presentation and dissemination, either in group workshops or individual counseling settings. A self-administered version of the program that relies exclusively on these materials is currently under study. We use professional-quality videotapes that present PREP's core ideas and demonstrate both problem patterns and skills. The program is also contained in a manual, and the instructor's manual provides detailed lecture outlines keyed to videotaped demonstrations and PowerPoint slides or overheads. For couples' further study, an audiotape series summarizing the program is available, as well as several books (see especially, Markman, Stanley, & Blumberg, 1994, which provides instructions for the skills and the material of each lecture).

Challenges in Program Implementation and Dissemination

Those interested in establishing community-based prevention programs face many challenges, and our experience with PREP is no exception. Challenges are presented by widespread cultural beliefs about marriage and couples, by mental health professionals, and by the larger social context. Bradbury and Fincham (1990) described a number of these challenges, including (a) general pessimism about the institution of marriage and the possibility of long-term happy relationships, resulting in a passive, fatalistic attitude; (b) low motivation of happy couples who typically believe the old adage, "if it ain't broke, don't fix it;" (c) a concern on the part of one or the other partner (typically the man) that programs will require group experiential exercises in which they are urged to "get in touch," cry, or express intimacy in public; (d) cultural myths, such as the notion that couples shouldn't reveal that they have problems (or even that they might needs skills for future problems) and the myth of "naturalism" (i.e., the belief that relationships should do well without any educational input or support, like in the movies and other media that portray romantic relationships as an effortless, consistently thrilling experience); (e) many mental health professionals' view that preventive work is less interesting than therapy, not lucrative enough, or is a threat to their livelihood; (f) beliefs of funders of mental health services that preventive work is less of a priority for limited funds than is money for treatment services; and (g) larger social issues, such as economic hardship and increased demands of the workplace, that may erect financial or temporal barriers to participation in such programs.

We believe that a core solution to these challenges is imaginative and persistent exposure of alternatives to the views listed above, including clearly presented research data that support these alternative views. Preventionists must use the media, short informational sessions and demonstrations, and other modalities to promote the ideas that all couples face problems at one time or another; that this should not be a reason for shame and secrecy but rather a reason for preventive skill-building and creating communities of care and support; and that marriage can be a challenging and enjoyable, long-lived adventure that with use of skills and a proactive attitude of teamwork will require some work but not necessarily "hard work." Useful would be advertisements and public service announcements that contrast the costs of marital distress and disruption with the costs of participating in prevention programs.

With respect to concerns about the activities within the workshop, we clearly describe PREP to prospective attendees as a course, not therapy. We also assure them that they will not need to discuss private material in a group setting and can choose whether and how much to discuss such material in the private coaching sessions.

Probably the best long-term approach to shifting the attitudes of the professional mental health community is to include prevention as a core topic in graduate training in psychiatry, psychology, pastoral counseling, social work, and allied professions. As we do in our respective doctoral programs, graduate students and interns can be involved as couple coaches and in conducting research and thereby hopefully become "hooked" on prevention. Post-graduate professionals can be encouraged to view conducting prevention workshops as one component of their career rather than as a substitute for clinical work. Periodic workshops with less distressed or nondistressed couples can provide a welcome change of pace from the challenges of working with more distressed couples. As an extra incentive, such workshops often generate private practice referrals.

Regarding the challenge of providing the program to those with limited financial resources, programs are already being offered in religious and community settings at little or no cost. We are clear that relationship-strengthening programs will not in themselves solve all the problems of economically and socially marginalized persons, but they may represent a useful component in assisting these couples to face multiple challenges presented by poverty. We agree with those (Bradbury & Fincham, 1990; Bradbury et al. 2000; Fraenkel, 1999) who maintain that other programs are needed to address the larger contextual forces that negatively affect the well-being of couples and families.

For couples who are "temporally challenged" and feel too busy to attend, short forms of the program are available. However, we hope that the above-described public education efforts will increase general enthusiasm for programs that require relatively little time commitment compared with the vast amount of time expended on relationship distress and disruption.

FUTURE DIRECTIONS

Although the empirical literature on determinants of distress and divorce has produced a wealth of rigorously derived and useful information to guide development of prevention efforts, and intervention studies to date generally support the efficacy of preventive programs, there are many areas for further work. We agree with the critique leveled by some (Bradbury & Fincham, 1990; Bradbury, et al. 2000; Kelly & Fincham 1999) that more attention needs to be placed on researching the impact of the beliefs, emotional vulnerabilities, and physiological-response sensitivities that each partner brings to the relationship, and on incorporating interventions that address these "enduring vulnerabilities" (Kelly & Fincham, 1999). For instance, given that, self-selection biases aside, approximately half of all people who enroll in preventive programs will be adult children of divorce, and that those individuals may have more insecurity about marriage, tend to experience more stress and have more anxiety and dissatisfaction with family and friends than adults from intact families (Glenn & Kramer, 1985; Kulka & Weingarten, 1979), programs might want to include special attention to these issues (Kelly & Fincham, 1999). The field of marital studies and prevention also needs to make use of the burgeoning developmental/personality literature on the impact of differing adult attachment styles (Klohnen & Bera, 1998; Kobak & Hazan, 1991) on relationship functioning and stability, as well as examine the related area of differences in temperament and their impact on thresholds for physiological flooding and overall tolerance for various forms of marital interaction and emotional expression. Likewise, it could be interesting to examine the impact on communication of differing cognitive styles (for example, divergent versus convergent thinking), or the impact of one partner having a learning disability (Walker & Shimmerlik, 1994). Findings could be translated into psychoeducational modules that guide effective coping with such biologically and developmentally determined differences in a manner that promotes resilience and acceptance (Jacobson & Christensen, 1996).

Kelly and Fincham (1999) also noted the seeming overemphasis of prevention programs on containment of conflict and avoidance of negative behavior, rather than promotion of positive behavior. They cited the growing literature showing the critical impact of such behaviors as agreement, empathy, identifying problems in a gentle fashion, creative and collaborative problem-solving, and spending enjoyable time together. We believe that both risk reduction and enhancement of protective factors are important. However, data (Behrens & Halford, 1994; Renick, Blumberg, & Markman, 1992; Stanley et al. 2001) suggest that with a limited amount of time in which to deliver a preventive service to couples, greater emphasis should be placed on helping couples master communication and problem-solving skills that can safeguard them from the primary intrarelationship risk factor of destructive interaction around the inevitable differences and problems that emerge when two people share a life.

It is also worth noting that many topics and activities primarily focused on reducing risk may simultaneously increase protective factors and vice versa. For instance, as couples learn effective, positive communication and problem-solving skills that help them manage conflict, they treat each other more gently (even in conflict) and come to take pride and have confidence in their joint capacities and teamwork, which Notarius and Vanzetti (1983) termed "relationship efficacy." Positive communication and pride in relationship efficacy then serve as protective factors by strengthening the couple's bond. Likewise, as couples build a "bank account" of good feeling through fun, friendship, and sensuality, they may be more inclined to approach discussing their inevitable differences more calmly and effectively—without disrupting the basic sense of "we-ness."

Some have suggested that preventive efforts need to be mounted to address larger contextual variables that affect marital outcomes (Bradbury & Fincham,

1990; Bradbury, Fincham, & Beach, 2000; Kelly & Fincham, 1999), such as unemployment (Aubry, Tefft, & Kinsbury, 1990), poverty, racism, and work pressures that lead to negative spillover and time away from family (Fraenkel & Wilson, 2000; Halford, Gravestock, Lower, & Scheldt, 1992). We agree, and one of us (Fraenkel) has developed a program in an urban setting to support homeless families and couples of color as they move from welfare to work (Fraenkel, Hameline, & Shannon, 2000; Fraenkel & Shannon, 1999). However, short of direct preventive efforts or public policy initiatives addressing these larger societal forces, existing distress prevention programs could include modules that help couples recognize the powerful impact of these forces on their stress levels and amount of time together (Fraenkel & Wilson, 2000).

Programs also could do more to recognize the larger cultural belief systems, shared to a greater or lesser degree by each particular couple, that inform common problematic patterns. For instance, the ubiquitous pursuer-distancer pattern, in which women typically pursue and become critical while men withdraw and become defensive (Christensen & Heavey, 1990), is partly the result of stereotyped gender beliefs, reinforced by such popular books as *Men Are From Mars, Women Are From Venus* (Gray, 1992), that women are more suited by nature to be the emotional "managers" of relationships and men are incapable of expressing their feelings. It might assist couples to become more flexible and equitable in their interactions if prevention programs included material that "deconstructs" or closely examines these powerful cultural messages and helps couples "externalize" or separate these beliefs from their own life narratives and preferred ways of being (White & Epston, 1990).

In addition, new challenges are emerging as prevention and enrichment programs are increasingly disseminated among specific cultural, ethnic, and religious groups (Crohn, Markman, Blumberg, & Levine, 2000; Stanley, Trathen, McCain, & Bryan, 1998; Whitfield, Markman, & Stanley, in press), specific social contexts in which couples share particular conditions and challenges (such as the armed forces), or whole societies different from the ones from which participants were drawn for the basic marital research and efficacy studies. It behooves us to conduct more research on marriage in these groups and societies, and to revise program formats and content to address the particular needs of marriages within them (Fraenkel, 1998, 1999). Likewise, more preventive programs should target couples at life-cycle stages known to involve increased risk, such as the transition to parenthood (Cowan & Cowan, 1992; Jordan, Stanley, & Markman, 1999; Matese, Shorr, & Jason, 1982), the "empty nest" (Arp, Stanley, Arp, Markman, & Blumberg, 2000), and the transition to retirement. More basic research is needed on the relationship between marital disorder and various forms of psychopathology, and preventive programs must be developed and tested to address the particular vulnerabilities of such couples.

Information such as that summarized in this chapter should be presented to those in positions to fund programs on a broad scale. In addition, marital distress prevention efforts must continue to be empirically evaluated and extended so that a steady stream of solid data supports their importance and viability.

In summary, much progress has been made over the past three decades in developing research-based programs for preventing marital disorder. Many challenges remain, however, particularly with regard to promoting prevention in the broader society. With the evergrowing body of data documenting the negative impact of distress and divorce, and the mounting evidence that skill-based educational programs for couples can make a difference, we believe social scientists, clinicians, community leaders, policy makers, and couples themselves would do well to invest time, money, and effort in prevention.

REFERENCES

Amato, P. R. (2000). The consequences of divorce for adults and children. *Journal of Marriage and the Family, 62,* 1269–1287.

Arp, C. S., Stanley, S. M., Arp, D. H., Markman, H. J., & Blumberg, S. L. (2000). *Fighting for your empty nest marriage: Reinventing your relationship when the kids leave home.* San Francisco: Jossey-Bass.

Aubry, T., Tefft, B., & Kingsbury, N. (1990). Behavioral and psychological consequences of unemployment in blue-collar couples. *Journal of Community Psychology, 18,* 99–109.

Barling, J. (1990). Employment and marital functioning. In F. D. Fincham & T. N. Bradbury (Eds.), *The psychology of marriage* (pp. 201–225). New York: Guilford.

Behrens, B., & Halford, K. (1994, August). *Advances in the prevention and treatment of marital distress.* Paper presented at the "Helping Families Change" Conference, University of Queensland, Brisbane, Australia.

Berger, R., & Hannah, M. T. (1999). Introduction. In R. Berger & M. T. Hannah (Eds.), *Preventive approaches in couples therapy* (pp. 1–27). Philadelphia, PA: Brunner/Mazel.

Bloom, B., Asher, S., & White, S. (1978). Marital disruption as a stressor: A review and analysis. *Psychological Bulletin, 85,* 867–894.

Bloom, B., Hodges, W. F., Caldwell, R. A., Systra, L., & Cedrone, A. R. (1977). Marital separation: A community survey. *Journal of Divorce, 1,* 7–19.

Bradbury, T. N., & Fincham, F. D. (1990). Preventing marital dysfunction: Review and analysis. In F. D. Fincham & T. N. Bradbury (Eds.), *The psychology of marriage* (pp. 375–401). New York: Guilford.

Bradbury, T. N., Fincham, F. D., & Beach, S. R. H. (2000). Research on the nature and determinants of marital satisfaction: A decade in review. *Journal of Marriage and the Family, 62*, 964–980.

Brody, G. H., Neubaum, E., & Forehand, R. (1988). Serial marriage: A heuristic analysis of an emerging family form. *Psychological Bulletin, 103*, 211–222.

Burman, B., & Margolin, G. (1992). Analysis of the association between marital relationships and health problems: An interactional perspective. *Psychological Bulletin, 112*, 39–63.

Cherlin, A. (1981). *Marriage, divorce, remarriage.* Cambridge, MA: Harvard University Press.

Cherlin, A. (1992). *Marriage, divorce, and remarriage* (2nd ed.). Cambridge, MA: Harvard University Press.

Christensen, A., & Heavey, C. L. (1990). Gender and social structure in the demand/withdraw pattern of marital conflict. *Journal of Personality and Social Psychology, 59*, 73–82.

Coie, J. D., Watt, N. F., West, S. G., Hawkins, J. D., Asarnow, J. R.., Markman, H. J., Ramey, S. L., Shure, M. B., & Long, B. (1993). The science of prevention: A conceptual framework and some directions for a national research program. *American Psychologist, 48*, 1013–1022.

Cowan, C. P., & Cowan, P. A. (1992). *When partners become parents: The big life change for couples.* Hillsdale, NJ: Erlbaum.

Crohn, J., Markman, H. J., Blumberg, S. L., & Levine, J. R. (2000). *Fighting for your Jewish marriage: Preserving a lasting promise.* San Francisco: Jossey-Bass.

DeMaria, R. (1998). *A national survey of married couples who participate in marriage enrichment*, No. 983–3080. Ann Arbor, MI: UMI Dissertation Services.

DeMaris, A. (2000). Til discord do us part: The role of physical and verbal conflict in union disruption. *Journal of Marriage and the Family, 62*, 683–692.

Durana, C. (1996). A longitudinal evaluation of the effectiveness of the PAIRS psychoeducational program for couples. *Family Therapy, 23*, 11–36.

Emery, R. E. (1982). Interparental conflict and the children of discord or divorce. *Psychological Bulletin, 92*, 310–330.

Fincham, F. D., Beach, S. R. H., Harold, G. T., & Osborne, L. N. (1997). Marital satisfaction and depression: Different causal relationships for men and women? *Psychological Science, 8*, 351–357.

Fincham, F. D., Bradbury, T. N., & Scott, C. K. (1990). Cognition in marriage. In F. D. Fincham & T. N. Bradbury (Eds.), *The psychology of marriage* (pp. 118–149). New York: Guilford.

Forthofer, M. S., Markman, H. J., Cox, M., Stanley, S. M., & Kessler, R. C. (1996). Associations between marital distress and work loss in a national sample. *Journal of Marriage and the Family, 58*, 597–605.

Fraenkel, P. (1995). The nomothetic-idiographic debate in family therapy. *Family Process, 34*, 113–121.

Fraenkel, P. (1997). Systems approaches to couple therapy. In W.K. Halford & H. Markman (Eds.), *Clinical handbook of marriage and couples interventions* (pp. 379–413). London: Wiley.

Fraenkel, P. (1998, June). *Guidelines to individually- and culturally-sensitive introduction of research-based prevention programs for couples.* Paper presented at the annual meeting of the American Family Therapy Academy, Montréal, Québec, Canada.

Fraenkel, P. (1999, Spring). Family therapy training in Hong Kong: Thoughts from a visiting colleague. *Family Therapy Forum*, pp. 5–11.

Fraenkel, P. (1999, April). *Last chance couple therapy.* Workshop presented at the Ackerman Institute for the Family, New York, New York.

Fraenkel, P., Hameline, T., & Shannon, M. (2000). *Collaborative family program development: Family support from welfare to work.* Manuscript in preparation.

Fraenkel, P., & Shannon, M. (1999). *Multiple family discussion group manual: Family Support from Welfare to Work Program (Fresh Start for Families).* Unpublished manual, Ackerman Institute for the Family, New York, New York.

Fraenkel, P., & Whittet, L. (1998, June). *How do couples use prevention skills? A qualitative study.* Poster presented at the annual research conference of the Society for Prevention Research, Park City, Utah.

Fraenkel, P., & Wilson, S. (2000). Clocks, calendars, and couples: Time and the rhythms of relationships. In P. Papp (Ed.), *Couples on the fault line: New directions for therapists* (pp. 63–103). New York: Guilford.

Giblin, P., Sprenkle, D. H., & Sheehan, R. (1985). Enrichment outcome research: A meta-analysis of premarital, marital, and family interventions. *Journal of Marital and Family Therapy, 11*, 257–271.

Glenn, N. D. (1991). The recent trend in marital success in the United States. *Journal of Marriage and the Family, 53*, 261–270.

Glenn, N. D., & Kramer, K. B. (1985). The psychological well-being of adult children of divorce. *Journal of Marriage and the Family, 47*, 905–912.

Glenn, N. D., & Weaver, C. N. (1981). The contribution of marital happiness to global happiness. *Journal of Marriage and the Family, 43*, 161–168.

Glenwick, D. S., & Jason, L. A. (1993). Behavioral approaches to prevention in the community: A historical and theoretical overview. In D. S. Glenwick & L. A. Jason (Eds.), *Promoting health and mental health in children, youth, and families* (pp. 3–13). New York: Springer Publishing.

Glick, P. C. (1984). How American families are changing. *American Demographics, 6*, 20–27.

Gotlib, I. H., & McCabe, S. B. (1990). Marriage and psychopathology. In F.

D. Fincham & T. N. Bradbury (Eds.), *The psychology of marriage* (pp. 226–257). New York: Guilford.

Gottman, J. M. (1993). A theory of marital dissolution and stability. *Journal of Family Psychology, 7*, 57–75.

Gottman, J. M. (1994a). *What predicts divorce?* Hillsdale, NJ: Erlbaum.

Gottman, J. M. (1994b). *Why marriages succeed or fail.* New York: Simon & Schuster.

Gottman, J. M. (1999). *The marriage clinic: A scientifically-based marital therapy.* New York: Norton.

Gottman, J. M., Coan, J., Carrere, S., & Swanson, C. (1998). Predicting marital happiness and stability from newlywed interactions. *Journal of Marriage and the Family, 60*, 5–22.

Gottman, J. M., & Gottman, J. S. (1999). The marriage survival kit: A research-based marital therapy. In R. Berger & M. T. Hannah (Eds.), *Preventive approaches in couples therapy* (pp. 304–330). Philadelphia: Brunner/Mazel.

Gottman, J. M., & Krokoff, L. J. (1989). Marital interaction and satisfaction: A longitudinal view. *Journal of Consulting and Clinical Psychology, 57*, 47–52.

Gottman, J. M., & Levenson, R. W. (1999a). How stable is marital interaction over time? *Family Process, 38*, 159–165.

Gottman, J. M., & Levenson, R. W. (1999b). What predicts change in marital interaction over time? A study of alternative models. *Family Process, 38*, 143–158.

Gottman, J. M., & Notarius, C. I. (2000). Decade review: Observing marital interaction. *Journal of Marriage and the Family, 62*, 927–947.

Gray, J. (1992). *Men are from Mars, women are from Venus: A practical guide for improving communication and getting what you want in your relationships.* New York: Harper Collins.

Grych, J., & Fincham, F. (1990). Marital conflict and children's adjustment. *Psychological Bulletin, 108*, 267–290.

Hahlweg, K., & Markman, H. J. (1988). Effectiveness of behavioral marital therapy: Empirical status of behavioral techniques in preventing and alleviating distress. *Journal of Consulting and Clinical Psychology, 56*, 440–447.

Hahlweg, K. Markman, H. J., Thurmaier, F., Engl, J., & Eckert, V. (1998). Prevention of marital distress: Results of a German prospective longitudinal study. *Journal of Family Psychology, 12*, 543–556.

Halford, W. K., Gravestock, F. M., Lowe, R., & Scheldt, S (1992). Toward a behavioral ecology of stressful marital interactions. *Behavioral Assessment, 14*, 199–217.

Halford, W. K., & Markman, H. J. (Eds.). (1997). *Clinical handbook of mar-*

riage and couples interventions. London: Wiley.

Howes, P., & Markman, H. J. (1984). Marital quality and child functioning: A longitudinal investigation. *Child Development, 60,* 1044–1051.

Jacobson, N. S., & Addis, M. E. (1993). Research on couple therapy: What do we know? Where are we going? *Journal of Consulting and Clinical Psychology, 61,* 85–93.

Jacobson, N. J., & Christensen, A. (1996). *Acceptance and change in couple therapy: A therapist's guide to transforming relationships.* New York: Norton.

Jacobson, N. S., & Gottman, J. M. (1998). *When men batter women.* New York: Simon & Schuster.

Jenkins, J. M. (2000). Marital conflict and children's emotions: The development of an anger organization. *Journal of Marriage and the Family, 62,* 723–736.

Jordan, P. L., Stanley, S. M., & Markman, H. J. (1999). *Becoming parents: How to strengthen your marriage as your family grows.* San Francisco: Jossey-Bass.

Julien, D., Arellano, C., & Turgeon, L. (1997). Gender issues in heterosexual, gay, and lesbian couples. In W. K. Halford & H. Markman (Eds.), *Clinical handbook of marriage and couples interventions* (pp. 107–127). London: Wiley.

Karney, B. R., & Bradbury, T. N. (1995). The longitudinal course of marital quality and stability: A review of theory, method, and research. *Psychological Bulletin, 118,* 3–34.

Karney, B. R., & Bradbury, T. N. (2000). Attributions in marriage: State or trait? A growth curve analysis. *Journal of Personality and Social Psychology, 78,* 295–309.

Kelly, A. B., & Fincham, F. D. (1999). Preventing marital distress: What does research offer? In R. Berger & M. T. Hannah (Eds.)., *Preventive approaches in couple therapy* (pp. 361–390). Philadelphia: Brunner/Mazel.

Kiecolt-Glaser, J. K., Malarkey, W. B., Chee, M., Newton, T., Cacioppo, J. T., Mao, H., & Glaser, R. (1993). Negative behavior during marital conflict is associated with immunological down-regulation. *Psychosomatic Medicine, 55,* 395–409.

Klohnen, E. C., & Bera, C. (1998). Behavioral and experiential patterns of avoidantly and securely attached women across adulthood: A 31-year longitudinal perspective. *Journal of Personality and Social Psychology, 74,* 211–223.

Kobak, R. R., & Hazan, C. (1991). Attachment in marriage: Effects of security and accuracy in working models. *Journal of Personality and Social Psychology, 60,* 861–869.

Kulka, R. A., & Weingarten, H. (1979). The long-term effects of parental divorce on adult adjustment. *Journal of Social Issues, 35*, 50–78.

Kurdek, L. A. (1998). Relationship outcomes and their predictors: Longitudinal evidence from heterosexual married, gay cohabiting, and lesbian cohabiting couples. *Journal of Marriage and the Family, 60*, 553–568.

Laird, J. (1999, Fall). The politics of "smart marriage." *American Family Therapy Newsletter*, 43–45.

Laird, J., & Green, R. J. (1996). *Lesbians and gays in couples and families: A handbook for therapists*. San Francisco: Jossey-Bass.

Luthar, S. S., & Zigler, E. (1991). Vulnerability and competence: A review of research on resilience in childhood. *American Journal of Orthopsychiatry, 61*, 6–22.

Mace, D., & Mace, V. (1980). Enriching marriages: The foundation stone of family strength. In N. Stinnett, B. Chesser, J. DeFrain, & P. Knaub (Eds.), *Family strengths: Positive models for family life* (pp. 89–110) Lincoln, NE: University of Nebraska Press.

Markman, H. J. (1981). Prediction of marital distress: A 5-year follow-up. *Journal of Consulting and Clinical Psychology, 49*, 760–762.

Markman, H. J., Floyd, F. J., Stanley, S. M., & Storaasli, R. D. (1988). Prevention of marital distress: a longitudinal investigation. *Journal of Consulting and Clinical Psychology, 56*, 210–217.

Markman, H. J., & Jones-Leonard, D. (1985). Marital discord and children at risk: Implications for research and prevention. In W. Frankenburg & R. Emde (Eds.), *Identification of the child at risk: An international perspective* (pp. 59–77). New York: Plenum.

Markman, H. J., Renick, M. J., Floyd, F. J., Stanley, S. M., & Clements, M. (1993). Preventing marital distress through communication and conflict management training: A four- and five-year follow-up. *Journal of Consulting and Clinical Psychology, 62*, 70–77.

Markman, H., Stanley, S., & Blumberg, S. L. (1994). *Fighting for your marriage*. San Francisco, CA: Jossey-Bass.

Martin, T. C., & Bumpass, L. (1989). Recent trends in marital disruption. *Demography, 26*, 37–51.

Matese, F., Shorr, S. I., & Jason, L. A. (1982). Behavioral and community interventions during transition to parenthood. In A. M. Jeger & R. J. Slotnick (Eds.), *Community mental health and behavioral ecology: A handbook of theory, research, and practice* (pp. 231–241). New York: Plenum.

National Center for Health Statistics (1996). *Advance report of final divorce statistics, 1989 and 1990*. Hyattsville, MD: National Center for Health Statistics.

Norton, A. J., & Miller, L. F. (1992). *Marriage, divorce, and remarriage in the 1990s*. Washington, DC: U.S. Department of Commerce.

Notarius, C., & Buongiorno, J. (1992). *Wait time until professional treatment in marital therapy.* Unpublished paper, Catholic University of America, Washington, D.C.

Notarius, C. I., & Markman, H. M. (1987). Coding marital and family interaction: Current status. In T. Jacob (Ed.), *Family interaction and psychopathology: Theories, methods, and findings* (pp. 329–390). New York: Plenum.

Notarius, C. I., & Markman, H. M. (1993). *We can work it out: Making sense of marital conflict.* New York: Putnam.

Notarius, C. I., & Vanzetti, N. (1983). The marital agenda protocol. In E. Filsinger (Ed.), *Marital and family assessment* (pp. 209–227). Beverly Hills, CA: Sage.

O'Leary, K. D., Barling, J., Arias, I., & Rosenbaum, A. (1989). Prevalence and stability of physical aggression between spouses: A longitudinal analysis. *Journal of Consulting and Clinical Psychology, 57,* 263–268.

Olson, D. H., & DeFrain, J. (1997). *Marriage and the family: Diversity and strengths* (2nd ed.). Mountain View, CA: Mayfield.

Papp, P. (2000). Gender differences in depression: His or her depression. In P. Papp (Ed.), *Couples on the fault line: New directions for therapists* (pp. 130–151). New York: Guilford.

Renick, M. J., Blumberg, S., & Markman, H. J. (1992). The Prevention and Relationship Enhancement Program (PREP): An empirically-based preventive intervention program for couples. *Family Relations, 41,* 141–147.

Roberts, L. J. (2000). Fire and ice in marital communication: Hostile and distancing behaviors as predictors of marital distress. *Journal of Marriage and the Family, 62,* 693–707.

Rogers, S. J., & Amato, P. R. (1997). Is marital quality declining? The evidence from two generations. *Social Forces, 75,* 1089–1100.

Rogge, R. M., & Bradbury, T. N. (1999). Recent advances in the prediction of marital outcomes. In R. Berger & M. T. Hannah (Eds.), *Preventive approaches in couples therapy* (pp. 331–360). Philadelphia: Brunner/Mazel.

Schmaling, K. B., & Sher, T. G. (1997). Physical health and relationships. In W. K. Halford & H. Markman (Eds.), *Clinical handbook of marriage and couples interventions* (pp. 323–345). London: Wiley.

Stanley, S. M. (1995, December). *How a marriage dies.* Paper presented at Focus on the Family Breakfast for Christian Counselors, Colorado Springs, Colorado.

Stanley, S. M., Blumberg, S. L., & Markman, H. J. (1999). Helping couples fight *for* their marriages: The PREP approach. In R. Berger & M. T. Hannah (Eds), *Preventive approaches in couples therapy* (pp. 279–303). Philadelphia: Brunner/Mazel.

Stanley, S. M., Bradbury, T. N., & Markman, H. J. (2000). Structural flaws in the bridge from basic research on marriage to interventions for couples. *Journal of Marriage and the Family, 62,* 256–264.

Stanley, S. M., Markman, H. J., Prado, L. M., Olmos-Gallo, P. A., Tonelli, L., St. Peters, M., Leber, B. D., Bobulinski, M., Cordova, A., & Whitton, S. (2001). Community-based premarital prevention: Clergy and lay leaders on the front lines. *Family Relations, 50*, 67–76.

Stanley, S. M., Markman, H. J., St. Peters, M., & Leber, D. (1995). Strengthening marriages and preventing divorce: New directions in prevention research. *Family Relations, 44*, 392–401.

Stanley, S. M., Trathen, D., McCain, S., & Bryan, M. (1998). *A lasting promise: A Christian guide to fighting for your marriage*. San Francisco: Jossey-Bass.

Straus, M., & Gelles, R. (1990). *Physical violence in American families: Risk factors and adaptations to violence in 8,145 families*. New Brunswick, NJ: Transaction Press.

Teachman, J. D., Tedrow, L. M., & Crowder, K. D. (2000). The changing demography of America's families. *Journal of Marriage and the Family, 62*, 1234–1246.

U.S. Bureau of the Census, (1998, March). Marital status and living arrangements (update). *Current Population Reports*, (Series P20–514).

Van Widenfelt, B., Hosman, C., Schaap, C., & Van Der Staak, C. (1996). The prevention of relationship distress for couples at risk: A controlled evaluation with nine-month and two-year follow-up. *Family Relations, 45*, 156–165.

Veroff, J., Kulka, R. A., & Douvan, E. (1981). *Mental health in America: Patterns of help-seeking from 1957 to 1976*. New York: Basic Books.

Walker, G., & Shimmerlik, S. (1994). The invisible battlefield. *Family Therapy Networker, 18*, 51–61.

White, M., & Epston, D. (1990). *Narrative means to therapeutic ends*. New York: Norton.

Whitfield, K., Markman, H. J., & Stanley, S. M. (in press). *Fighting for your African-American marriage*. San Francisco: Jossey-Bass.

ACKNOWLEDGMENT

Support for the first author during preparation of this chapter was provided in part by a generous grant from the Robert Goelet Foundation to the Family Studies Program of the New York University Child Study Center.

CHAPTER 13

Promoting Mental Health in Later Life

*Margaret Gatz, Michael Crowe, Amy Fiske,
Wendy Fung, Christopher Kelly, Boaz Levy,
Michele Maines, Gia Robinson, Derek D. Satre,
Juan Pedro Serrano Selva, Kristen Suthers,
Kecia Watari, and Julie Loebach Wetherell*

DESCRIPTION OF THE PROBLEM

Older adults should be prime targets for preventive interventions because increasing numbers of individuals are living into their seventies, eighties, nineties, and beyond. In the United States in 1996, 16.5% of the population was age 60 or older (Day, 1996). By 2020, the "baby boomer" generation will have reached old age, leading to a marked increase in numbers of older adults. Life expectancy will continue to climb, projected to reach 82 years in 2050 (Day, 1996). Among older adults and future older adults, however, not just length of life but quality of life is a prime concern. Preventive programs are vehicles for improving the healthy lifespan by reducing disability and helping

The literature reviews discussed herein were carried out as a class project: relaxation (Satre), meditation (Fung), stress management (Robinson), physical exercise (Fiske and Levy), volunteerism (Kelly and Maines), life review (Serrano), memory training (Crowe and Watari), widow support groups (Robinson), caregiver support groups (Fung), and psychosocial interventions with medical patients (Wetherell). Tables summarizing studies for each intervention are available from the respective authors.

people cope with the various problems that dictate the landscape of old age, such as the deaths of loved ones and limitations imposed by health conditions. At the same time, older adults present special issues for prevention, such as the frequent comorbidity of physical and mental dysfunction, and the importance of cognitive impairment as well as emotional disorders in the spectrum of psychopathology of old age.

Existing literature provides a strong rationale for prevention. Among older adults with medical illnesses, depressive symptoms can compound the disability and lead to increased mortality and morbidity (Bruce, Seeman, Merril, & Blazer, 1994). Preventing depression speeds recovery and improves physical functioning (Oslin, Streim, Katz, Edell, & TenHave, 2000). Among those providing care to a physically frail or demented elderly family member, stress can be associated with negative physical and psychological consequences for the caregiver (Aneshensel, Pearlin, Mullan, Zarit, & Whitlatch, 1995). Preventing a build-up of stress supports the caregiver and thereby enables the demented older adult to live for longer in the community (Mittelman, Ferris, Shulman, Steinberg, & Levin, 1996).

REVIEW AND CRITIQUE OF THE LITERATURE

In this chapter we summarize the results of randomized clinical trials for preventive interventions with older adults. Systematic selection of studies involved the following criteria: (a) a sample consisting of older adults (or a mixed-age sample with separate analysis of an older adult subsample), (b) a sample not recruited on the basis of psychiatric disorder, (c) a noninstitutionalized sample, (d) random assignment to treatment and control conditions, (e) intervention including some defined behavioral aspect, (f) pre- and posttest data using objective measures, (g) at least one outcome measure that was psychological (e.g., improved life satisfaction, optimism, sense of personal control, social ties, or reduced symptoms of depression or anxiety, sleep difficulties, or pain). Where possible, we preferred studies that included a follow-up assessment after the posttest. Where there was sufficient literature, we focused on more recent research. For one type of intervention reviewed (volunteerism), it was not possible to find any studies that met the criteria, and we relaxed the random assignment requirement.

Our review is, by necessity, selective. We include interventions that have been used in adults of various ages but may have special rationale or procedures with older adults (i.e., relaxation training, stress management, physical exercise, volunteerism) and interventions that are age-specific or that are directed to at-risk groups that often include older adults (i.e., life review, memory training, outreach to bereaved older adults, caregiver support groups, interventions with older medical patients).[1] For each preventive intervention, we include: the rationale for the intervention; a description of the intervention, including the settings and population where it is typically practiced; and a summary of studies supporting the efficacy of the preventive intervention.

Relaxation Training

Rationale

Older adults appear to be particularly likely to exhibit subsyndromal levels of psychological distress, including anxiety and depression, and to face consensually stressful situations. Relaxation often is included as a component in multicomponent "wellness programs" for older adults. Physiologically, the state of relaxation serves to lower blood pressure and decrease levels of stress hormones associated with negative physical health outcomes (see DeBerry, 1982, for a review).

Description

Progressive relaxation entails tensing and relaxing different muscle groups while focusing on physiological sensations (see manual by Bernstein & Borkovec, 1973). Individuals are instructed to skip over any muscle group in which they are likely to feel pain or discomfort. Relaxation training may be conducted in either group or individual sessions, with audiotaping of training sessions sometimes used to assist in practicing the techniques at home. Imaginal relaxation procedures are relatively less standardized, do not require the actual tensing and relaxing of muscles, and may include instructions to imagine the tensing and relaxing of muscles or to imagine pleasant scenes. This method has been advocated for use with older adults who may have physical problems such as arthritis (Lichstein, 1988).

   We found no separate evaluations of meditation as a preventive intervention. However, in two studies (DeBerry, 1982; DeBerry, Davis, & Reinhard, 1989), meditation—specifically, visualization of a calming scene—was combined with progressive relaxation.

Outcome Studies

Seven randomized controlled trials were found. Progressive muscle relaxation training appears to be effective in reducing levels of anxiety as well as self-reported psychiatric symptoms among community-dwelling samples of older adults. DeBerry (1982), DeBerry, Davis, and Reinhard (1989), Yesavage (1984), and Rankin, Gilner, Gfeller, and Katz (1993) all found that relaxation training significantly reduced trait and/or state anxiety. Scogin, Rickard, Keith, Wilson, and McElreath (1992) found that progressive muscle relaxation and imaginal relaxation techniques were equally effective in increasing relaxation level as well as reducing anxiety and psychiatric symptoms, with gains maintained at one-year follow-up (Rickard, Scogin, & Keith, 1994). Other studies (DeBerry, 1982; DeBerry et al. 1989) have suggested that the continued practice of relaxation techniques is necessary to maintain anxiety symptom reduction.

Positive effects of relaxation training are quite broad. DeBerry (1981–82) found that a group of anxious widows reported less anxiety, less muscle tension, better sleep, and fewer headaches following combined progressive muscle relaxation and guided visual imagery, with reduction in anxiety maintained at follow-up. Use of relaxation with older medical patients is discussed in a later section. Furthermore, relaxation may improve the effectiveness of memory training (Yesavage, 1984).

Stress Management

Rationale and Description

Various programs for older adults have the general goal of promoting positive mental health, increasing self-esteem, and optimizing a sense of personal control. Components of these interventions include: cognitive restructuring (Lachman, Weaver, Bandura, Elliot, & Lewkowicz, 1992); effective problem solving; exercise; and educational topics, such as nutrition and safety. Interventions categorized as stress inoculation (Meichenbaum, 1977) encompass relaxation, information about stressors and coping strategies, and self-statements concerning one's ability to master the situation. Programs tend to be conducted as classes, often in retirement communities or senior housing.

Outcome Studies

Results are promising for stress management interventions using stress inoculation. Stress inoculation led to increases in effective strategies to handle stress and decreases in anxiety compared with placebo controls or no treatment (Lopez & Silber, 1991). Compared with an alternative form of training and a control group, stress inoculation led to more lasting gains in inductive reasoning

(Hayslip, 1989) and to superior performance 3 years later among those reminded to use the skills they had learned (Hayslip, Maloy, & Kohl, 1995). Finally, an omnibus program of stress management, nutritional awareness, physical fitness, and spirituality led to improvements in perceived control and spirituality compared with the placebo control (Slivinske & Fitch, 1987).

Physical Exercise

Rationale

Cross-sectional and epidemiological evidence suggests that physical activity in older adults may be positively related to cognitive functioning (for a review, see Emery & Blumenthal, 1991) and psychological well-being (for a review, see McAuley & Rudolph, 1995). Furthermore, exercise has been shown to reduce depressive symptoms among adults with clinically significant depression (reviewed by Craft & Landers, 1998). These findings have encouraged the hypothesis that promoting physical fitness in nonclinical populations of sedentary older adults may enhance cognitive capacities and psychological well-being and attenuate age-related psychological decrements.

Description

Exercise programs included in outcome studies typically consist of 1-hour sessions, including aerobic exercise, warm-up and cool-down periods, and possibly strength and flexibility training. Sessions are typically three times per week; duration of the interventions ranges from 3 weeks to 1 year. Most programs are conducted in groups.

Outcome Studies

The review of experimental research indicates that results are mixed for both cognitive and mood outcome measures. Some (Dustman et al., 1984; Williams & Lord, 1997), but not all (Kramer et al. 1999; Madden, Blumenthal, Allen, & Emery, 1989) studies find that simple reaction time improves after involvement in an exercise program. It appears that improvement in reaction time cannot be explained by changes in psychomotor speed, which either did not improve (Emery & Gatz, 1990; Emery, Schein, Hauck, & MacIntyre, 1998) or actually deteriorated (Blumenthal, Emery, Maddem, and Schiedore, 1991) with exercise. Measures of attention show mixed results as well. Several investigators (e.g., Hawkins, Kramer, & Capaldi, 1992) have reported improved attentional processes, but others have not (e.g., Hill, Storandt, & Malley, 1993). Most studies find no evidence that exercise improves memory (Blumenthal et al. 1989; Hill, Storandt, & Malley, 1993; Perri & Templer, 1984–85), but there are exceptions. One study with a small convenience sample found broad improvement in memory (Fabre et al. 1999). Hill and colleagues et al. (1993) found that memory for text was better in the exercise than in the control group at follow-up, due to decline in the control group. In tests of both reaction time and memory, Kramer et al. (1999) found improvement only on tasks that involved executive functioning. No evidence was found of improvement in fluid intelligence as a result of exercise (Dustman et al. 1984; Williams & Lord, 1997).

Most randomized controlled trials have found that exercise does not significantly improve depressive symptoms among nonclinical populations of older adults (e.g., Emery, Schein, Hauck, & MacIntyre, 1998; Williams & Lord, 1997). An exception is the Blumenthal et al. (1989) study, which reported reduced depressive symptoms, but only among men. Wallace et al. (1998) found that a multifaceted intervention with exercise as a central component led to decreased depressive symptoms in a normal older adult sample, but the effects could have been due to other components of the intervention. Results show a similar mixed pattern with regard to the effects of an exercise program on anxiety symptoms. Williams and Lord (1997) found improvement on measures of depression and anxiety for those who had the highest levels of symptoms at baseline. In summary, there is some evidence that exercise may enhance well-being, although the strongest evidence tends to appear on subjective perceptions (Emery & Blumenthal, 1990; Fabre et al. 1999; Williams & Lord, 1997).

Volunteering

Rationale and Description

Retirees are often viewed as an untapped service resource; at the same time, volunteer work often is seen as a way to help the older volunteers themselves. Studies (Aquino, Russell, Cutrona, & Altmaier, 1996; Kuehne & Sears, 1993; Musick, Herzog, & House, 1999) have shown correlations between volunteering and such variables as self-esteem, life satisfaction, and decreased mor-tality. Volunteering can take many forms: (a) paraprofessional activities, with older adults serving as peer counselors, community educators, legal advisors, or mediators, (b) intergenerational programs (e.g., in schools); and (c) com-munity service, using the older adults' life skills (e.g., at community libraries).

Outcome Studies

A meta-analysis (Wheeler, Gorey, & Greenblatt, 1998) concluded that volun-teering does bolster well-being in the older volunteer. However, virtually all evidence is based on collecting data before volunteers begin and after some period of time as a volunteer. With no comparison groups, change cannot unequivocally be attributed to the effects of volunteering. In two evaluations of peer programs, both using a pre-post design, Gatz et al. (1982) found that serving as an indigenous community worker led to improvements in problem-solving abilities and increased life satisfaction, while Petty and Cusack (1989) found that peer counselors increased in helping skills and in the ability to com-pensate for sensory losses.

In programs in school classrooms, Newman, Karip, and Faux (1995) found that especially among the oldest volunteers (i.e., age 70 and older) memory performance and subjective memory improved, while Carney, Dobson, and Dobson (1987) reported improvement in purpose of life scores. Booz, Allen, and Hamilton (1985) evaluated the federally sponsored Retired Seniors Volunteer Program (RSVP) using a randomly selected sample of volunteers from sites around the country. Experienced volunteers reported fewer psy-chological symptoms as well as higher functioning and morale compared with new volunteers and dropouts.

Life Review

Rationale and Description

Life review is the process by which people evaluate and reorganize past expe-riences in order to come to terms with their lived lives (Butler, 1963). Life review can be conducted on an individual or group basis. Groups may allow for older persons to find common ground with others and thereby engage in a process of mutual social support (Thorsteim & Roberts, 1996). There is a great deal of variety in the types of experiences that are called life review or reminiscence groups, possibly reflecting a lack of conceptual clarity. Haight and Webster (1995) is the best source for a systematic overview of how to conduct life review. Another source is Birren and Birren's (1996) description of their class in guided autobiography; members write and share their autobiographies, using a variety of sensitizing materials to structure the writing process.

Outcome Studies

There have been few randomized controlled trials with nondepressed older adults or with noninstitutionalized samples. Compared with a friendly visitors intervention and to a nontreatment control group, Haight (1988, 1992) found that participants in a program of structured life review demonstrated improved life satisfaction and psychological well-being. Neither Haight (1992), with home-bound older adults, nor Stevens-Ratchford (1993), in a retirement community setting, found changes in symptoms of depression.

Life review also has been used with an elderly medical population. One large-scale study (McWilliam et al. 1999) found positive effects on some variables for an intervention featuring nurse-facilitated critical reflection on life and health in chronically ill older people newly discharged from the hospital. In patients facing surgery or other invasive medical procedures, a structured life review intervention focused on life challenges resulted in reduced anxiety and enhanced coping self-efficacy, significantly different from an untreated control group, although for the most part not better than general reminiscence or relaxation (Rybarczyk & Auerbach, 1990; Rybarczyk, Auerbach, Jorn, & Lofland, 1993).

Memory Training

Rationale

Many older adults fear that they will lose their memory, especially given the current level of media attention to Alzheimer's disease. Tests of memory functioning typically show age-related decline, although this decline often does not affect daily living. Memory training research, therefore, has focused on improving older adults' subjective memory perceptions, in addition to improving objective memory skills.

Description

Traditional memory training programs are mainly didactic, teaching mnemonic techniques such as visualization, chunking information (i.e., using rules to combine the information to be remembered into smaller units), pegword (i.e., associating items to be remembered with nouns that rhyme with numbers), or method of loci (i.e., visualizing items to be remembered in specific, well-known locations). Some programs include pretraining, such as relaxation or imagery (Brooks, Friedman, Pearman, Gray, & Yesavage, 1999; Yesavage, 1984). Comprehensive manuals are now available, including information about memory and aging, training in mnemonic techniques, and cognitive restructuring (i.e., altering pessimistic beliefs about memory abilities) (Caprio-Prevette & Fry, 1996a). Duration of the training varies from one session to 12 weekly sessions. Formats range from group or individual sessions to self-instruction. Participants are generally community-dwelling older adult volunteers with subjective memory complaints, who are screened to rule out dementia, severe medical or neurological conditions, psychopathology, or use of medications that could affect memory or cognition.

Outcome Studies

A meta-analysis by Verhaeghen, Marcoen, and Goossens (1992) concluded that mnemonic training was superior to control or placebo groups in improving objective memory performance. A subsequent meta-analysis by Floyd and Scogin (1997) established that memory training led to improved subjective memory functioning when compared with no treatment. However, the effect size for subjective memory functioning (.19) in Floyd and Scogin (1997) was less than that for objective memory measures (.66) in Verhaegen et al. (1992).

   We identified another 13 randomized controlled trials since Verhaegen et al. (1992), generally demonstrating that memory training groups lead to improved performance on assorted objective tests, such as recall, encoding, and attention (e.g., Brooks, et al., 1995). Scogin and his colleagues (Scogin & Prohaska, 1992; Scogin, Prohaska, & Weeks, 1998) reported that a self-taught memory training manual was more effective than a waiting list control group and as effective as a group format, although not more effective than attention placebo; the self-taught manual also improved subjective memory functioning relative to both waiting-list and attention placebo control conditions.

Lachman, Weaver, Elliot, and Lewkoxwicz (1992) found that combined cognitive restructuring and memory skills training led to greater subjective improvement, while the combined intervention and separate components were equivalent on improving performance on various memory tasks. Caprio-Prevette and Fry (1996b) reported that cognitive restructuring was more effective than traditional memory training in improving objective memory. Cognitive restructuring also increased perceived control over memory, while reducing concerns about memory, anxiety, and depression.

Memory training has been found to be more effective than education alone, at least on some outcome measures, with changes maintained at follow-up of 3 to 6 months (Andrewes, Kinsella, & Murphy, 1996; Mohs et al., 1998; Schmidt, Sijkstra, Berg, & Deelman, 1999). Rebok, Rasmusson, Bylsma, and Brandt (1997) found that two widely advertised memory audiotapes did not improve memory performance compared with a control group; however, participants felt more confident and perceived more control over their memory abilities.

Combined memory training and pharmacotherapy (with pramiracetam, from a class of drugs known as nootropics which improve the operation of the neurotransmitter acetylcholine) has been found to improve both objective and subjective memory more than drug treatment alone or memory training alone (De Vreese et al., 1996). Greater objective gains were registered among older adults diagnosed with age-associated cognitive decline compared with those who had subjective memory complaints (De Vreese, Belloi, Iacono, Finelli, & Neri, 1998).

In summary, there has been accumulating evidence that memory training, particularly if it encompasses cognitive and behavioral techniques, does lead to some significant improvements for cognitively unimpaired, nondepressed older adults. With new drugs available to treat cognitive loss associated with Alzheimer's disease and trials underway to test whether drugs or other agents (e.g., vitamin E, nerve growth factor, gingko biloba) can delay the onset of dementia among those with mild cognitive impairment, further studies contrasting and combining these treatments and memory training would be of special note.

Support Groups for Bereaved and Lonely Older Adults

Rationale and Description

Bereaved individuals are at elevated risk for a variety of emotional and physical problems. Support groups are seen as strengthening participants' social support network, providing opportunities for social comparison, and encouraging coping (Vachon & Stylianos, 1988). Topics addressed in bereavement groups include grief and adjusting to an environment without the deceased. Silverman's (1988) Widow-to-Widow program emphasizes mutual help, using widow aides to connect new widows with practical resources and to conduct discussion groups. Building on this model, the AARP Widowed Persons Service provides training materials and consultation.[2]

Outcome Studies

In two randomized controlled trials of bereavement groups, Vachon, Lyall, Rogers, Freedman-Letofsky, and Freeman (1980) found less distress and quicker resolution of grief among participants compared with the control group, especially among those initially more distressed. Caserta and Lund (1993) found reduced depression and grief among participants with lower intrapersonal resources at baseline. Those with higher competencies had elevated symptoms at the 1-year posttest but decreased depression at the 2-year follow-up. Andersson (1985) randomly assigned lonely elderly women who lived alone (63% widows) to social support meetings or a control condition. At follow-up, the social support group was more socially engaged and less lonely, although there were no significant differences on measures of self-esteem or powerlessness.

Caregiver Support Groups

Rationale and Description

Caregivers of older adults with dementia are targeted for preventive interventions because family caregiving is seen as an important source of burden and stress that can threaten the caregivers' quality of life and physical health and leave them at risk for developing symptoms of psychological distress (Aneshensel, Pearlin, Mullan, Zarit, & Whitlatch, 1995). Caregiver interventions generally entail eight to ten weekly sessions; however, some last up to 6 months, and many support groups in nonresearch settings are open-ended. Some groups target either adult children or spousal caregivers, while other groups are mixed.

Caregiver interventions are extremely eclectic. Components may include: (a) provision of information about dementia and/or caregiving, (b) training in problem-solving skills (e.g., Roberts, Browne, Streiner, Gafni, & Pallister, 1994) and discussion of specific behavior management problems and solutions, (c) cognitive behavioral training (e.g., assertiveness training, cognitive restructuring), (d) stress management techniques and (e) emotional support.

Outcome Studies

A meta-analysis of caregiver interventions (Knight, Lutzky, Macofsky-Urban, 1993) indicated modest effectiveness. For the present review, seven randomized controlled trials with caregivers age 60 and older were identified, including support groups or workshops (Gendron, Poitras, Dastoor, & Perodeau, 1996; Ostwald, Hepburn, Caron, Burns, & Mantell, 1999; Toseland, Labreque, Goebel, & Whitney, 1992[3]); individualized interventions (Chang, 1999[4]; Roberts et al., 1999; Zarit, Anthony, & Boutselis, 1987); and multicomponent interventions (Mittelman et al., 1997; Mohide et al., 1990[5]). Key outcome variables examined included depression, burden, and marital satisfaction.

Changes in depressive symptoms favoring caregivers in the intervention condition were found by Chang (1999) and Mittelman et al., (1997). Toseland Labreque, Goebel, & Whitney (1992) reported improvement in depressive symptoms favoring the control group, while the other studies found no differences. Decreases in burden favoring participants in the intervention were found in only two studies (Ostwald, Hepburn, Caron, Burns, & Mantell, 1999; Toseland et al., 1992). However, other indications of decreased burden were reported by Mohide et al. (1990), Toseland et al., (1992), and Ostwald et al., (1999), who found that participants evidenced a decrease in how upset they were by their relatives' problem behaviors. Subjective rating of support increased for participants in the Zarit et al., (1987) individual problem-solving condition and for participants in Mittelman et al., (1997). With respect to marital outcome measures, Toseland et al., (1992) found that participants in their support group condition registered benefit, while Gendron et al., (1996) found improvement in their information-support group but a decrease in their cognitive-behavioral intervention group. Finally, compared with modest effects on these quantitative outcomes, all studies noted that participants rated the intervention very positively.

Friendly Visitors and Other Interventions Designed to Change the Social Environment

Rationale and Description

Older adults experience social loss due to retirement (which reduces contact with coworkers), deaths of friends and family, and physical illness (which restricts ability to participate in activities). A number of preventive interventions are premised on the idea that increasing social activities and informal social support should enhance well-being. These ideas are included in the rationale for wellness classes, widow-to-widow programs, and caregiver support groups. Interventions that explicitly aim to increase social ties include group activities in senior centers (Krout, 1985), friendly visitor programs where students or other volunteers visit homebound elderly (Bogat & Jason, 1983), telephone support (Heller, Thompson, Trueba, Hogg, & Vlachos-Weber, 1991), and, most recently, the internet (White et al. 1999).

Outcome Studies

Bogat and Jason (1983) randomly assigned enrollees in Friendly Visitors to be visited using a social network building protocol, in which the visitors used various behavioral approaches to encourage greater involvement in social activities, or a standard relationship-oriented protocol. There was also a nonrandom control group of homebound individuals not enrolled in Friendly Visitors. After three months, analyses generally showed nonsignificant differences among the three groups, although those in the social network building protocol tended to improve more in life satisfaction, sense of personal control, and number of activities accomplished, while those in the standard relationship-oriented visitation condition tended to improve more in number of telephone calls. Heller, Thompson, Trucba, Hogg, & Vlachos-Weber (1991) randomly assigned community-residing, low-income, elderly women with low perceived social support to a 10-week program of staff telephone contact or to a control group. Subsequently, those in the experimental condition were randomly assigned to continued staff contact, peer telephone contact, or no contact. There were no significant differences on measures of social support and depression between the control and intervention groups, or between the two intervention groups (i.e., staff initiated and peer dyad). Heller et al. (1991) observed that those who did remain in contact with peers tended to be those who already had more friends and higher perceived social support.

One lesson from these studies is the need for those designing interventions to be sensitive to lifespan differences in the nature of social support. Although maintaining longstanding social ties may be psychologically important for older adults, an intervention largely entailing exposure to social interaction, especially among individuals with a long history of social isolation, may be ineffectual or even counterproductive (Tornstam, 1989).

Interventions with Older Medical Patients

Rationale

Medical patients, many of whom are older adults, are considered targets for preventive efforts because they are at elevated risk for psychological disorders and symptoms such as depression and anxiety. Psychological interventions also can be used in those undergoing unpleasant diagnostic or treatment regimens such as cardiac catheterization or knee or hip replacement (Anderson & Masur, 1989; Daltroy, Morlino, Eaton, Poss, & Liang, 1998; Gammon & Mulholland, 1996; Ludwick-Rosenthal & Neufeld, 1993).

Description

Interventions with older medical patients typically are administered in a group format, except for programs targeting home-bound or hospitalized elderly. Interventions are variously delivered by professionals, trained volunteer therapists, and videotapes. They usually comprise a variety of elements, making evaluation of any specific component difficult. Education, problem solving, and cognitive restructuring tend to be directed toward improved management of a chronic condition, such as heart disease, diabetes, sensory impairment, or arthritis, or to lifestyle changes to prevent disease recurrence (Toobert, Glasgow, Nettekoven, & Brown, 1998). Relaxation has been used to reduce anxiety and breathing problems in older medical patients (Gift, Moore, & Soeken, 1992). Because of the group format, mutual support and information sharing is undoubtedly an important feature of many interventions.

Outcome Studies

In medical patients, evidence for the efficacy of this cluster of interventions is generally favorable. Several randomized, controlled trials, some with impressively large samples, have demonstrated improvements relative to waiting list or usual care control groups for general medical patients given disease management or relaxation classes (Lorig et al. 1999; Rybarczyk, DeMarco, DeLaCruz, & Lapidos, 1999) and for patients with cardiovascular conditions (Clark et al. 1997; Trzcieniecka-Green & Steptoe, 1996). Generally, smaller studies have not found significant differences, suggesting a modest effect size. In research designs in which interventions were tested against attention placebos or education-only control groups, results have been less impressive (Calfas, Kaplan, & Ingram, 1992; Jongbloed & Morgan, 1991), and it has been difficult to demonstrate significant differences between different psychosocial treatments (Montovani et al. 1996). The lack of a follow-up assessment period is a weakness of most investigations.

Although some studies have shown reduction in symptoms of anxiety and depression (Henry, Wilson, Bruce, Chisholm, & Rawling, 1997; Trzcieniecka-Green & Steptoe, 1996), effects have tended to be stronger for specific disease-related outcomes than for broad outcome measures such as depressive symptoms (Andersson, Melin, Scott, & Lindberg, 1994; Gilden, Hendryx, Clar, Casia, & Singh, 1992; Glasgow et al., 1992). Interventions with older adults identified as frail have not yet demonstrated efficacy on psychological outcomes (Coleman, Grothaus, Sandhu, & Wagner, 1999; Hall et al., 1992).

Pain is another frequent target of intervention. An intervention in which patients received information, relaxation training, both, or neither the day before knee or hip replacement surgery produced no effects on anxiety or pain, suggesting that a single-session intervention may be insufficient (Daltroy, Morlino, Eaton, Poss, & Liang, 1998). One very large-scale intervention for pain that offered one session of assessment and education actually increased pain relative to the usual care condition, suggesting that heightening awareness of pain without teaching coping skills might be detrimental for patients (Desbiens et al. 1998). Other studies with longer interventions, including relaxation, were successful in reducing pain (Appelbaum, Blanchard, Hickling, & Alfonso, 1988; Subramanian, 1991).

There is evidence that a more collaborative, patient-directed approach works better than a traditional lecture format (Thomas, 1995). Treatment matching based on patient characteristics such as preference for information and coping style also may be beneficial (Ludwick-Rosenthal & Neufeld, 1993).

CASE EXAMPLE

We have experience with older adult volunteers answering a telephone helpline at a university-based older adult counseling center and with older adult community outreach workers. Four implementation issues are salient:

1. Some volunteers are gifted interpersonally and/or have relevant work experience, while other volunteers are not naturally talented at helping roles

but may be very enthusiastic. Our approach has been to find a way to use each volunteer rather than to screen people out. For example, one male volunteer accepted the task of promoting the program rather than working directly as a peer counselor. This issue illustrates the tension inherent in the question of whether the program's primary goal is helping the older adult volunteer or helping the people who call the helpline for information.

2. Older adult volunteers may have competing commitments (e.g., extended trips out of town to visit family). In our experience, we simply had to work around these absences. For example, at each supervision meeting, we made a calendar of when different volunteers would be available or away, and we did not question their sense of priorities.

3. Several times we found ourselves dealing with other issues in the volunteers' lives. For instance, two women volunteers had husbands with Parkinson's disease. In both cases, the husbands became physically abusive, and we chose to intervene. Volunteers are not immune to physical illnesses that often accompany old age; one male peer counselor, for example, had physical mobility limitations and occasional emotional lability as consequences of a stroke. Supervisors and other volunteers accommodated him in a fairly matter-of-fact way and assured him that we were not made uncomfortable by his emotions.

4. Working with older adults introduces special transference and countertransference issues. Typically the peer counselor is older than the supervisor. Some have retired from prominent managerial or professional positions; all have accumulated substantial life experience. Parent-child or grandparent-grandchild transference-countertransference relationships would be easy to fall into. We found it useful to take advantage of being from the university, where the supervisors were professors or professors-in-training, simultaneously stressing that all of us—peer counselors and supervisors alike—were both teachers and learners. Consistent with our approach, the peer counselors initiated the habit of referring to our weekly supervision time as "going to class."

FUTURE DIRECTIONS

We have reviewed preventive intervention programs aimed at improving the emotional and cognitive well-being of community-dwelling older adults. Some of these programs are universal; others are aimed at groups who may be at greater risk of psychological distress. Research evidence supports teaching relaxation to older adults, to those who view themselves as anxious, as a component of memory training, and as part of a psychoeducational package for medical patients. Stress management interventions using stress inoculation have demonstrated utility. Life review appears to improve life satisfaction in nondepressed, noninstitutionalized older samples. Evidence for psychological benefits from physical exercise programs in nondepressed older adults is inconclusive. The most consistent results are for subjective perceptions. Research on volunteerism is limited but shows promise. With respect to memory training, there is accumulating evidence for its circumscribed effectiveness among cognitively unimpaired, nondepressed older adults. Although many people advocate the importance of support groups for bereaved older adults and older caregivers, evidence for their usefulness remains sparse. In the main, strategies that work best are those that start with a specific conceptualization with respect to the risk factor or behavior being targeted, and that train intensively in the intended skill.

Implications for the future include the need routinely to build evaluation into preventive intervention programs in the community in order to ensure better information about what programs work, when interventions may have negative effects, and how to connect older adults to programs best suited for them. We were struck by the disparity between participants' subjective evaluations and the evidence obtained from more objective measures. In part, the discrepancy may reflect the unsuitability of the measures that were chosen; for example, it may not be realistic to use a decrease in depressive symptoms as a criterion for program success in individuals who were not depressed. In addition, evidence generally lags behind public enthusiasm for many of these programs. Combining traditional randomized controlled trials with other methodologies may permit better understanding of this disparity. Other methodologies might include behaviorally oriented time-series designs, which have been employed with older adults in institutional settings and might profitably be extended to community designs, as well as various combinations of quantitative and qualitative methods.

In conclusion, there is a place for strategies to prevent psychological problems in older individuals. Older adults should not be excluded by those planning prevention programs, by those evaluating preventive interventions, or by those summarizing the literature about prevention. In the coming decades, there will be greater numbers of older adults, and these elderly will have grown up with different life experiences from today's elderly. Preventive interventions can productively address inevitable age-associated stresses and promote emotional, cognitive, and physical well-being.

NOTES

[1]   Because we excluded studies in which participants were selected based on psychiatric conditions and studies predominantly concerned with institutionalized populations (where a large proportion of participants are cognitively compromised), the focus of the interventions is predominantly individual, including the individual's social

environment. Interventions involving the physical environment or public policy were beyond the scope of this review.

2   Online: *http://www.aarp.org/griefprograms/wps.html*

3   "Caregiver's Support Group Manual" is available from Terry Harbert, Chief, Social Work Service (122), Colmery-O'Neil Department of Veterans Affairs Medical Center, 2200 Gage Boulevard, Topeka, KN 66622.

4   To obtain the Nurseline Video-Assisted Modeling Program (NVAMP) video, contact Dr. Betty Chang, School of Nursing, UCLA, 700 Tiverton Drive, Box 956918, Los Angeles, CA 90095-6918. E-mail: *bchang@sonet.ucla.edu.*

5   The outline of the intensive 80-hour training program for Caregiver Support Nurses is available from E. Ann Mohide, M.Sc., McMaster University, Faculty of Health Sciences, 1200 Main Street W., Room 2J40f, Hamilton, Ontario, L8N 3Z5, Canada.

REFERENCES

Anderson, K., & Masur, F. (1989). Psychological preparation for cardiac catheterization. *Advances, 6*, 8–10.

Andersson, G., Melin, L., Scott, B., & Lindberg, P. (1994). Behavioural counselling for subjects with acquired hearing loss: A new approach to hearing tactics. *Scandinavian Audiology, 23*, 249–256.

Andersson, L. (1985). Intervention against loneliness in a group of elderly women: An impact evaluation. *Social Science and Medicine, 20*, 355–364.

Andrewes, D. G., Kinsella, G., & Murphy, M. (1996). Using a memory handbook to improve everyday memory in community-dwelling older adults with memory complaints. *Experimental Aging Research, 22*, 305–322.

Aneshensel, C. S., Pearlin, L. I., Mullan, J. T., Zarit, S. H., & Whitlatch, C. J. (1995). *Profiles in caregiving: The unexpected career.* New York: Academic Press.

Appelbaum, K. A., Blanchard, E. B., Hickling, E. J., & Alfonso, M. (1988). Cognitive behavioral treatment of a veteran population with moderate to severe rheumatoid arthritis. *Behavior Therapy, 19*, 489–502.

Aquino, J. A., Russell, D. W., Cutrona, C. E., & Altmaier, E. M. (1996). Employment status, social support, and life satisfaction among the elderly. *Journal of Counseling Psychology, 43*, 480–489.

Bernstein, D. A., & Borkovec, T. D. (1973). *Progressive relaxation training: A manual for the helping professions.* Champaign, IL: Research Press.

Birren, J. E., & Birren, B. A. (1996). Autobiography: Exploring the self and encouraging development. In J. E. Birren, G. M. Kenyon, J.-E. Ruth, J. J. F. Schroots, & T. Svensson (Eds.) *Aging and biography: Explorations in adult development* (pp. 283–299). New York: Springer Publishing.

Blumenthal, A. J., Emery, C. F., Madden, D. J., George, L. K., Coleman, R. E.,

Walsh-Riddle, M., McKee, D. C., Reasoner, J., & Williams, R. S. (1989). Cardiovascular and behavioral effects of aerobic exercise training in healthy older men and women. *Journal of Gerontology, 44*, M147–M157.

Blumenthal, A. J., Emery, C. F., Madden, D. J., Schniedore, S. (1991). Long-term effects of exercise on psychological functioning in older men and women. *Journal of Gerontology, 46*, 352–361.

Bogat, G. A., & Jason, L. A. (1983). An evaluation of two visiting programs for elderly community residents. *International Journal of Aging and Human Development, 17*, 267–280.

Booz, Allen, & Hamilton, Inc. (1985). *National Retired Senior Volunteer program participant impact evaluation: Round two*. Report prepared for ACTION, Office of Policy and Planning/Evaluation Division. Washington, DC: ACTION.

Brooks, J. O., Friedman, L., Pearman, A. M., Gray, C., & Yesavage, J. A. (1999). Mnemonic training in older adults: Effects of age, length of training, and type of cognitive pretraining. *International Psychogeriatrics, 11*, 75–84.

Bruce, M. L., Seeman, T. E., Merrill, S. S., & Blazer, D. G. (1994). The impact of depressive symptoms on physical disability: MacArthur Studies of Successful Aging. *American Journal of Public Health, 84*, 1796–1799.

Butler, R. N. (1963). The life review: An interpretation of reminiscence in the aged. *Psychiatry, 26*, 65–76.

Calfas, K. J., Kaplan, R. M., & Ingram, R. E. (1992). One-year evaluation of cognitive-behavioral intervention in osteoarthritis. *Arthritis Care and Research, 5*, 202–209.

Carney, J. M., Dobson, J. E., & Dobson, R. L. (1987). Using senior citizen volunteers in the schools. *Journal of Humanistic Education and Development, 25*, 136–143.

Caprio-Prevette, M. D., & Fry, P. S. (1996a). *Memory enhancement program for community-based older adults: A guide for practitioners*. Gaithersburg, MD: Aspen Publishers.

Caprio-Prevette, M. D., & Fry, P. S. (1996b). Memory enhancement program for community-based older adults: Development and evaluation. *Experimental Aging Research, 22*, 281–303.

Caserta, M. S., & Lund, D. A. (1993). Intrapersonal resources and the effectiveness of self-help groups for bereaved older adults. *Gerontologist, 33*, 619–629.

Chang, B. L. (1999). Cognitive-behavioral intervention for homebound caregivers of persons with dementia. *Nursing Research, 48*, 173–182.

Clark, N. M., Janz, N. K., Dodge, J. A., Schork, M. A., Wheeler, J. R. C., Liang, J., Seteyian, S. J., & Santinga, J. T. (1997). Self-management of heart disease by older adults. *Research on Aging, 19*, 362–382.

Coleman, E. A., Grothaus, L. C., Sandhu, N., & Wagner, E. H. (1999). Chronic care clinics: A randomized controlled trial of a new model of primary care for frail older adults. *Journal of the American Geriatrics Society, 47*, 775–783.

Cox, E. O., & Parsons, R. J. (1992). Senior-to-senior mediation service project. *Gerontologist, 32*, 420–422.

Craft, L. L., & Landers, D. M. (1998). The effect of exercise on clinical depression and depression resulting from mental illness: A meta-analysis. *Journal of Sport & Exercise Psychology, 20*, 339–357.

Daltroy, L. H., Morlino, C. I., Eaton, H. M., Poss, R., & Liang, M. H. (1998). Preoperative education for total hip and knee replacement patients. *Arthritis Care and Research, 11*, 469–478.

Day, J. C. (1996). *Population projections of the United States by age, sex, race, and Hispanic origin: 1995 to 2050*. U.S. Bureau of the Census, Current Population Reports, P25–1130. Washington, DC: U.S. Government Printing Office.

DeBerry, S. (1981–82). An evaluation of progressive muscle relaxation on stress related symptoms in a geriatric population. *International Journal of Aging and Human Development, 14*, 255–269.

DeBerry, S. (1982). The effects of meditation-relaxation on anxiety and depression in a geriatric population. *Psychotherapy: Theory, Research and Practice, 19*, 512–521.

DeBerry, S., Davis, S., & Reinhard, K. E. (1989). A comparison of meditation-relaxation and cognitive/behavioral techniques for reducing anxiety and depression in a geriatric population. *Journal of Geriatric Psychiatry, 22*, 231–247.

Demers, A., & Lavoie, J. (1996). Effect of support groups on family caregivers to the frail elderly. *Canadian Journal on Aging, 15*, 129–144.

Desbiens, N. A., Wu, A. W., Yasui, Y., Lynn, J., Alzola, C., Wenger, N. S., Connors, A. F., Phillips, R. S., & Fulkerson, W. (1998). Patient empowerment and feedback did not decrease pain in seriously ill hospitalized adults. *Pain, 75*, 237–246.

De Vreese, L. P., Belloi, L., Iacono, S., Finelli, C., & Neri, M. (1998). Memory training programs in memory complainers: Efficacy on objective and subjective memory functioning. *Archives of Gerontology and Geriatrics* (Suppl. 6), 141–154.

De Vreese, L. P., Neri, M., Boiardi, R., Ferrari, P., Belloi, L., & Salvioli, G. (1996). Memory training and drug therapy act differently on memory and metamemory functioning: Evidence from a pilot study. *Archives of Gerontology and Geriatrics* (Suppl. 5), 9–22.

de Vries, S. (1968). Immediate and long-term effects of exercise upon resting muscle action potential level. *Journal of Sports Medicine and Physical fitness, 8*, 25–28.

Dustman, R. E., Ruhling, R. O., Russell, E. M., Shearer, D. E., Bonekat, H. W., Shigeoka J. W., Wood, J. S., & Bradford, D. C. (1984). Aerobic exercise training and improved neuropsychological function of older individuals. *Neurobiology of Aging, 5*, 35–42.

Emery C. F., & Blumenthal J. A. (1990). Perceived changes among participants in an exercise program for older adults. *Gerontologist, 30*, 516–521.

Emery, C. F., & Blumenthal, J. A. (1991). Effects of physical exercise on psychological and cognitive functioning of older adults. *Annals of Behavioral Medicine, 13*, 99–107.

Emery, C. F., & Gatz, M. (1990). Psychological and cognitive effects of an exercise program for community-residing older adults. *Gerontologist, 30*, 184–188.

Emery, C. F., Schein, R. L., Hauck, E. R., & MacIntyre, N. R. (1998). Psychological and cognitive outcomes of a randomized trial of exercise among patients with chronic obstructive pulmonary disease. *Health Psychology, 17*, 232–240.

Fabre, C., Masse-Biron, J., Chamari, K., Varray, A., Mucci, P., & Prefaut, C. (1999). Evaluation of quality of life in elderly healthy subjects after aerobic and/or mental training. *Archives of Gerontology and Geriatrics, 28*, 9–22.

Floyd, M., & Scogin, F. (1997). Effects of memory training on the subjective memory functioning and mental health of older adults: A meta-analysis. *Psychology and Aging, 12*, 150–161.

Gammon, J., & Mulholland, C. W. (1996). Effect of preparatory information prior to elective total hip replacement on post-operative physical coping outcomes. *International Journal of Nursing Studies, 33*, 589–604.

Gatz, M., Barbarin, O. A., Tyler, F. B., Mitchell, R. E., Moran, J. A., Wirzbicki, P. J., Crawford, J., & Engelman, A. (1982). Enhancement of individual and community competence: The older adult as community worker. *American Journal of Community Psychology, 10*, 291–303.

Gendron, C., Poitras, L., Dastoor, D. P., & Perodeau, G. (1996). Cognitive-behavioral group intervention for spousal caregivers: Findings and clinical considerations. *Clinical Gerontologist, 17*(1), 3–19.

Gift, A. G., Moore, T., & Soeken, K. (1992). Relaxation to reduce dyspnea and anxiety in COPD patients. *Nursing Research, 41*, 242–246.

Gilden, J. L., Hendryx, M. S., Clar, S., Casia, C., & Singh, S. P. (1992). Diabetes support groups improve health care of older diabetic patients. *Journal of the American Geriatrics Society, 40*, 147–150.

Glasgow, R. E., Toobert, D. J., Hampson, S. E., Brown, J. E., Lewinsohn, P. M., & Donnelly, J. (1992). Improving self-care among older patients with type II diabetes: The "sixty something . . ." study. *Patient Education and Counseling, 19*, 61–74.

Haight, B. K., (1988). The therapeutic role of a structured life review process in homebound, elderly subjects. Journal of *Gerontology, 43*, 40–44.

Haight, B. K. (1992). Long-term effects of a structured life review process. *Journal of Gerontology, 47*, 312–315.

Haight, B., & Webster, J. (1995) *The art and science of reminiscing: Theory, research, methods, and applications.* London: Taylor & Francis.

Hall, N., De Beck, P., Johnson, D., Mackinnon, K., Gutman, G., & Glick, N. (1992). Randomized trial of a health promotion program for frail elders. *Canadian Journal on Aging, 11*, 72–91.

Hawkins, H. L., Kramer, A. F., & Capaldi, D. (1992). Aging, exercise, and attention. *Psychology and Aging, 7*, 643–653.

Hayslip, B. (1989). Alternative mechanisms for improvements in fluid ability performance among older adults. *Psychology and Aging, 4*, 122–124.

Hayslip, B., Maloy, R. M., & Kohl, R. (1995). Long-term efficacy of fluid ability interventions with older adults. *Journal of Gerontology: Psychological Sciences, 50B*, P141–P149.

Heller, K., Thompson, M. G., Trueba, P. E., Hogg, J. R., & Vlachos-Weber, I. (1991). Peer support telephone dyads for elderly women: Was this the wrong intervention? *American Journal of Community Psychology, 19*, 53–74.

Henry, J. L., Wilson, P. H., Bruce, D. G., Chisholm, D. J., & Rawling, P. J. (1997). Cognitive-behavioural stress management for patients with non-insulin dependent diabetes mellitus. *Psychology, Health, and Medicine, 2*, 109–118.

Hill, R. D., Storandt, M., & Malley, M. (1993). The impact of long-term exercise training on psychological function in older adults. *Journal of Gerontology, 48*, P12–P17.

Jongbloed, L., & Morgan, D. (1991). An investigation of involvement in leisure activities after a stroke. *American Journal of Occupational Therapy, 45*, 420–427.

Knight, B. G., Lutzky, S. M., & Macofsky-Urban, F. (1993). A meta-analytic review of interventions for caregiver distress: Recommendations for future research. *Gerontologist, 33*, 240–248.

Kramer, A. F., Hahn, S., Cohen, N. J., Banich, M. T., McAuley, E., Harrison, C. R., Chason, J., Vakil, E., Bardell, L., Boileau, R. A., & Colcombe, A. (1999). Ageing, fitness and neurocognitive function. *Nature, 400*, 418–419.

Krout, J. A. (1985). Senior center activities and services: Findings from a national study. *Research on Aging, 7*, 455–471.

Kuehne, V. S., & Sears, H. A. (1993). Beyond the call of duty: Older volunteers committed to children and families. *Journal of Applied Gerontology, 12*, 425–438.

Lachman, M. E., Weaver, S. L., Bandura, M., Elliot, E., & Lewkowicz, C.

(1992). Improving memory and control beliefs through cognitive restructuring and self-generated strategies. *Journal of Gerontology: Psychological Sciences, 47*, P293–P299.

Lichstein, K. L. (1988). *Clinical relaxation strategies.* New York: Wiley.

Lopez, M. A., & Silber, S. (1991). Stress management for the elderly: A preventive approach. *Clinical Gerontologist, 10*(4), 73–76.

Lorig, K. R., Sobel, D. S., Stewart, A. L., Brown, B. W., Bandura, A., Ritter, P., Gonzalez, V. M., Laurent, D. D., & Holman, H. R. (1999). Evidence suggesting that a chronic disease self-management program can improve health status while reducing hospitalization: A randomized trial. *Medical Care, 37*, 5–14.

Ludwick-Rosenthal, R., & Neufeld, R. W. J. (1993). Preparation for undergoing an invasive medical procedure: Interacting effects of information and coping style. *Journal of Consulting and Clinical Psychology, 61*, 156–164.

Madden, D. J., Blumenthal, J. A., Allen, P. A., & Emery, C. F. (1989). Improving aerobic capacity in healthy older adults does not necessarily lead to improved cognitive performance. *Psychology and Aging, 4*, 307–320.

McAuley, E., & Rudolph, D. (1995). Physical activity, aging, and psychological well-being. *Journal of Aging and Physical Activity, 3*, 67–96.

McWilliam, C. L., Stewart, M., Brown, J. B., McNair, S., Donner, A., Desai, K., Coderre, P., & Galajda, J. (1999). Home-based health promotion for chronically ill older persons: Results of a randomized controlled trial of a critical reflection approach. *Health Promotion International, 14*, 27–41.

Meichenbaum, D. H. (1977). *Cognitive behavior modification: An integrative approach.* New York: Plenum.

Mittelman, M. S., Ferris, S. H., Shulman, E., Steinberg, G., Ambinder, A., & Mackell, J. (1997). Effects of a multicomponent support program on spouse-caregivers of Alzheimer's disease patients: Results of a treatment/control study. In L. L. Heston (Ed.), *Progress in Alzheimer's disease and similar conditions* (pp. 259–275). Washington, DC: American Psychiatric Press.

Mittelman, M. S., Ferris, S. H., Shulman, E., Steinberg, G., & Levin, B. (1996). A family intervention to delay nursing home placement of patients with Alzheimer's disease. *Journal of the American Medical Association, 276*, 1725–1731.

Mohide, E. A., Pringle, D. A., Steiner, D. L., Gilbert, J. R., Muir, G., & Tew, M. (1990). A randomized trial of family caregiver support in the home management of dementia. *Journal of the American Geriatric Society, 38*, 446–454.

Mohs, R. C., Ashman, T. A., Jantzen, K., Albert, M., Brandt, J., Gordon, B., Rasmusson, X., Grossman, M., Jacobs, D., & Stern, Y. (1998). A study of the efficacy of a comprehensive memory enhancement program in healthy elderly persons. *Psychiatry Research, 77*, 183–195.

Montovani, G., Astara, G., Lampis, B., Bianchi, A., Curreli, L., Orru, W., Carpiniello, B., Carta, M. G., Sorrentino, M., & Rudas, N. (1996). Impact of psychosocial intervention on the quality of life of elderly cancer patients. *Psycho-oncology, 5*, 127–135.

Musick, M. A., Herzog, A. R., & House, J. S. (1999). Volunteering and mortality among older adults: Findings from a national sample. *Journals of Gerontology: Social Sciences, 54B*, S173–S180.

Neely, A. S., & Bäckman, L. (1995). Effects of multifactorial memory training in old age: Generalizability across tasks and individuals. *Journal of Gerontology: Psychological Sciences, 50B*, P134–P140.

Newman, S., Karip, E., & Faux, R. B. (1995). Everyday memory function of older adults: The impact of intergenerational school volunteer programs. *Educational Gerontology, 21*, 569–580.

Oslin, D. W., Streim, J., Katz, I. R., Edell, W. S., & TenHave, T. (2000). Change in disability follows inpatient treatment for late life depression. *Journal of the American Geriatrics Society, 48*, 357–362.

Ostwald, S. K., Hepburn, K. W., Caron, W., Burns, T., & Mantell, R. (1999). Reducing caregiver burden: A randomized psychoeducational intervention for caregivers of persons with dementia. *Gerontologist, 39*, 299–309.

Perri, S., II., & Templer, D. I. (1984–85). The effects of aerobic exercise program on psychological variables in older adults. *International Journal of Aging and Human Development, 20*, 167–172.

Petty, B. J., & Cusack, S. A. (1989). Assessing the impact of a seniors' peer counselor program. *Educational Gerontology, 15*, 49–64.

Rankin, E. J., Gilner, F. H., Gfeller, J. D., & Katz, B. M. (1993). Anxiety states and sustained attention in a cognitively intact elderly sample: preliminary results. *Psychological Reports, 75*, 1176–1178.

Rebok, G. W., Rasmusson, D. X., Bylsma, F. W., & Brandt, J. (1997). Memory improvement tapes: How effective for elderly adults? *Aging, Neuropsychology, and Cognition, 4*, 304–311.

Rickard, H. C., Scogin, F., & Keith, S. (1994). A one-year follow-up of relaxation training for elders with subjective anxiety. *Gerontologist, 34*, 121–122.

Roberts, J., Browne, G., Milne, C., Spooner, L., Gafni, M., Drummond-Young, M., LeGris, J., Watt, S., LeClair, K., Beaumont, L., & Roberts, J. (1999). Problem-solving counseling for caregivers of the cognitively impaired: Effective for whom? *Nursing Research, 48*, 162–172.

Roberts, J., Browne, G., Streiner, D., Gafni, A., & Pallister, R. (1994). A RCT to determine the effectiveness and efficiency of either a problem-solving intervention or phone call support in promoting adjustment to chronic illness and reducing health service utilization. Appendix A. *Final Report*. NHRDP Grant #6606–407861.

Rybarczyk, B., & Auerbach, S. (1990). Reminiscence interviews as stress management interventions for older patients undergoing surgery. *Gerontologist, 30*, 522–528.

Rybarczyk, B., Auerbach, S., Jorn, M. L., & Lofland, K. R. (1993). Using volunteers and reminiscence to help older adults cope with an invasive medical procedure: A follow-up study. *Behavior, Health, and Aging, 3*, 147–162.

Rybarczyk, B., DeMarco, G., DeLaCruz, M., & Lapidos, S. (1999). Comparing mind-body wellness interventions for older adults with chronic illness: Classroom versus home instruction. *Behavioral Medicine, 24*, 181–190.

Schmidt, I. W., Dijkstra, H. T., Bert, I. J., & Deelman, B. G. (1999). Memory training for remembering names in older adults. *Clinical Gerontologist, 20*(2), 57–73.

Scogin, F., & Prochaska, F. (1992). The efficacy of self-taught memory training for community-dwelling older adults. *Education Gerontology, 18*, 751–766.

Scogin, F., Prochaska, F., & Weeks, E. (1998). The comparative efficacy of self-taught and group memory training for older adults. *Journal of Clinical Geropsychology, 4*, 301–314.

Scogin, F., Rickard, H. C., Keith, S., Wilson, J., & McElreath, L. (1992). Progressive and imaginal relaxation training for elderly persons with subjective anxiety. *Psychology and Aging, 7*, 419–424.

Silverman, P. R. (1988). Widow-to-Widow: A mutual help program for the widowed. In R. H. Price, E. L. Cowen, R. P. Lorion, & J. Ramos-McKay (Eds.), *Fourteen ounces of prevention: A casebook for practitioners* (pp. 175–186). Washington, DC: American Psychological Association.

Slivinske, L. R., & Fitch, V. L. (1987). The effect of control enhancing interventions on the well-being of elderly individuals living in retirement communities. *Gerontologist, 27*, 176–181.

Stevens-Ratchford, R. G. (1993). The effect of life review reminiscence activities on depression and self-esteem in older adults. *American Journal of Occupational Therapy, 47*, 413–420.

Subramanian, K. (1991). Structured group work for the management of chronic pain: An experimental investigation. *Research on Social Work Practice, 1*, 32–45.

Thomas, J. J. (1995). Reducing anxiety during phase I cardiac rehabilitation. *Journal of Psychosomatic Research, 39*, 295–304.

Thorsteim, H. & Roberts, B. (1996). Praxis through shared lifestories: A design process for community empowerment through social elaboration of learning. In W. W. Gasparsky, M. K. Mlicki, & B. B. Banathy (Eds.), *International annual of practical philosophy and methodoloy; Vol. 4. Social agency: Dilemmas and education praxology* (pp.233–250). New Brunswick, NJ: Transactions Publishers.

Toobert, D. J., Glasgow, R. E., Nettekoven, L. A., & Brown, J. E. (1998). Behavioral and psychosocial effects of intensive lifestyle management for women with coronary heart disease. *Patient Education and Counseling, 35*, 177–188.

Tornstam, L. (1989). Gero-transcendence: A reformulation of disengagement theory. *Aging, 1*, 55–63.

Toseland, R. W., Labreque, M. S., Goebel, S. T., & Whitney, M. H. (1992). An evaluation of a group program for spouses of frail elderly veterans. *Gerontologist, 32*, 382–390.

Trzcieniecka-Green, A., & Steptoe, A. (1996). The effects of stress management on the quality of life of patients following acute myocardial infarction or coronary bypass surgery. *European Heart Journal, 17*, 1663–1670.

Vachon, M. L. S., Lyall, W. A., Rogers, J., Freedman-Letofsky, K., & Freeman, S. J. (1980). A controlled study of self-help intervention for widows. *American Journal of Psychiatry, 137*, 1380–1384.

Vachon, M. L. S., & Stylianos, S. K. (1988). The role of social support in bereavement. *Journal of Social Issues, 44*, 175–190.

Verhaeghen, P., Marcoen, A., & Goossens, L. (1992). Improving memory performance in the aged through mnemonic training: A meta-analytic study. *Psychology and Aging, 7*, 242–251.

Wallace, J. I., Buchner, D. M., Grothaus, L., Leveille, S., Tyll, L., LaCroix, A. Z., & Wagner, E. H. (1998). Implementation and effectiveness of a community-based health promotion program for older adults. *Journal of Gerontology: Medical Sciences, 53A*, M301–M306.

Wheeler, J. A., Gorey, K. M., & Greenblatt, B. (1998). Beneficial effects of volunteering for older volunteers and the people they serve: A meta-analysis. *International Journal of Aging and Human Development, 47*, 69–79.

White, H., McConnell, E., Clipp, E., Bynum, L., Teague, C., Navas, L., Craven, S., & Halbrecht, H. (1999). Surfing the Net in later life: A review of the literature and pilot study of computer use and quality of life. *Journal of Applied Gerontology, 18*, 358–378.

Williams, P., & Lord, S. R. (1997). Effects of group exercise on cognitive functioning and mood in older women. *Australian and New Zealand Journal of Public Health, 21*, 45–52.

Yesavage, J. (1984). Relaxation and memory training in 39 elderly patients. *American Journal of Psychiatry, 141*, 778–781.

Zarit, S. H., Anthony, C. R., & Boutselis, M. (1987). Interventions with care givers of dementia patients: Comparison of two approaches. *Psychology and Aging, 2*, 225–232.

PART IV

Community and Societal Issues

CHAPTER 14

Preventing Racist, Sexist, and Heterosexist Behavior

Doreen D. Salina and
Linda M. Lesondak

Racism, sexism, and heterosexism are negative social processes that consist of prejudicial attitudes and discriminatory practices toward members of targeted communities. Their impact is pervasive and results in significant economic, social, and psychological costs to those who are victims of these negative attitudes and to society as a whole. Individuals and communities who are the targets of such attitudes and actions experience significant stress which impacts on physical and mental health as well as on economic opportunities (Byrd, 1990; Clark, Anderson, Clark, & Williams, 1999; Hubler & Silverstein, 1993; Jackson, 1990; Jones, 1981; Skillings & Dobbins, 1991). Brooks (1981) concluded that individuals of an oppressed group in society experience more negative life events and daily struggles due solely to membership in a particular community or because of their minority group status. These include overt and covert environmental stressors, hostility from the majority group, and various forms of oppression embedded within society's institutional structures (Thomas & Miles, 1995).

The goals of this chapter are both (a) to provide a brief overview of these social issues and resulting consequences and (b) to assist the reader in better conceptualizing these problems in order to reduce and prevent the negative consequences of sexism, racism, and heterosexism. We provide a case example of how one community-based agency addresses these negative social forces both internally and within the general society and conclude with suggestions on how one might develop prevention programs that address and ameliorate these complex social forces.

DESCRIPTION OF THE PROBLEM

Social psychologists, educators, and community activists have utilized different yet parallel theories to understand the impact of oppression. The perspectives presented here emphasize the operation of these social influences within an ecological and prevention framework. An ecological perspective provides a number of salient features which facilitate the understanding of these social responses and their prevention. Such a perspective conceptualizes the individual's needs within a larger context (Kelly, 1971) and takes into account the unique contributions of diverse cultures to the communities as a whole (Wolff, 1987). Some key components include understanding environmental contexts, promoting empowerment, and valuing diversity. The concept of preventing or reducing the effects of social oppression through promoting a sense of community is an essential component of an ecological framework. Effective prevention programs target multiple levels of a social issue to better address the complex interactions that perpetuate problems of oppression, discrimination, and barriers to equality.

Heterosexism, racism, and sexism are learned behaviors to specific stimuli and as such are open to modification. Individuals who engage in various types of racist, sexist, and heterosexist behaviors come from families and communities in which these beliefs and behaviors are supported by implicit or explicit group norms (Ponterotto & Pedersen, 1993). From a social learning theory point of view (Bandura, 1977, 1986) many of these individuals have seen these behaviors modeled by peers and family members during their childhood and have viewed the positive reinforcement of the expression and enactment of these prejudicial beliefs.

The relationships among racism, heterosexism, and sexism are complex, especially when one is a member of more than one minority group. Although members in each of these affected groups differ and the form of the resulting oppression may differ, commonalties do exist. Individuals who belong to more than one minority community struggle with multiple sources of stress and discrimination, while having potentially less access to needed resources (Stokes & Peterson, 1998). This interaction of negative social factors, increased stress, and barriers to resources may place them at greater risk for developing stress-related illnesses or result in less adaptive coping. People of color who also are members of other minority groups (i.e., women or gay or lesbian communities) are often victimized in multiple and pervasive ways (Thomas & Miles, 1995). Members of multiple minority communities (for example, Latinas or gay men of color) are especially targeted with prejudicial attitudes and misperceptions and may experience significant oppression in a multitude of forms. This is especially true if there are conflicting cultural values regarding specific aspects of individual identity within the communities to which the individual belongs.

The perception that an individual is a member of one of these minority groups often includes beliefs that the perceived individual is in some way inferior or deficient in some important key qualities. These perceptions form a cognitive framework for the biased perceiver and provide a rationale for denying members of these groups the same civil rights and access to resources as the majority group that holds the power. Depending on which oppressed community one holds membership in, this differential treatment may take varied forms. Yet the results are the same: decreased access to resources, additional stressors related to group membership, and increased violence directed at the individual member.

Stereotypes, Prejudice, and Discrimination

Allport (1954) suggested that cognitive categorization of people into groups was necessary for adaptive functioning. Forming groups by identifying some common attributes or characteristics serves to reduce the amount of information to be managed and thereby reduces the complexity of the social world. Allport (1954) did not believe this categorization necessarily led to a devaluing of dissimilar others, but served as a cognitive strategy of organizing large amounts of information about dissimilar others.

Unfortunately, this type of cognitive organization may lead to a biased evaluation and negative attributions about members of these groups. Stereotypes are a set of beliefs about members of a particular group (Ashmore & Del Boca, 1981); they do not necessarily have to be negative in nature, but those that are not benign may lead to prejudicial beliefs. Members of minority groups are often perceived via stereotypes, which an individual has learned within the family or community or through stereotypical portrayal of members through mass media (Winett, King, & Altman, 1989).

Prejudice is not benign. It also consists of belief systems about members of particular groups but includes negative attitudes about and evaluations of qualities of all members of that group (Fishbein & Azjen, 1975). These attitudes and beliefs are cognitive components of prejudice. There appears to be a universal tendency for people to dislike groups with dissimilar values and beliefs; the more dissimilar and unlike the perceiver's perspective, the more likely that prejudice will develop (Ponterotto & Pedersen, 1993).

Discrimination is the behavioral manifestation of stereotyping and prejudicial beliefs (Allport, 1954; Ashmore & DelBoca, 1981). It is an individual or majority group's ability to deny another's access to various resources because of group membership or specific salient characteristics of that group's membership. These resources include jobs, housing, money, medical treatment, and fair and equal treatment. Discrimination is a set of behaviors that create physical, psychological, and societal barriers that prevent members of minority groups from achieving parity with members of the majority culture or group. Discrimination includes the negative attitudes and beliefs that accompany negative stereotypes and prejudice.

Sexism

Sexism is defined as prejudice, discrimination, or bias against people based on their gender (Frieze, Parsons, Johnson, Ruble, & Zellman, 1978). Sexist practices include differential rates of pay for equivalent work, denial of reproductive rights, and numerous forms of sexual violence, including harassment, rape, and child sexual abuse (Biglan et al., 1990; Myers, 1993; Ostertag & McNamara, 1991). Sexism is established through the relationship between gender and power, and serves to deny women economic, political, and legal equality (Biglan et al., 1990; Myers, 1993). It is utilized frequently to characterize the experiences of women as less important or relevant than the experiences of men. Sexism is maintained through denial of economic and legal advancement so that the patriarchal society may maintain its traditional power bases.

Women have less access to such tangible resources such as food, housing, childcare, and medical services (U.S. Bureau of the Census, 1995). Sexist attitudes are maintained and promoted through strict adherence to beliefs about the appropriateness of traditional, rigid gender roles within relationships and within society (Bem, 1993; Bem & Bem, 1973). Patriarchal beliefs such as female gender inferiority, as well as the frequency of domestic violence, wage inequity, and institutional support for women to remain less powerful than men, potentiate the effects of poverty, racism, heterosexism, and discrimination, and often victimize women in multiple ways (Thomas & Miles, 1995).

Sexist practices begin in childhood through differential socialization of girls and boys (Gilligan, 1982). Through gender role stereotyping, boys are taught and reinforced to be more aggressive and dominant when interacting with others, and are more likely to resolve conflict with force than are girls (Maccoby, 1990). In a landmark article, Maccoby (1990) reviewed significant differences in the ways girls and boys are socialized. According to Maccoby (1990) and others (Biglan, 1995; Gilligan, 1982), girls are socialized to be more compliant and more focused on others' perspectives, and to experience more pressure to accommodate to these demands. These differences affect how girls view the world and what they conclude are appropriate roles and behaviors for women. Biglan (1995) connected sexist practices and childrearing with increased rates of sexual violence, including women's inability to resist sexual coercion by men.

Heterosexism

Heterosexism has been defined as the social system which "denies, denigrates, and stigmatizes any nonheterosexual form of behavior, identity, relationship, or community" (Dean et al. 2000, p.152). Laws and programs designed within a heterosexist perspective generally exclude the experiences of homosexual people by implicitly or explicitly promoting the superiority of heterosexual relationships compared with same-gender relationships. Homophobia is the irrational fear and hatred of those who love and sexually desire other individuals of the same sex. There is evidence that suggests that people who react negatively toward homosexuals are also intolerant of many other types of interpersonal or social interactions. Homophobic individuals have been found to be more cognitively (MacDonald & Games, 1974) and sexually (Brown & Amoroso, 1975) rigid, more negative about their own sexual impulses (Dunbar, Brown, & Amoroso, 1973), more prejudicial toward persons with AIDS, and generally less accepting of others (Salina, 1989).

Empirical data on the impact of heterosexism and homophobia are far from complete. According to the National Gay and Lesbian Task Force (NGLTF, 1993), lesbians and gay men make up approximately 10% to 20% of the United States population. This is considered an estimate because government-sponsored databases routinely ignore the question of sexual identity or orientation as an important demographic category (Laumann, Gagnon, Michael, & Michael, 1994; NGLTF, 1993). Many interventions that target specific social or health concerns may not take into account gay and lesbian perspectives because most programs and services are developed within a heterosexist framework. In addition, the lack of specific tailoring of services designed specifically for gays and lesbians of color results in both heterosexism and racism. This lack of cultural responsiveness may prevent targeted individuals from reporting problems such as discrimination or violence that may have their genesis in both heterosexism and racism (Comstock, 1991).

Lesbian, gay, bisexual, and transgendered (LGBT) youth are especially vulnerable to the effects of stereotyping, prejudice, and discrimination. Many LGBT youth are rejected by their families and their heterosexual friends (Ryan & Futterman, 1998). According to Ryan and Futterman (1998), 25% to 35% of homeless youth who receive services in Los Angeles are lesbian or gay, and in Seattle 40% of homeless youth are estimated to be lesbian or gay. Homeless teenagers are significantly more likely to contract HIV through unprotected intercourse, intravenous drug use, and engagement in survival sex (Rotheram-Borus, Hunter, & Rosario, 1994). Gay and lesbian youth are two to three times more likely than heterosexual youths to have attempted suicide (D'Augelli & Hershberger, 1993). These findings are generally understood to be a result of expressed homophobia on the part of youths' peer groups, families, and communities.

Racism

Racism is prejudice against people of a different race, often accompanied by discriminatory behaviors (Jones, 1972). Racism consists of attitudes and beliefs of perceived superiority that may be overt or covert, but that result in the systematic oppression of an entire group of individuals based on their race or ethnicity. Jones (1981) defined racism as the exercise of power against a racial group that has been defined as inferior by society through beliefs supported by the dominant society. He further separated racism into three types and outlined how each serves to deny access to power and resources. Individual racism is racial prejudice based on biological or visual differences between people that are expressed through behavior that is observable or measurable. This includes both verbal and nonverbal behavior that the targeted person experiences as demeaning, discriminating, or bigoted. Institutional racism is the tolerance or promotion of organizational, legal, or political policies that unfairly prohibit various groups from having access to resources and opportunity. Some examples are discriminatory hiring processes resulting in lower-paying jobs, or discrimination in a bank's policies for awarding home ownership mortgages (Hubler & Silverstein, 1993; Jackson, 1990).

Finally, cultural racism pervasively affects both the individual and the community. This form of racism is the most subtle and potentially the most damaging because it promotes the dominant culture as superior and desirable. Such ethnocentric beliefs are covertly embedded in the societal structure so that they become difficult to measure or change. Cultural racism denies the experience of people in these communities, rendering them less able to maintain cultural traditions, including language, food, clothing, and belief systems.

Hate Crimes

Although prejudice and discrimination have significant psychological, social, and economic costs, the most violent expression of prejudicial beliefs and discrimination is the perpetration of hate crimes. Hate crimes are violent crimes perpetrated against individuals of minority communities due solely to their perceived membership in those subcultures. Hate crimes influence substantial numbers of individuals to fear victimization due to some personal attribute or group membership (Herek & Berrill, 1992). Documented rates of bias-related crimes have increased significantly since the federal Hate Crime Statistics Act was signed into law in 1990 (Herek & Berrill, 1992; NGLTF, 1993). Hate crimes can be defined as those in which prejudice based on gender, race, religion, sexual orientation, and/or ethnicity plays a role in the perpetration of violence. Estimates of the number of victims of bias-related crimes vary greatly because of inconsistent reporting methods, different definitions of the severity of the crime, and reluctance on the part of some crime victims to come forward and report the event (Finn & Taylor, 1987). Verbal intimidation, assault, and vandalism are the most commonly reported hate crimes (D'Augelli, 1989; Finn & Taylor, 1987; Herek & Berrill, 1992). Because they are intended to intimidate an entire group, these types of crimes are far more psychologically harmful than comparable crimes that do not involve prejudice (Garnets, Herek, & Levy, 1992; Herek, 1990). According to Garofalo and Martin (1991), victims of bias-related crime suffer further psychological consequences (e.g., anger and vulnerability) because the crime that was committed against them was not random. As a result, many victims require additional psychological resources to assist in their recovery process (Garnets, 1992; Garnets et al., 1992).

REVIEW AND CRITIQUE OF THE LITERATURE

Programs that reduce the incidence and impact of prejudice and discriminatory behaviors should be comprehensive and should conceptualize the problem at the individual, community, and social infrastructure levels (Hobfoll, 1988). Unfortunately, few programs designed to reduce or prevent sexism, racism, and heterosexism have been scientifically designed and evaluated for effectiveness. In an American Psychological Association (APA)-sponsored annotated bibliography on psychology and racism (Bernard, Holliday, Crump, & Sanchez, 1998) compiled from reviews of psychlit journals, chapters, and books (1974–1996) as well as medline searches from 1990 to 1996, 293 citations were included. Of these abstracts, only three empirical studies were directly designed to prevent or reduce racism. A similar dearth of research on the prevention of sexism, heterosexism, and homophobia also was found in literature searches conducted by the current authors. Searches of the social sciences databases yielded similar results. The absence of prevention programs may stem from the multiple components involved in the formation and expression of racism, sexism, and heterosexism. These include cognitive, affective, and behavioral components which are present and reinforced through multiple and covert sources. Most of the articles and studies highlighted the effects of these social oppressions on the targeted individuals and communities, concluding with suggestions for future prevention-oriented research. Thus, little is known empirically regarding the prevention of sexism, racism, and heterosexism.

Individual-Level Strategies

It appears that in order to prevent the formation of prejudicial beliefs and to reduce discriminatory behavior, prevention ideally should occur in the early developmental years when children are still forming key understandings about diversity. Individual-based programs focus on both increasing minority individuals' abilities to cope effectively with the stress of prejudice and discrimination, and decreasing or preventing the formation of prejudicial attitudes and beliefs in biased or potentially biased individuals. Rooney-Rebeck and Jason (1986) found that first graders were better able than third graders to gain from diverse ethnic/racial tutoring relationships in school, perhaps due to less overt ingrained prejudice. In a series of classroom experiments (Presser, Stephan, Kennedy, & Aronson, 1978; Stephan, Kennedy, & Aronson, 1977), Aronson and his colleagues reduced competition and increased interdependence in young children of diverse backgrounds. Their results indicated that the children demonstrated an increased ability to understand other student's perspectives and experiences after these exercises. The researchers concluded that, through the promotion of mutual interdependence, the children were able to better comprehend the experiences of others and relate to the children who were different from themselves. These findings suggest that the earlier prejudice-reducing activities are introduced to children to prevent biased attitudes from forming, the more effective they may be in promoting acceptance of diversity.

A number of interventions have been used to combat racism among individuals in various settings. Barnard and Benn (1988) reported that the creation of dialogues between European Americans and African Americans concerning prejudice reduced prejudicial attitudes expressed toward the other group. Another study (Batts, 1983) attempted to affect how individuals responded to cultural scripts by implementing behavioral skill exercises between European Americans and African Americans. A number of educators (Sapon-Shevin, 1988; Sonnenschein, 1988) have developed curricula for school-age children and adolescents which utilize the cognitive strengths of young people to reduce prejudicial attitudes and beliefs. These programs, although not empirically validated, serve to challenge prejudicial beliefs through the development of critical thinking. Such curricula also encourage a more complete discussion of historical and cultural events to accurately include indigenous perspectives and the role of people of color.

Prejudice and discrimination may be considered stressors that impact on individual well-being. As stressors, they exact a cost on the recipients' physical and mental health, and they must be addressed by members of the targeted minority community. Individuals who are the targets of prejudice and discrimination may utilize a variety of coping styles that generally can be categorized as adaptive or maladaptive. Maladaptive coping responses are presumed to be ineffective in decreasing the amount of distress experienced by the targeted individual or group. Adaptive coping responses are methods utilized by the targeted individual or group which help reduce the stress of the prejudicial or discriminatory behavior and may serve a positive health promotion function. One intriguing method of coping with racism has been highlighted within a larger model of examining the biopsychosocial effects of racism (Clark, Anderson, Clark, & Williams, 1999). It consists of identifying and modifying thoughts and behaviors used in processing racist stimuli and effectively resolving the situation in an adaptive manner. It is consistent with the social cognitive theory (Bandura, 1986, 1990) that if individuals who are the targets of prejudice and discrimination can cognitively address the stress and enact adaptive responses, then the impact of these stressors will be reduced.

Watts and his colleagues (Watts & Abdul-Adil, 1997; Watts, Griffith, & Abdul-Adil, 1999) have promoted adaptive coping with oppression through the increased development of critical consciousness within small groups of African-American men. Critical consciousness can be thought of as increased awareness of how power unequally distributed serves to disenfranchise entire communities. Their programs used culturally relevant media such as music videos to promote individual empowerment and critical analyses of political mechanisms that foster social injustices related to prejudice and discrimination. Through these culturally specific strategies, Watts et al. (1999) stimulated increased understanding of the sociopolitical messages inherent in society that serve as a barrier to social equality and that may serve a depersonalizing function to the targeted individual. Although Watts et al. (1999) focused their work within the African-American community, their approach has relevance for other disenfranchised groups targeted by the same mechanisms of oppression.

Community Level Strategies

Prevention or intervention programs are most likely to be effective and reach significant numbers of persons when they are conducted in community settings where people spend most of their time (Shinn, 1987). Potential sites include primary health clinics, churches and other faith-based organizations, and sites that are easily accessible by public transportation and provide childcare. In addition, to be successful, community-based programs need to be sensitive to the culture and language of the targeted populations and include key members of the community in their formation and implementation.

For an intervention to be successful, one must first identify how various members of the community experience these problems and what resources already exist to address them (Rappaport, 1977). The creation of a continuous dialogue among community groups, schools, and community opinion leaders is critical to effectively identify complex community needs and potential solutions. Such dialogues promote an understanding of diverse perspectives within the community and can lead to solutions that tend to be more inclusive (Rappaport, 1981). These solutions tend to be more respectful of the perspectives of different segments of the community and more efficacious in reducing the impact of the social problem. This interactive dialogue promotes acceptance of diverse opinions and uses them to develop more comprehensive and effective solutions. Through this type of interactive process, more members are included and individual differences may become less important as the community unites toward developing solutions.

Empowering Communities

Community-level interventions often include an empowerment component to assist targeted individuals in coping and processing prejudicial or discriminatory conditions. Empowerment programs can help facilitate the identification and use of existing resources in the community to eliminate or combat the effects of racism, sexism, and heterosexism. Wolff (1987) defined empowerment as a process by which individuals, organizations, and communities gain mastery over their lives. Rappaport, Davidson, and Wilson (1975) discussed the importance of "cultural amplifiers" in empowerment activities. These amplifiers may be considered the natural resources that are present in a particular a group and that can be further developed to effectively address the impact of sexism, racism, and heterosexism. For example, many individuals participate in faith-based organizations which can effectively mobilize the community to demand more equitable access to resources and reduce negative situations.

One example of how community resources were identified and utilized to fight homophobia was the development of the National Gay and Lesbian Task Force (NGLTF) Incidence of Violence Survey. In order to measure and reduce the amount of discrimination and violence occurring in the LGBT community, the NGLTF conducted an eight-city survey that investigated the incidence of hate crimes against gays and lesbians in the United States (NGLTF, 1993). This study yielded data indicating that more than 50% of gays and lesbians who participated in some form of gay and lesbian community organization had experienced some form of general violence related to their sexual orientation. There were no significant differences related to social class or income level. With respect to race, women of color experienced violence more frequently than did White women in the sample.

This survey resulted in a collaborative, multisite effort, entitled the "Campaign to Count and Counter Hate Crimes: Document, Educate, and Advocate." Every year five major American cities—Chicago, Boston, New York, Minneapolis, and San Francisco—simultaneously announce their hate crime statistics, and members of various communities join together to facilitate social change by fighting for legal and social justice. These activities include increased community organizing to patrol targeted communities, lobbying for the passage of legal statutes that punish hate-motivated criminal acts, and addressing the needs of victims of hate crimes. These data also have facilitated systemic changes in some cities in the way hate crimes are handled by law enforcement, including more accurate documentation of violent acts as hate crimes, and appropriate investigation. In addition, many police departments now offer sensitivity training to more accurately identify hate crimes and appropriately respond to victims.

Use of Social Support

The development of effective social support systems can help facilitate systemic change within communities to reduce prejudice and discrimination. There is consensus that social support typically includes a number of common factors, including understanding of the experience by key individuals in the person's life, a perception of available social resources, and access to tangible resources within the community (e.g., Cutrona & Russell, 1987; Sarason, Shearin, Pierce, & Sarason, 1987). Klaw and Rhodes (1995) found that the presence of a natural or nonprofessional mentor in the lives of pregnant, teenage African-American women resulted in increased life optimism and more positive beliefs in future career opportunities. Community-based institutions can enable members to make more of shared collective resources by recognizing how social oppressions serve to alienate members from resources and from each other. Forming networks can help provide cohesiveness within the community and improve access to resources. The impact of prejudice can be reduced and discrimination addressed through cooperative programs that provide comprehensive support to community members through the development of explicit social support networks that buffer the complex effects of unequal access to resources.

Use of Media in Community Interventions

An additional method of altering beliefs, attitudes, and behavior at the community level is through the use of social marketing involving the media. Winett, king, and Altman (1989) emphasized the tailored use of media channels to target specific segments of the population. By being specifically designed to reach individuals who are the targets of prejudice and discrimination, media-based messages can both heighten the awareness of the issue and stimulate cognitive awareness of possible solutions. The media also can be utilized to influence key opinion leaders within communities who then can help modify behavior through diffusion and interaction with others (Bandura, 1986; Winett, Leckliter, Chinn, Stahl, & Love, 1985). Because social cognitive theory identifies modeling by important others as an effective method of behavior change, watching others who are admired engage in nondiscriminatory and inclusive behaviors can help modify the viewer's biased responses.

The media, which perpetrates stereotypes that often lead to prejudicial expression, can be used to promote campaigns that are inclusive and diverse. Such campaigns can reduce or eliminate stigma through appropriate design of the message and by destimatizing an issue or a particular group. One study, entitled "Families in Touch—Understanding AIDS," was conducted fairly early in the AIDS epidemic (Crawford, Jason, & Salina, 1990; Salina, Crawford, & Jason, 1992). This project was designed to promote the understanding that anyone can be at risk for HIV infection and to increase community awareness about HIV prevention. Since AIDS was first identified in the gay community, increases in gay-related violence and discrimination have increased (NGLTF, 1993). Indeed, the HIV virus was first identified as GRID or Gay-Related Immune Deficiency (Shilts, 1987), but also was known informally in some medical circles as WOG or "Wrath of God" (Douglas, Kalman, & Kalman, 1985). By presenting a media campaign that focused on how HIV can affect all people, including children and families, the "Families in Touch" program concentrated on the disease and its transmission routes, and not on the community which was most affected by its presence. Employment of the media in this manner can play a significant role in facilitating changes in attitude and behavior. In addition, appropriately designed media campaigns can, through the use of role models and culturally specific messages, target groups who experience discrimination and prejudice. These campaigns can use appropriate role models to demonstrate effective methods of coping with these social ills and promote perceived self-efficacy in effective problem solving and overcoming barriers to resources.

CASE EXAMPLE

Many community-based organizations encounter the acute and chronic effects of institutionalized racism, sexism, and heterosexism from society, and internalized effects from within the specific agency. Both authors have previously worked at Howard Brown Health Center (HBHC) in Chicago. HBHC actively addresses racism, sexism, and heterosexism specifically at HBHC, and within the larger society in general. HBHC's message is to address specific health disparities within lesbian, gay, bisexual, and transgendered (LGBT) communities that are due to heterosexism and to combat race and gender biases present in the health care system and society in general.

HBHC was founded in 1974 by a group of concerned medical students and volunteers to provide low-cost, confidential testing and treatment of sexually transmitted diseases (STDs) to the gay community in Chicago. It was established as a small volunteer clinic because expressed heterosexism on the part of medical professionals was perceived as a barrier for infected gay men to receive appropriate medical care for STDs. It has since grown into a federally qualified health center, and its programs are dedicated to promoting the well-being of LGBT persons through general and HIV primary care and wellness programs, including clinical, educational, social services, and research activities. Currently, the clinic administers a range of services with sliding-scale rates to ensure that underserved populations meet their essential health care needs within a culturally appropriate framework.

Over time, HBHC staff recognized that its clients were primarily gay, European-American men. Recognizing that not effectively serving women was an expression of sexism, the Women's Program was developed in 1993 to address the differing needs of lesbian and bisexual women. Initially, the program's function was to encourage women to use existing services, but it soon evolved and expanded because of the recognition that women faced additional barriers to health care because of sexism and heterosexism. Current empirical research has begun to highlight the specific health care needs of lesbian and bisexual women (Solarz, 1999). Lesbians and bisexual women remain a relatively hidden and poorly understood group of heterogeneous women, with relatively little known regarding the impact of such factors such as age, race, socioeconomic status, and sexual identity on healthcare access and utilization.

The Women's Program was designed to alter biases stemming from sexism and heterosexism through two major foci. First, all staff are expected to be culturally competent in order to effectively address the diversity of women's experiences. The Women's Program Director is a matrix position (participating in all departments). She ensures that the specific needs of women are addressed in new programs and that program staff actively represent lesbians and bisexual women at community venues in order to challenge assumptions of sexism and heterosexism. Second, specific personnel within each department are identified as belonging to the Women's Program, with more extensive training and expertise to ensure the highest quality of services.

Rainbow Families, a collaborative community program designed to address the multiple needs of alternative families, is administered through the Women's Program to help provide social support to families likely to experience heterosexism and homophobia. Rainbow Families meets regularly to discuss the unique challenges involved in raising children with same-gendered parents and also to provide social support through events, networking, and community mobilization. A lesbian-identified physician also performs alternative insemination to women who are denied insemination services because of their sexual orientation or who are uncomfortable with disclosing information because of fear of heterosexist responses and discrimination.

Besides providing health services, the two authors have developed a behavior-based HIV prevention program targeted at finding women who have sex with women (WSW) in the community and providing them with important information and behavior strategies for reducing the risk of HIV/STD transmission. In addition, issues of sexism within the health center are being directly addressed through a sexism reduction task force. The task force is designed to promote dialogue between male and female staff, with discussion of specific instances of perceived sexism and development of specific recommendations for their elimination.

HBHC staff also recognized that the health needs of many people of color were not being adequately addressed. Over time, dialogues with key leaders of communities of color identified a number of factors preventing LGBT people of color from utilizing HBHC services. Some were logistical; for example, Chicago is a very large city, with heavy concentrations of ethic found in specific parts of the city. Others were based on perceptions that programs were Euro-Americanocentric, that is, not representing people of Latino, Asian, or African-American descent. To address these perceptions of institutionalized racism, changes in policies were made regarding the nature and content of media and advertising materials. In general, these materials are now developed with input from diverse groups and use volunteers from the targeted communities as media models.

A community advisory board meets monthly to advise HBHC on issues of concern within communities of color. The advisory board is an independent group of leaders from diverse communities of color whose function is to ensure appropriate program diversity. In addition to the above committees, a cultural competency task force, consisting of various staff members who represent diverse cultures, has been created to evaluate how institutionalized racism can be addressed more effectively. Recommendations have included posting bilingual signs and displaying more diverse artwork in the clinic.

As a result of its forums held within communities of color, HBHC leadership recognized that additional changes were needed to address racial disparities within the LGBT community with regard to healthcare access. To this end, Harambee Wellness Center was created specifically to serve people of color who were unable or unwilling to come to HBHC's primary northside location. The word "Harambee" means "coming together" in Swahili, the most common language of East Africa. Harambee Wellness Center was opened to offer people of African descent accessible primary care, prevention, and HIV and STD testing services in an Afrocentric environment. Although Harambee is part of HBHC, its staff, location, and service provision are designed to meet the particular needs of gay and bisexual African Americans and same-gender-loving men and women of African descent who do not identify as gay or bisexual. This is an important distinction because cultural variations also exist among the LGBT community, and there are differing levels of acceptance of same-sex relationships across cultures.

In addition to addressing specific concerns of racism and sexism within the health center, HBHC has worked collaboratively with other direct service providers to ensure that the LGBT community is adequately represented in other areas of society. In recent years, in an effort to reduce heterosexism and homophobia, the agency has created partnerships targeting specific, underserved, hard-to-reach populations. For instance, to reduce homophobia, HBHC has established formal linkages with organizations to enhance social services offered to HIV-positive individuals and those at high risk for the disease. We have also developed a year-long certificate program for mental health providers to gain experience in working with LGBT clients. These types of activities help HBHC better serve LGBT clients through linkage with a comprehensive health care network and allows for prejudice and discrimination to be reduced through the overt presence of sexual, gender, and racial minorities in all aspects of the agency.

FUTURE DIRECTIONS

It is unlikely that our diverse society will be able to entirely eliminate racism, sexism, or heterosexism. Members of a diverse society hold both individual attitudes and behaviors that are formed through customs, norms, and institutions. However, it is logical to assume that attitudes and beliefs can be changed or attenuated through the same mechanisms by which they are formed. Infrastructure support for the elimination of discrimination is often sporadic and subject to the influences of the existing political climate. Local, state, and federal government can implicitly support discriminatory behavior by the lack of legislation prohibiting such behavior. Discriminatory practices also can be supported through the failure to collect crucial data related to the frequency and quality of these behaviors. For example, since the 1990 Hate Crimes Act statistics were released, only 34 states had passed hate crime laws, and 14 of these did not include crimes based on sexual orientation (NGLTF, 1993).

Community-based projects that attempt to prevent or reduce prejudice and discrimination should include advocating changes in city and state legislation to eliminate prejudicial language and discriminatory practices. Prevention specialists and community psychologists can work collaboratively with members of minority communities to more effectively address these issues. Barriers to equality can be reduced through mobilizing members to vote, contacting their political representatives, and economically supporting agencies which lobby the federal government to make legislative changes to guarantee equal access to resources.

Prevention specialists can provide consultation to community members aimed at facilitating systemic change through the development of more effective strategies for utilizing the legal system. Legal mechanisms to help combat illegal discrimination can empower disenfranchised communities to address some of the issues inherent in inequities among genders, races, and sexual minorities. Such mechanisms include access to city contracts for specific minority businesses, domestic partnership policies that include same-gender relationships, and legal organizations such as tenants rights groups. Organizations which challenge existing discriminatory legal practices, such as Operation PUSH, the American Civil Liberties Union, the Lambda Legal Defense Fund, and the National Organization for Women, can affect policy. When prevention specialists work with agencies to achieve parity for their constituents and reduce discrimination by empowering leaders in the community to mount legal challenges to discriminatory practices, they maximize their impact in facilitating systemic change.

Sexist assumptions are imbedded within the context of societal institutions and treat the male perspective as normative. Bem (1993) called this perspective "androcentrism" and argued that it functions to exclude the unique experience of women. Biglan (1995) recommended involving men in the active reduction of sexist practices through the modification of normative support for coercive sexual practices. By including men in programs designed to reduce sexism, prevention specialists work to challenge group norms supporting rigid gender roles and sexual violence toward women. In addition, secondary gains include reducing prejudice and discrimination by weakening the androcentric framework and providing mechanisms for inclusion.

Strategies to address inequalities stemming from racism, sexism, and heterosexism should involve both (a) direct interventions that reduce prejudicial beliefs and discriminatory behavior and (b) the general inclusion of diversity in all activities and experiences. Future prevention programs should include as a goal the promotion of open and honest communication about differences for all persons (Strickland, 2000). Community psychologists can help facilitate communication between parents and children about diversity of race, gender, sexual orientation, culture, and religion. Prevention programs can cognitively stimulate challenges to stereotypical thinking which may be activated when individuals encounter people or groups different from them. Through such programs, all segments of society are involved in ensuring that our society continues to value the contribution that multiculturalism brings (Jackson, 2000).

Community psychologists can both provide information about diverse members of our society and promote acceptance of the value of diversity and multipluralism within community based interventions. To accomplish this, we must first create more rigorously designed methodological studies that are theoretically driven and that evaluate the programs' effectiveness. Community-based programs must establish both process and outcome evaluations in order to identify which norms, attitudes, and behaviors are contributing to the formation and maintenance of sexism, racism and heterosexism. Community psychologists can provide feedback to community organizations regarding realistic strategies that members can incorporate into prevention programs. These activities should include multilevel components for attitude and behavior change in already existing prevention programs. Ideally, such programs should cut across multiple settings and provide a consistent, theoretical message about the value of diversity and the desirability of tolerance and inclusion. These efforts can target not only individuals and institutions but also neighborhoods and local community-based agencies.

Community psychologists and media specialists can contribute to these societal changes through developing alternative positive portrayals of various members of oppressed groups in the media. If stereotypes portrayed in various forms of the media are challenged, differences between communities may not be easily perceived as negative. Community psychologists should begin to evaluate these strategies on a local level by monitoring inappropriate portrayals of minority group members on local television programs and in public service announcements. A final, and perhaps more controversial, role for the community psychologist is as an advocate using various media outlets (e.g., television interviews, local newspapers, and national conferences) to promote attitude and behavioral change in their neighborhoods or institutions.

As community members and trained professionals, we have the ability to assist communities in recognizing existing tangible resources that can be used to promote intergroup acceptance and respect. As community psychologists, we can form collaborative relationships and provide assistance in fighting prejudice and discrimination by making our collective skills part of the community advocacy. These activities can promote the well-being of individuals and groups who have been systematically denied access to life-sustaining and life-enhancing institutional resources such as quality medical care, adequate housing, safe child care, and basic commodities such as food. Through activism and community mobilization, and through confronting discrimination and stereotypical beliefs when we encounter them individually and collectively, we can reduce the costs to ourselves, our families, our communities, and our country.

REFERENCES

Allport, G. W. (1954). *The nature of prejudice*. Reading, MA: Addison-Wesley.

Ashmore, R., & Del Boca, F. (1981). Conceptual approaches to the understanding of intergroup conflict. In D. L. Hamilton (Ed.), *Cognitive processes in stereotyping and intergroup behavior* (pp. 1–35). Hillsdale, NJ: Erlbaum.

Bandura, A. (1977). *Social learning theory*. Englewood Cliffs, NJ: Prentice-Hall.

Bandura, A. (1986). *Social foundations of thought and action: A social cognitive theory*. Englewood Cliffs, NJ: Prentice-Hall.

Bandura, A. (1990). Perceived self-efficacy in the exercise of control over AIDS. *Evaluation & Progam Planning*, 3, 9–17.

Barnard, W., & Benn, M. (1988). Belief congruence and prejudice reduction in an interracial contact setting. *Journal of Social Psychology, 128*, 125–134.

Batts, V. (1983). Knowing and changing the cultural script component of racism. *Transactional Analysis Journal, 13*, 255–257.

Bem, S. (1993). *The lenses of gender: Transforming the debate on sexual inequality*. New Haven, CT: Yale.

Bem, S., & Bem, D. (1973). Does sex-biased job advertising "aid and abet" sex discrimination? *Journal of Applied Social Psychology, 3*, 6–18.

Bernard, N., Holliday, B., Crump, S., & Sanchez, N. (1998). *Psychology and racism: Annotated bibliography*. Washington DC: American Psychological Association.

Biglan, A. (1995). *Changing cultural practices: A contextual framework for intervention research*. Reno, NV: Context Press.

Biglan, A., Metzler, C., Wirt, R., Ary, D., Noell, J., Ochs, L., French, C., & Hood, D. (1990). Social and behavioral factors associated with high-risk sexual behavior among adolescents. *Journal of Behavioral Medicine, 13*, 245–262.

Brooks, V. (1981). *Minority stress and lesbian women*. Lexington, MA: D. C. Heath.

Brown, M., & Amoroso, D. (1975). Attitudes towards homosexuality among West Indian male and female college students. *Journal of Social Psychology, 97*, 163–168.

Byrd, W. M. (1990). Race, biology, and health care: Reassessing the relationship. *Journal of Health Care for the Poor and Underserved, 1*, 278–296.

Clark, R., Anderson, N. B., Clark, V. R., & Williams, D. R. (1999). Racism as a stressor for African Americans: A biopsychosocial model. *American Psychologist, 54*, 805–816.

Comstock, G. D. (1991). *Violence against lesbians and gay men*. New York: Columbia University Press.

Crawford, I., Salina, D. D., & Jason, L. A. (1990). The use of behavioral strategies in a multi-media based AIDS prevention program. *The Community Psychologist, 23*, 9–11.

Crawford, I., Salina, D. D., & Jason, L. A. (1992). Recommendations for implementing a media-based AIDS prevention program, *Prevention Update, 3*, 6.

Cutrona, S. & Russell, D. (1987). The provisions of social relationships and adaptation to stress. In W. H. Jones & D. Perlman (Eds.), *Advances in personal relationships* (vol. 1). Greenwich, Connecticut: JAI Press.

Cutrona, S. & Russell, D. (1990). Type of social support and specific stress: Toward a theory of optimal matching. In B. R. Sarason, I. G. Sarason, & G. R. Pierce (Eds.), *Social support: An interactional view* (pp. 319–366). New York: Wiley.

D'Augelli, A. (1989). Lesbians and gay men's experiences of discrimination and harassment in a university community. *American Journal of Community Psychology, 17*, 317–320.

D'Augelli, A., & Hershberger, S. (1993). Lesbian, gay, and bisexual youths in community settings: Personal challenges and mental health problems. *American Journal of Community Psychology, 21*, 421–448.

Dean, L., Meyer, I., Robinson, K., Sell, R., Sember, R., Silenzio, V., Bowen,

D., Bradford, J., Rothblum, E., Scout, White, J., Dunn, P., Lawrence, A., Wolfe, D., Xavier, J., Carter, D., Pittman, J., & Tierney, R. (2000). *Journal of the Gay and Lesbian Medical Association, 4,* 101–151.

Douglas, D., Kalman, C., & Kalman, T. (1985). Heterosexism among physicians and nurses: An empirical study. *Hospital and Community Psychiatry, 36,* 1309–1311.

Dunbar, J., Brown, M., & Amoroso, D. (1973). Some correlates of attitudes towards homosexuality. *Journal of Social Psychology, 89,* 271–279.

Finn, P., & Taylor, M. (1987). *The response of the criminal justice system to bias crime.* Cambridge, MA: Abt Associates, Inc.

Fishbein, M. & Ajzen, I. (1975). *Belief, attitude, intention and behavior: An introduction to theory and research.* Reading, MA: Addison-Wesley.

Frieze, I., Parsons, J., Johnson, P., Ruble, D., & Zellman, G. (1978). *Women and sex roles: A social psychological perspective.* New York: W.W. Norton & Company.

Garofalo, J., & Martin, S. (1991). The law enforcement response to bias-motivated crimes. In J. Kelly (Ed.), *Bias crime* (pp. 30–42). Chicago: Office of International Criminal Justice.

Garnets, L. (1992, August). *The psychological treatment of survivors of anti-gay violence.* Paper presented at the annual meeting of the American Psychological Association, Washington, D.C.

Garnets, L., Herek, G., & Levy, B. (1992). Violence and victimization of lesbians and gay men: Mental health consequences. In G. M. Herek & K. T. Berrill (Eds.), *Hate crimes: Confronting violence against lesbians and gay men* (pp. 207–226). Newbury Park, CA: Sage.

Gilligan, C. (1982). *In a different voice.* Cambridge, MA: Harvard University Press.

Herek, G. (1990). The context of anti-gay violence. *Journal of Interpersonal Violence, 5,* 274–294.

Herek, G. (Ed.) (1998). *Stigma and sexual orientation.* Newbury Park, CA: Sage.

Herek, G. M. & Berrill K. T. (Eds.) (1992). *Hate crimes: Confronting violence against lesbians and gay men.* Newbury Park, CA: Sage.

Hobfoll, S. E. (1988). *The ecology of stress.* New York: Hemisphere.

Hubler, S., & Silverstein, S. (1993, July 13). Schooling doesn't close minority earning gap. *Los Angeles Times,* pp. A1, A16.

Jackson, A. M. (1990). Evolution of ethnocultural psychotherapy. *Psychotherapy, 27,* 428–435.

Jackson, J. (2000). What ought psychology to do? *American Psychologist, 55,* 328–330.

Jones, J. M. (1972). *Prejudice and racism.* Reading, MA: Addison Wesley.

Jones, J. M. (1981). The concept of racism and its changing reality. In B. J. Bowser & R. G. Hunt (Eds.), *Impacts of racism on White Americans* (pp. 27–49). Beverly Hills, CA: Sage.

Kelly, J. (1971). Qualities for the community psychologist. *American Psychologist, 26*, 897–903.

Klaw, E., & Rhodes, J. (1995). Mentor relationships and the career development of pregnant and parenting African-American teenagers. *Psychology of Women Quarterly, 19*, 551–562.

Laumann, O., Gagnon, J. H., Michael, R. T., & Michael, S. (1994). *The social organization of sexuality: Sexual practices in the United States*. Chicago, IL: University of Chicago Press.

Maccoby, E. E. (1990). Gender and relationships: A developmental account. *American Psychologist, 45*, 513–520.

MacDonald, A., & Games, R. (1974). Some characteristics of those who hold positive and negative attitudes towards homosexuals. *Journal of Homosexuality, 1*, 23–33.

Myers, D. L. (1993). Participation by women in behavior analysis II. *The Behavior Analyst, 16*, 75–86.

National Gay and Lesbian Task Force. (1993). *1993 updated fact sheets of the NGLTF Policy Institute*. Washington, DC: Author.

Ostertag, P. A., & McNamara, J. R. (1991). Feminization of psychology: The changing sex ratio and its implications for the profession. *Psychology of Women Quarterly, 15*, 349–369.

Ponterotto, J., & Pedersen, P. (1993). *Preventing prejudice: A guide for counselors and educators*. Newbury Park, CA: Sage.

Presser, N., Stephan, C., Kennedy, J., & Aronson, E. (1978). Attributions to success and failure in cooperative, competitive, and interdependent interaction. *European Journal of Social Psychology, 8*, 269–274.

Rappaport, J. (1977). *Community psychology*. New York: Holt, Rhinehart & Winston.

Rappaport, J. (1981). In praise of paradox: A social policy of empowerment over prevention. *American Journal of Community Psychology, 9*, 1–25.

Rappaport, J., Davidson, W., & Wilson, J. (1975). Alternatives to blaming the victim or the environment: Our places to stand have not moved the earth. *American Psychologist, 30*, 525–528.

Rooney-Rebeck, P., & Jason, L. (1986). Prevention of prejudice in elementary school students. *Journal of Primary Prevention, 7*, 63–73.

Rotheram-Borus, M. J., Hunter, J., & Rosario, M. (1994). Suicidal behavior and gay-related stress among gay and bisexual male adolescents. *Journal of Adolescent Research, 9*, 498–508.

Ryan, C., & Futterman, D. (1998). *Lesbian and gay youth: Care and counseling*. New York: Columbia University Press.

Salina, D. D. (1989). *The impact of knowledge and level of homophobia on prejudice towards persons with AIDS*. Unpublished doctoral dissertation, DePaul University, Chicago, Illinois.

Salina, D. D., Crawford, I. C., & Jason, L. A. (1992). AIDS prevention: Using mass media to increase communications between parents and children. *The Community Psychologist, 23*, 9–11.

Sapon-Shevin, M. (1988). A minicourse for junior high students. *Social Education, 52*, 272–275.

Sarason, B., Shearin, E., Pierce, G., & Sarason, I. (1987). Interrelations of social support measures: Theoretical and practical implications. *Journal of Personality and Social Psychology, 52*, 813–832.

Shilts, R. (1987). *And the band played on: Politics, people, and the AIDS epidemic*. New York: St. Martin's Press.

Shinn, M. (1987). Expanding community psychology's domain. *American Journal of Community Psychology, 15*, 555–574.

Skillings, J. & Dobbins, J.E. (1991). Racism as a disease: Etiology and treatment implications. *Journal of Counseling and Development, 70*, 206–212.

Solarz, A. (Ed.) (1999). *Lesbian health care: Current assessment and directions for the future*. Washington, DC: Institute of Medicine, National Academy Press.

Sonnenschein, F. (1988). Countering prejudiced beliefs and behaviors: The role of the social studies professional. *Social Education, 52*, 264–266.

Stephan, C., Kennedy, J., & Aronson, E. (1977). Attribution of luck or skill as a function of cooperating or competing with a friend or acquaintance. *Sociometry, 40*, 107–111.

Stokes, J., & Peterson, J. (1998). Heterosexism, self-esteem, and risk for HIV among African-American men who have sex with men. *AIDS Education and Prevention, 10*, 278–292.

Strickland, B. (2000). Misassumptions, misadventures and the misuse of psychology. *American Psychologist, 55*, 333–338.

Thomas, V., & Miles, S. (1995). Psychology of Black women: Past, present, and future. In H. Landrine (Ed.), *Bringing cultural diversity to feminist psychology* (pp. 303–330). Washington, DC: American Psychological Association.

U.S. Bureau of the Census (1995). *Statistical abstracts of the United States: 1995* (115th ed.). Washington, DC: Author.

Watts, R., & Abdul-Adil, J. (1997). Promoting critical consciousness in young, African-American men. *Journal of Prevention and Intervention in the Community, 16*, 63–86.

Watts, R., Griffith, D., & Adul-Adil, J. (1999). Sociopolitical development as an antidote for oppression-theory and action. *American Journal of Community Psychology, 27*, 255–271.

Winett, R., King, A., & Altman, D. (1989). *Health psychology and public health: An integrative approach*. New York: Pergamon.

Winett, R., Leckliter, I., Chinn, D., Stahl, B., & Love, S. (1985). Effects of television modeling on residential energy conservation. *Journal of Applied Behavior Analysis, 18*, 33–44.

Wolff, T. (1987). Community psychology and empowerment: An activist's insights. *American Journal of Community Psychology, 15*, 149–165.

CHAPTER 15

Promoting Healthy Communities Through Community Development

Maury Nation,

Abraham Wandersman, and

Douglas D. Perkins

Child abuse, risky adolescent behaviors (e.g., unprotected sex, pregnancy), delinquency, and substance abuse have been the topics of numerous treatment and prevention studies (e.g., Choi & Coates, 1994; Shedler & Block, 1990; Webster-Stratton & Hammond, 1997). Typically, these studies have focused on the individual and intrapsychic conceptualizations of problems, and they have proposed and tested many therapies and programs based on those conceptualizations. Although these efforts are laudable, they often ignore many important factors that contribute to the development and perpetuation of these problems. Community problems, including poverty, dilapidated housing, and social isolation, have been implicated in the development of many "individual" problems, including child abuse and neglect (Coulton, Korbin, & Su, 1999), domestic violence (Miles-Doan, 1998), crime and delinquency (Morenoff & Sampson, 1997; Sampson & Lauritsen, 1994), poor prenatal care and early child development (Duncan, Brooks-Gunn, & Klebanov, 1994; Perloff & Jaffee, 1999), low birth weight babies (Roberts, 1997), adolescent mental health problems (Aneshensel & Sucoff, 1996), and risky adolescent sexual behavior and pregnancy (Ku, Sonenstein, & Pleck, 1993; Mayer & Jencks, 1989).

Bronfenbrenner (1979) proposed that ecological variables, including family, school, neighborhood, and community could affect an individual's behavior. Recent research continues to support Bronfrenbrenner's ideas about the importance of environmental context on the healthy development of individuals. In fact, reviews of this research (e.g., Gephart, 1997; Wandersman & Nation, 1998) leave little doubt that a community's social, physical, political, and economic qualities play important roles in producing healthy individuals who, in turn, create a healthy, vibrant community life. These reviews also raise doubts about the sufficiency of individual-focused models to address psychological and social problems.

The gap between individual-focused models of intervention and our understanding of the impact of community problems suggests the need for community models to supplement individual- and family-level models (Goodman & Wandersman, 1994). Goodman and Wandersman (1994) proposed that a comprehensive causal model for many psychological and health problems, such as substance abuse, is one that includes risk factors at the individual, family, and community levels. Therefore, interventions must also involve all three levels.

In this chapter, we consider a community model of social problems and interventions. These models supplement individual and family models and are based on community development and public health perspectives. There are four sections to the chapter: (a) a description of the problem that is focused on a multidimensional conceptualization of community problems, and on the link between community problems and individual outcomes, (b) a review of the literature related to community development and public health approaches to intervention in distressed communities, (c) a case example of a program in which family and community development are central components, and (d) recommendations to guide the development of new interventions and future directions for research and practice in troubled communities.

DESCRIPTION OF THE PROBLEM

Proposing a community model for intervening in psychological problems requires that we define two central concepts, namely *community* and *community problems*. There are numerous phenomenological definitions of community. Here we define community as a residential area with limited geographic boundaries, such as a neighborhood or a street block. History and attachment to a physical place is a vital element of what builds and sustains community in our definition.

Because all communities have problems that vary from minor annoyances to profound distress, building consensus on comprehensive indicators of community problems is difficult. We approach community problems as a multidimensional construct that includes the economic, social, physical, and political conditions within a community. Communities vary in these dimensions, with some experiencing serious problems, including poverty (as measured by various indices), large numbers of disrupted families, residential instability, physical and social disorder, and political marginalization.

Economic Problems

The impact of poverty on health and mental health outcomes is well documented. Early ecological studies (e.g., Faris & Dunham, 1939; Shaw & McKay, 1969) documented the tendency for poverty to be concentrated in specific communities, and suggested that living in these communities adds to one's risk of poor outcomes, such as juvenile delinquency and psychiatric hospitalization. Most of the subsequent ecological analyses of health and developmental outcomes have validated poverty as a powerful predictor of poor outcomes, including school dropout, juvenile delinquency, low birth weight, and child maltreatment (e.g., Figueira-McDonough, 1991; Roberts, 1997; Zuravin, 1989). Such neighborhood measures as poverty status, high rates of unemployment, and low per capita income are among the structural characteristics commonly used to indicate economic decline.

Physical Problems

Neighborhood disorder refers to the decline in the physical and ambient conditions, called incivilities, that are common in distressed neighborhoods. During the 1970s and 1980s, changes in urban neighborhoods such as the emergence of the underclass and the gentrification of some urban neighborhoods highlighted the plight of disordered neighborhoods (Taylor & Covington, 1988; Wilson, 1987). Skogan (1990) included dilapidated houses, abandoned buildings, vandalism, litter, and garbage as physical incivilities of neighborhoods. This category of incivilities symbolizes visual indicators of negligence and decay that, if left unchecked, might lead to serious crimes (Wilson & Kelling, 1982).

Research (e.g., Taylor, Shumaker, & Gottfredson, 1985) has confirmed that both subjective and objective indicators of disorder do have an impact on residents' perceptions of their neighborhoods. Covington and Taylor (1991) and Perkins and Taylor (1996) introduced a multilevel analysis strategy that compared individual, individual-within-block/neighborhood, and between-neighborhood effects of social and physical disorder (using multiple measures) on fear of crime. The results indicated that both physical and social incivilities were positively related to levels of fear of crime. Taylor and Covington's (1993) study of 66 Baltimore neighborhoods found that incivilities and fear were high in those areas that experienced significant increases in the proportion of youth and African Americans in the past decade. This suggests that there may be a relationship between neighborhood disorder and the neighborhood's structural characteristics.

Other types of ambient conditions such as building design, crowding, and noise have been associated with poor outcomes as well, including children's behavioral problems and low academic achievement (see Wandersman & Nation, 1998, for a review). For example, exposure to toxic hazards (e.g., lead, PCBs) has been associated with such outcomes as birth defects, academic problems, and cancer (e.g., Edelstein, 1988; Marshall, Grensburg, Deres, Geary, & Cayo, 1997). Such toxins tend to be concentrated in poor ethnic communities (United Church of Christ Commision on Racial Justice, 1987).

Social Problems

The presence of social incivilities and the disruption or dissolution of social networks is another aspect of the community that portends poor social and developmental outcomes. Social incivilities include public drunkenness, corner gangs, street harassment, drug trading, and noisy neighbors (Skogan, 1990). The importance of social networks has been illustrated clearly in studies of child abuse and neglect, which have found that neighborhoods having a heavy child care burden (i.e., a high ratio of children to adults, with low percentages of male and elderly residents) and residential instability had higher rates of child maltreatment (Coulton, Korbin, Su, & Chow, 1995; Garbarino & Kostelny, 1992).

The importance of social structure is not limited to child maltreatment outcomes. Social disorganization theory has emerged as one of the most influential theories linking communities to crime and delinquency. In its purest form, social organization refers to a community's ability to realize a common set of values and to mobilize to internally solve its commonly experienced problems (Kornhauser, 1978). There is high social organization to the degree that informal social networks, neighborhood institutions (e.g., schools and churches), and other formal organizations (e.g., civic clubs and homeowners associations) can exert social control from within a community (Bursik & Grasmick, 1993). Tests of this theory have found high community transience to be related to poor neighborhood networks and property crimes, including vandalism and auto theft (Sampson & Groves, 1989). Connell and Halpern-Felsher (1997) tapped into a similar construct which they termed "symbolic and social exchange processes." Investigations of these processes, which include the development of social networks and supervision of children, provide further support for the impact of social decline, particularly when it is paired with poverty. For example, McLoyd (1990) suggested that parents respond to the physical danger of poor neighborhoods by using more punitive and coercive parenting styles. Social disorganization theory predicts that the quality of social networks may be a powerful mediator of the impact of community conditions on individual outcomes.

Political Problems

Political problems are indicated by the disempowering of a community (i.e., a general lack of hope, participation, and control over local decision-making). Causal factors may include macroeconomic factors, such as national and regional economic and employment structure, institutional policies and practices (both public and private) that are undemocratic or ignore citizen concerns, and social conditions (e.g., unchecked disorder and discrimination). A primary issue here is how these factors may differentially have an impact on neighborhoods in ways that cause or perpetuate the lack of political power.

Examination of discriminatory housing practices demonstrates how the continued ghettoization of minorities and the poor occurs. Despite fair housing laws, subtle discriminatory practices of banks and real estate professionals still have a significant effect on the distribution of racial and ethnic populations. Housing audits using black and white agents as prospective renters are used to determine the presence of discrimination. Galster and Keeney's (1988) review of 71 audit studies led them to conclude that racial discrimination was a dominant feature for both housing rental and sales markets in metropolitan areas. Practices such as racial steering (i.e., guiding black and white clients to neighborhoods that differ in key economic or racial characteristics) were common. Massey and Denton (1993) reported that the practice of informal redlining (i.e., refusing to underwrite mortgages in areas that contained black residents, were adjacent to predominantly black areas, or were at risk to attract black residents) by the Federal Housing Administration (FHA) and private lenders continued to discourage integration of racial and ethnic groups. Farley and Frey (1994) documented several factors that have perpetuated segregation and the concentration of poverty, including federal housing policies that encouraged the isolation of public housing from middle-class communities. Racial disparity is carried over into home ownership rates and home equity. In fact, Oliver and Shapiro (1995) reported that White high school dropouts on average have more home equity wealth (this wealth is based on property values, which, in turn, are based on desirability of neighborhood) than Black professionals.

Population shifts (e.g., the onset of suburbanization and the shift from traditional manufacturing to service and high-technology industries) also have contributed to the isolation of urban neighborhoods, with high-skilled and higher paying jobs tending to be located in the suburban areas of cities. Consequently, middle-class residents (and everyone else who could afford to) moved out of urban areas for these jobs, with the residents who remained frequently being minorities, who were poor, unskilled, and lacked transportation (Sassen, 1990).

REVIEW AND CRITIQUE OF THE LITERATURE

Because community problems are often systemic, proposed solutions (both prevention and rehabilitation) should be comprehensive and systemic. Two professional traditions that often take such an approach in communities are community development and public health. Historically, these traditions have been somewhat distinct in their ideology and goals. Both traditions provide insight into effective methods of addressing community problems, and both have produced collaborations with psychologists to develop interventions that improve individual outcomes.

Community Development

Although there has been some controversy about the definition of community development (see Ferguson & Dickens, 1999), it may be broadly defined as government policies, nonprofit organizations, citizen voluntary associations, or public-private partnerships working to improve a community's environment (Perkins, Crim, Silberman, & Brown, in press; for a list of community development and community organizing resources, see *http://www.people.vanderbilt.edu/~douglas.d.perkins/cdwebsites.htm* on the internet). Although there are many potential interventions that may come under the rubric of this definition, community development has been associated largely with community development corporations (CDCs). Typically, CDCs are private, nonprofit organizations designed to meet residents' needs within a designated geographic area. In turn, CDCs have become associated with two interventions: the development of affordable housing and the development of community-based businesses.

There have been several successful CDCs. The most famous example may be the Bedford-Stuyvesant Restoration Corporation. Started in the 1960s in a community that had all of the stereotypic characteristics of decline, this CDC implemented an economic and political action plan that eventually resulted in new housing, new retail stores, and increased social services (Ferguson & Dickens, 1999). Since the development of this CDC, the political and economic environments of the community have changed substantially. Shrinking federal funding has shrunk the vision of many CDCs and forced the specialization and professionalization of many of these organizations (Stoutland, 1999). Therefore, despite these positive examples, the eventual impact of CDCs is still unknown.

Broader definitions of community development have included everything from neighborhood clean-ups and community policing, to national policies such as empowerment and enterprise zones (i.e., programs in which federal monies are used to create incentives for economic development in poor communities). Like the CDCs, these have had varying degrees of success. For example, Palen (1997) noted that for a variety of reasons, including the residential instability of the targeted communities and the difficulty in attracting and staffing high-wage and high-skill jobs, empowerment zones have not been sufficient to turn around distressed neighborhoods. The end result is that their sustained impact on distressed communities may be negligible.

Community policing is another intervention that is associated with a broad definition of community development. This method of crime prevention emphasizes improving the social environment by increasing police visibility through interventions such as foot patrols and neighborhood-based police stations. In their discussion of a national survey of police departments, Breci and Erickson (1998) reported that more than half of the police departments that served large communities (50,000 or more) had implemented some form of community-oriented policing. Thus far, however, it appears that community policing has been most effective in middle-class communities (Skogan, 1990). Furthermore, some case studies suggest that many of these initiatives fail because of a failure to communicate effectively with residents in the affected neighborhoods (Schneider, 1999).

Public Health

Initially, public health was a field focused on the control of communicable diseases and prevention of disease and injury (Tulchinsky & Varavikova, 2000). However, public health has evolved from a singular focus on individuals' health to a multifaceted mission that encompasses the promotion of the health and welfare of individuals and communities. Today, a public health concern may be broadly defined as any problem that affects the health of a population (Freudenberg & Manoncourt, 1998). The concentration of many poor outcomes in troubled communities has made health promotion a priority in urban areas. There may be minor differences between the orientation of some health promotion interventions and some community development interventions. Most notably, public health urban interventions are sometimes focused on specific health problems affecting community residents (e.g., Kass & Freudenberg, 1997). Despite this health-related focus, public health practitioners have recognized that the community context is important for effective intervention (Leviton, Snell, & McGinnis, 2000).

Commensurate with the evolution of the field of public health has been a change in the tools used to improve outcomes. In 1995, the Centers for Disease Control (CDC) convened a meeting to determine the important factors in increasing the capacity of communities to deal with public health problems (for a summary, see Goodman et al., 1998). Among the conclusions was an emphasis on the importance of including community members in the development of interventions and in understanding the social context of the neighborhood. Furthermore, the CDC funded urban research centers to specifically investigate problems and evaluate interventions in urban communities (Speers & Lancaster, 1998).

There are many examples of effective community interventions. Barton and Tyska (1999) described the impact of community-based health centers in a predominantly African American community in Chicago. This health center emphasized primary health care and encouraged residents to become partners in their health-related decision making. In addition to health-specific issues, the center staff worked with residents to encourage the completion of high school and the development of interpersonal and job skills. Another example is a program focused on improving cardiovascular health in a poor urban community in New York (Shea, Basch, Wechsler, & Lantigua, 1996). The project involved several components, including an education campaign (focused on promoting low-fat milk), health screenings, and participant-led exercise clubs. Although the impact of the intervention on heart disease is unclear, the intervention did result in some positive health-related behaviors, including exercise and dietary changes.

For the last several years, Comprehensive Community Initiatives (CCIs) have been the preferred approach to health-related urban interventions (Aspen Institute, 1997; McNeely, 1999). CCIs consist of coalitions of community agencies, institutions (e.g., schools and churches), and concerned citizens who unite to address health problems. Community initiatives have been developed to address several outcomes, including alcohol and drug abuse, smoking, heart disease, violence, and immunizations. Some examples of community coalition-based interventions are the community partnerships funded through the Center for Substance Abuse Prevention (CSAP), Johnson & Johnson's SAFEKIDS, and the National Cancer Institute's COMMIT program (e.g., COMMIT Research Group, 1995). Butterfoss et al. (1998) described an urban community-based coalition aimed at increasing children's immunization. The program provided a number of interventions, including increased access to services and support for families. The ultimate result was a nearly 20% increase in the percentage of children receiving immunizations. Evaluations (e.g., Butterfoss, Goodman, & Wandersman, 1993; COMMIT Research Group, 1995; Davidson, Durkin, Kuhn, & O'Connor, 1994) suggest that coalitions are a promising strategy for addressing a variety health-related problems.

Both community development and public health practitioners are recognizing the importance of comprehensive intervention. Perkins, Grim, Silberman, and Brown (in press) for example, proposed a comprehensive community development framework for attacking community problems at multiple levels and on all four dimensions (i.e., social, political, environmental, and economic; see Figure 15.1). In addition to the typical focus on housing and economic issues, this framework suggests that efforts should be focused simultaneously on (a) local and national policies that affect neighborhoods and (b) organized efforts at improving a neighborhood's physical environment. In the realm of public health, Leviton, Snell, and McGinnis (2000) argued that problems in urban communities are so intertwined that effective intervention requires the joining of public services, community organizations, and residents to build the capacity to address the array of problems facing urban communities.

As illustrated in Figure 15.1, this ecological framework emphasizes intervention in all four areas of community problems. The large-scale policy column highlights how public community development policy can be used to improve community and individual problems through direct intervention (e.g., providing community programs and jobs) and indirectly by supporting the empowerment of individuals within their communities. Likewise, small-scale community development interventions provide the settings and opportunities for empowerment and work to improve the immediate economic (Perkins et al., in press), social (Butterfoss et al., 1998), political (Speer & Hughey, 1995), and physical (Perkins & Brown, 1996) environments. Our review indicates that intervention at each level can have a positive influence on social and psychological problems. Putting these strategies together has the potential for creating a dynamic community development process that supports continued positive community and individual outcomes.

CASE EXAMPLE

Free to Grow is a national initiative (Jones, Gutman, & Kaufman, 1999) funded by a partnership that includes the Robert Wood Johnson Foundation, the Doris Duke Charitable Foundation, and the local communities participating in the

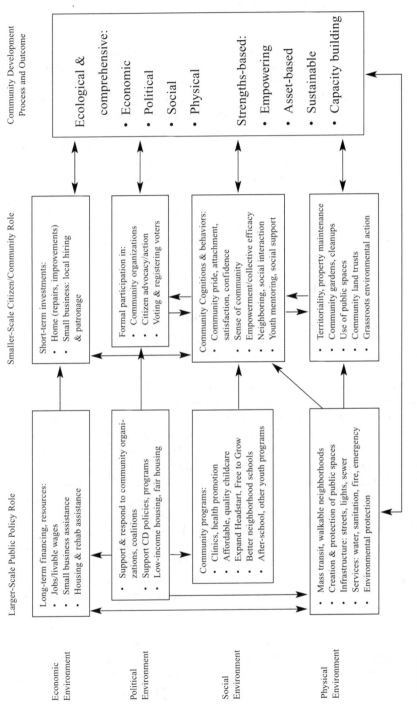

FIGURE 15.1 An ecological framework for community development.

Adapted from Perkins, Grim, Silberman, & Brown, (in press)

project. The United States Department of Justice's Office of Juvenile Justice and Delinquency Prevention is also a partner in the evaluation of the program. Free to Grow combines features of the public health and community development perspectives, and has many social scientists, including psychologists, involved in its design and implementation. Its aim is the reduction of young children's vulnerability to substance abuse and other high-risk behaviors as they grow older.

Free to Grow is based on a causal model that suggests that there are both family and neighborhood risk factors that predict substance abuse (e.g., Kumpfer, Molgaard, & Spoth, 1996; Peterson, Hawkins, Abbott, & Catalano, 1995), as well as protective factors at the family and neighborhood levels that reduce the probability of substance abuse (Hawkins & Catalano, 1992). It uses Head Start centers as a catalyst and organizer of family and neighborhood interventions to reduce risk factors and increase protective factors. Jones Gutman, and Kaufman (1999) stated:

> The national Head Start program is a natural partner in this initiative, not only because it enrolls large numbers of preschool children from below poverty level families, but it establishes a positive relationship with the child and the family, is well-regarded in the community, and its mission is to assist with the child's total development (p. 283).

The successful grantee applicant builds a collaboration with other agencies and groups in the community, performs a needs and resource assessment to determine priorities, and designs interventions that will enhance family functioning *and* the neighborhood or community in which the families live. Family-strengthening strategies include peer mentoring, support groups, and case management. Community-strengthening strategies include civic organizing, leadership development, and community education. There is a concern with the community's economic vitality and the job opportunities available to families, as well as a strong interest in community development. The emphasis on risk and protective factors and on community viability presents an example of the integration of the public health and community development traditions.

Four distinctive Free to Grow models have been offered for adaptation to sites funded in the second phase of the Free to Grow grant program. One model is the Audubon Area Community Services model which was developed in Owensboro, Kentucky, and integrates multiple components. For example:

> A revised family service structure is designed to allow staff to assess a family's level of need so that intensive case management services can be provided to the agency's high-risk families. Stronger families join other community residents for leadership development training that builds crit-

ical skill areas to support prevention-focused Community Action Groups, who work in collaboration with community leaders to create strategies to address key risk and protective factors within the community (Robert Wood Johnson Foundation, 2000, pp. 22–23).

A scaled Family Partnership Plan provides guidelines for assessing families in order to determine an appropriate level of intervention. Family Advocates are trained to gear their interventions based upon a family's "service level," working with families on a broad range of issues, including education, job training, effective parenting skills, behavior management and discipline, and access to social services. Those families who are assessed to be at highest risk are targeted for participation in intensive case management activities.

Each year, high-functioning families (both Head Start families and other families and residents from the community) are identified to participate in community development activities. These trained Head Start families, working in collaboration with other neighborhood residents, as well as with key institutions and organizations, form a Community Action Group. As the priority prevention issues are defined, the Community Action Groups develop strategic plans to bring about the desired changes at the community level. These projects might include cleaning up local vacant lots, launching a drug and alcohol awareness campaign in collaboration with a local school, or organizing an alcohol-free high-school event. As residents build skills and strengthen relationships with key stakeholders, collaboratively they begin to take on more complicated prevention activities, such as improving local policing practices, reducing youth access to alcohol, improving enforcement of drug-free school zones, or seeking stronger sentences for repeat drug-dealing offenses (Robert Wood Johnson Foundation, 2000).

FUTURE DIRECTIONS

There are many effective interventions that have made a difference in communities. Nevertheless, we still are confronted with the question of how to improve the plight of communities. It is clear that the problems are complex and that no one program will work for all communities. However, we believe that the literature of community development and public health outlines themes important to sustained and effective intervention in urban community decline. Based on this literature, we recommend that the next generation of interventions for neighborhoods and communities emphasize four factors: comprehensiveness, empowerment, identification and utilization of assets, and sustainability.

Comprehensiveness

The lack of comprehensive interventions may be an overarching reason for the absence of widespread improvement in community problems. Although we conceptualize community-based problems as multifaceted, the typical intervention (whether community development or public health) addresses only one or two of the dimensions central to the development and maintenance of community problems. Such a piecemeal approach rarely produces the critical mass needed to turn around distressed communities. Highlighting this fact, Stoutland (1999) concluded that even the larger and well-established CDCs did not engage in comprehensive intervention. In the case of successful CCIs, there is also recognition (Butterfoss et al.. 1998) that these interventions will be somewhat limited in their impact unless attention is focused on building neighborhoods' overall capacity to detect and respond to problems.

Empowerment

Throughout the community development and public health literature there is an emphasis on the importance of grassroots involvement in producing positive outcomes. Shea, Barch, Wechsler, and Lantigua's (1996) summary of effective interventions in their heart disease prevention initiative found that a citizen participation component was a distinguishing factor between effective and ineffective interventions. Empowerment builds community residents' and service providers' capacity to identify and address problems and, eventually, to sustain interventions beyond traditional funding cycles (e.g., Butterfoss et al. 1998). Goodman et al. (1998) suggested that building capacity leads to skills, resources, and social networks that become a part of the community and become assets for future interventions.

In community development, grassroots involvement has been important in interventions in virtually all types of neighborhood problems. Empowerment requires little financial investment but provides great returns in energizing and/or stabilizing communities (Perkins et al., in press; Zimmerman & Perkins, 1995). The most effective examples of empowerment have not emphasized the prototypical top-down (i.e., expert driven) or bottom-up (i.e., exclusively grassroots driven) models of intervention. Rather, the inclusion of citizens has meant that projects are collaborative in ways that value both the outsider's technical expertise and residents' experiential expertise and resources (Maton & Salem, 1995). The power of this collaboration was illustrated in a public housing neighborhood in San Francisco where a community-based pilot program was started to prevent tobacco use (El-Askari et al., 1998). In addition to being energized to address tobacco-related problems, residents were so empowered that they successfully advocated for general neighborhood improvements including improved street lighting and speed bumps. It seems likely that neighborhood interventions that fail to involve neighborhood residents in meaningful ways (e.g., planning and implementation) are limited at best and will have little chance of surviving beyond the time frame of parties external to the neighborhood.

Identifying and Utilizing Assets

With respect to community development, Kretzmann and McKnight (1993) argued for a change in the way we think about neighborhoods. Specifically, they suggested an emphasis on a community's strengths as a way of supporting distressed neighborhoods. That is, rather than focusing on remediating problems, intervention should focus on identifying, mapping, developing, and using indigenous social, physical, and economic assets. The importance of assets also has affected public health theory and practice. Freudenberg and Manoncourt (1998) noted that often a community's strengths (including the residents themselves and community organizations) are overlooked in health promotion interventions in urban neighborhoods.

Assets are broadly defined and overlap well with our ecological conceptualization of the problem. They may be physical (e.g., land), social (e.g., cohesion, volunteers), economic (e.g., consumers, entrepreneurs and workers, funding agencies), and political (e.g., voters, advocates, local officials, and community leaders). Perkins and colleagues (in press) described, for example, an asset-based intervention in Arizona. In the Building a Healthier Mesa-Neighborhood Development Initiative, residents responded to a need for youth activities by using the backyard of one of the residents as the site for a program. From a meager beginning, the neighborhood developed collaborations with the Chamber of Commerce, the United Way, and other local organizations. As illustrated in this example, utilizing the resources indigenous to a community can provide the initial energy needed to advocate for more comprehensive intervention.

Sustainability

The idea that development must be sustainable has become axiomatic in response to failed urban renewal policies in the United States and international economic development policies. Economic sustainability, or the development of a self-sustaining local economy that does not require regular infusions of outside capital or credit, is an important application of the idea of sustainability. Development also must be environmentally, politically, and socially sustainable. Environmental sustainability has gained considerable international support and implies developing a means of production that does not contaminate the ecosystem or exhaust natural resources. Perkins et al. (in press) expanded the concept of sustainability to include the political and social domains of community development as well:

> Political sustainability can be thought of as the maintaining of momentum and active participation among members of a grassroots organization by avoiding leader burnout and developing new leaders. Social sustainability might be considered the degree to which communities can develop and maintain social capital and avoid delinquency, crime, drugs, racism, and other social problems. Sustainability is strengths-based in its emphasis on ecologically healthy development based on renewable community resources (Perkins et al., in press).

CONCLUSION

It is no longer a question of *whether we can* effectively intervene in community problems. The more salient question is *how do we do it* in a way that provides substantial and sustainable gains that restore the viability of targeted communities? As with psychological treatment of individual disorders, conceptualization of the problem is critical to directing the intervention. Simplistic conceptualizations may lead to short-term behavioral change, but rarely address the underlying problems. Community problems are complex and require a conceptualization that acknowledges their complexity. Our approach emphasizes the multiple systems that are involved in many community problems and suggests interventions for each dimension. We do not attempt to recommend specific, one-size-fits-all interventions because it is unlikely that any one type of intervention will easily or successfully be transferred to different neighborhoods with different conditions and characteristics. However, our conceptualization of the problem does raise the kinds of issues likely to be important in any neighborhood problem, and our recommendations provide a place to look for the solutions.

This multidimensional conceptualization may make the task seem overwhelming. Both professionals and community members may believe that it may not be worth becoming involved if they cannot bring about large-scale change. However, the recommendations described here apply not only to communitywide interventions but also may be useful in creating pockets of health within communities. Identifying and utilizing assets can apply as easily to a family or block as to a neighborhood or community. In a qualitative study of what keeps families and neighborhoods healthy, Hadden (2000) found that a family's ability to identify and utilize its strengths, and its connection with resources already available in the neighborhood, were the factors associated with healthy families. Both distressed people and distressed neighborhoods have strengths and assets to identify, develop, and bring to bear in solving community problems. Small problems may be amenable to direct action by a community group. Larger problems may require pressuring the public and/or private sectors for assistance. However, if the process is grassroots led, the outcome is more likely to be comprehensive (as residents raise related problems), empowering, asset-based, and sustainable.

REFERENCES

Aneshensel, C. S., & Sucoff, C. A. (1996). The neighborhood context of adolescent mental health. *Journal of Health and Social Behavior, 37*, 293–310.

Aspen Institute (1997). *Voices from the field: Learning from the early work of comprehensive community initiatives*. Washington, DC: Author.

Barton, E., & Tyska, C. (1999). Primary health care in an urban community teaching center. In B. J. McElmurry, C. Tyska, & R. S. Parker (Eds.), *Primary health care in urban communities* (pp. 165–174). Sudbury, MA: Jones and Bartlett.

Breci, M. G., & Erickson, T. E. (1998). Community policing: The process of transitional change. *FBI Law Enforcement Bulletin, 67*, 16–21.

Bronfrenbrenner, U. (1979). *The ecology of human development: Experiments by nature and design*. Cambridge, MA: Harvard University Press.

Bursik, R. J. Jr., & Grasmick, H. G. (1993). *Neighborhoods and crime: The dimensions of effective community control*. New York: Lexington.

Butterfoss, F. D., Goodman, R. M., & Wandersman, A. (1993). Community coalitions for prevention and health promotion. *Health Education Research, 8*, 315–330.

Butterfoss, F. D., Morrow, A., Rosenthal, J., Dini, E., Clinton, R., Webster, J., & Louis, P. (1998). CINCH: An urban coalition for empowerment and action. *Health Education and Behavior, 25*, 212–225.

Choi, K. H., & Coates, T. J. (1994). Prevention of HIV infection. *AIDS, 8*, 1371–1389.

COMMIT Research Group (1995). Community intervention trial for smoking cessation (COMMIT): I. Cohort results from a four-year community intervention. *American Journal of Public Health, 85*, 183–192.

Connell, J. P., & Halpern-Felsher, B. L. (1997). How neighborhoods affect educational outcomes in middle childhood and adolescence: Conceptual issues and an empirical example. In J. Brooks-Gunn, G. J. Duncan, & J. L. Aber (Eds.), *Neighborhood poverty: Context and consequences for children* (pp. 174–199). New York: Sage.

Coulton, C. J., Korbin, M., & Su, M. (1999). Neighborhoods and child maltreatment: A multi-level study. *Child Abuse and Neglect, 23,* 1019–1040.

Coulton, C. J., Korbin, M., Su, M., & Chow, J. (1995). Community level factors and child maltreatment rates. *Child Development, 66,* 1262–1276.

Covington, J., & Taylor, R. B. (1991). Fear of crime in urban residential neighborhoods: Implications of between and within-neighborhood sources for current models. *Sociological Quarterly, 32,* 231–249.

Davidson, L. L., Durkin, M. S., Kuhn, L., & O'Connor, P. (1994). The impact of the Safe Kids/Healthy Neighborhoods Injury Prevention Program in Harlem, 1988 through 1991. *American Journal of Public Health, 84,* 580–586.

Duncan, G. J., Brooks-Gunn, J., & Klebanov, P. K. (1994). Economic deprivation and early childhood development. *Child Development, 65,* 296–318.

Edelstein, M. R. (1988). *Contaminated communities: The social and psychological impacts of residential toxic exposure.* Boulder, CO: Westview Press.

El-Askari, G., Freestone, J., Irizarry, C., Kraut, K. L., Mashiyama, S. T., Morgan, M. A., & Walton, S. (1998). The healthy neighborhoods project: A local health department's role in catalyzing community development. *Health Education and Behavior, 25,* 146–159.

Faris, R. E. L., & Dunham, W. H. (1939). *Mental disorders in urban areas: An ecological study of schizophrenia and other psychoses.* New York: Hafner Publishing.

Farley, R., & Frey, W. H. (1994). Changes in the segregation of Whites from Blacks during the 1980s: Small steps toward a more integrated society. *American Sociological Review, 59,* 23–45.

Ferguson, R. F., & Dickens, W. T. (1999). Introduction. In R. F. Ferguson & W. T. Dickens (Eds.), *Urban problems and community development* (pp. 1–32). Washington, DC: Brookings Institution.

Figueira-McDonough, J. (1991). Community structure and delinquency: A typology. *Social Service Review, 65,* 68–91.

Freudenberg, N., & Manoncourt, E. (1998). Urban health promotion: Current practices and new directions. *Health Education and Behavior, 25,* 138–145.

Galster, G. C., & Keeney, W. (1988). Race, residence, discrimination, and economic opportunity: Modeling the nexus of urban racial phenomena. *Urban Affairs Quarterly, 24,* 87–117.

Garbarino, J., & Kostelny, K. (1992). Child maltreatment as a community problem. *Child Abuse and Neglect, 16,* 455–464.

Gephart, M. A. (1997). Neighborhoods and communities as context for development. In J. Brooks-Gunn, G. J. Duncan, & J. L. Aber (Eds.), *Neighborhood poverty: Context and consequences for children, Vol 1: Context and consequences for children* (pp. 1–43). New York: Sage.

Goodman, R. M., Speers, M. A., McLeroy, K., & Fawcett, S., Kegler, M., Parker, E., Smith, S. R., Sterling, T.D., & Wallerstein, N. (1998). Identifying and defining the dimensions of community capacity to provide a basis for measurement. *Health Education and Behavior, 25*, 258–278.

Goodman, R. M., & Wandersman, A. (1994). FORECAST: A formative approach to evaluating community coalitions and community-based initiatives. In S. Kaftarian & W. Hansen (Eds.), Improving methodologies for evaluating community-based partnerships for preventing alcohol, tobacco, and other drug use. *Journal of Community Psychology Monograph Series, (CSAP Special Issue)*, 6–25.

Hadden, L. (2000). The community as co-producer of health. *Health Forum Journal, 43*, 44–49.

Hawkins, J. D., & Catalano, R. (1992) *Communities that care: Action for drug abuse prevention*. San Francisco: Jossey-Bass.

Jones, J. E., Gutman, M. A., & Kaufman, J. (1999). Free to Grow: Translating substance abuse research and theory into preventive practice in a national Head Start initiative. *Journal of Primary Prevention, 19*, 279–296.

Kass, D., & Freudenberg, N. (1997). Coalition building to prevent childhood lead poisoning: A case study from New York City. In M. Minkler (Ed.), *Community organizing and community building for health* (pp. 278–290). New Brunswick, NJ: Rutgers University Press.

Kornhauser, R. (1978). *Social sources of delinquency*. Chicago: University of Chicago Press.

Kretzmann, J. P., & McKnight, J. L. (1993). *Building communities from the inside out: A path toward finding and mobilizing a community's assets*. Chicago: ACTA.

Ku, L., Sonenstein, F. L., & Pleck, J. H. (1993). Neighborhood, family, and work: Influences on the premarital behaviors of adolescent males. *Social Forces, 72*, 479–503.

Kumpfer, K. L., Molgaard, V., & Spoth, R. (1996) The Strengthening Families Program for the prevention of delinquency and drug use. In R. D. Peters & R. J. McMahon (Eds.), *Preventing childhood disorders, substance abuse and delinquency* (pp. 241–267). Thousand Oaks, CA: Sage.

Leviton, L., Snell, E., & McGinnis, M. (2000). Urban issues in health promotion strategies. *American Journal of Public Health, 90*, 863–866.

Marshall, E. G., Gensburg, L. J., Deres, D. A., Geary, N. S., & Cayo, M. R. (1997). Maternal residential exposure to hazardous wastes and risk of central nervous system and musculoskeletal birth defects. *Archives of Environmental Health, 52*, 416–425.

Massey, D. S., & Denton, N. (1993). *American apartheid: Segregation and the making of the underclass.* Cambridge, MA: Harvard University Press.

Maton, K. L., & Salem, D. A. (1995). Organization characteristic of empowering community settings: A multiple case study approach. *American Journal of Community Psychology, 23*, 631–656.

Mayer, S. E., & Jencks, C. (1989). Growing up in poor neighborhoods: How much does it matter? *Science, 243*, 1441–1445.

McLoyd, V. C. (1990). The impact of economic hardship on black families and development. *Child Development, 61*, 311–346.

McNeely, J. (1999). Community building. *Journal of Community Psychology, 27*, 741–750.

Miles-Doan, R. (1998). Violence between spouses and intimates: Does neighborhood context matter? *Social Forces, 77*, 623–645.

Morenoff, J. D., & Sampson, R. J. (1997). Violent crime and the spatial dynamics of neighborhood transition: Chicago, 1970–1990. *Social Forces, 76*, 31–64.

Oliver, M. L., & Shapiro, T. M. (1995). *Black wealth, White wealth.* New York: Routledge.

Palen, J. J. (1997). *The urban world* (5th ed.). New York: McGraw-Hill.

Perkins, D. D., & Brown, B. B. (1996, August). The psychology of urban community development. In A. Wandersman (Chair), *Tale of new cities—psychology's response to urban america: Our urban neighborhoods and our mental health.* Presidential mini-convention symposium conducted at the annual convention of the American Psychological Association, Toronto, Ontario, Canada.

Perkins, D. D., Grim, B., Silberman, P., & Brown, B. B. (in press). Community development as a response to community-level adversity: Ecological research and strengths-based policy. In K. Maton, C. Schellenbach, B. Leadbeather, & A. Solarz (Eds.), *Strengths-building research and policy: Investing in children, youth, families, and communities.* Washington, DC: American Psychological Association.

Perkins, D. D., & Taylor, R. B. (1996). Ecological assessments of community disorder: Their relationship to fear of crime and theoretical implications. *American Journal of Community Psychology, 24*, 63–108.

Perloff, J. D., & Jaffee, K. D. (1999). Late entry into prenatal care: The neighborhood context. *Social Work, 44*, 116–128.

Peterson, P. L., Hawkins, J. D., Abbott, R. D., & Catalano, R. F. (1995) Disentangling the effects of parental drinking, family management, and parental alcohol norms on current drinking by Black and White adolescents. In G. M. Boyd, J. Howard, & R. A. Zucker (Eds.), *Alcohol problems among adolescents: Current directions in prevention research* (pp. 33–57), Hillsdale, NJ: Erlbaum.

Robert Wood Johnson Foundation (2000). *Free to Grow grant application instructions.* Princeton, NJ: Author.

Roberts, E. M. (1997). Neighborhood social environments and the distribution of low birthweight in Chicago. *American Journal of Public Health, 87,* 597–603.

Sampson, R. J., & Groves, W. B. (1989). Community structure and crime: Testing social-disorganization theory. *American Journal of Sociology, 94,* 774–802.

Sampson, R. J., & Lauritson, J. L. (1994). Violent victimization and offending: individual-, situational-, and community-level risk factors. In A. J. Reiss Jr. & J. A. Roth (Eds.), *Understanding and preventing violence, Vol. 3: Social Influences* (pp. 1–114). Washington, DC: National Academy Press.

Sassen, S. (1990). Economic restructuring and the American city. *Annual Review of Sociology, 16,* 465–490.

Schneider, S. R. (1999). Overcoming barriers to communication between police and socially disadvantaged neighbourhoods: A critical theory of community policing. *Crime, Law and Social Change, 30,* 347–377.

Shaw, C. R., & McKay, H. D. (1969). *Juvenile delinquency in urban areas.* Chicago: University of Chicago Press.

Shea, S., Basch, C. E., Wechsler, H., & Lantigua, R. (1996). The Washington Heights-Inwood healthy heart program: A 6–year report from a disadvantaged urban setting. *American Journal of Public Health, 86,* 166–175.

Shedler, J., & Block, J. (1990). Adolescent drug use and psychological health: A longitudinal inquiry. *American Psychologist, 45,* 612–630.

Skogan, W. G. (1990). *Disorder and Decline.* New York: Free Press.

Speer, P. W., & Hughey, J. (1995). Community organizing: An ecological route to empowerment and power. *American Journal of Community Psychology, 23,* 729–748.

Speers, M. A., & Lancaster, B. (1998). Disease prevention and health promotion in urban areas: CDC's perspective. *Health Education and Behavior, 25,* 226–233.

Stoutland, S. E. (1999). Community development corporations: Mission, strategy, and accomplishments. In R. F. Ferguson, & W. T. Dickens (Eds.) *Urban problems and community development* (pp. 193–240). Washington, DC: Brookings Institute.

Taylor, R. B., & Covington, J. (1988). Neighborhood changes in ecology and violence. *Criminology, 26,* 553–590.

Taylor, R. B., & Covington, J. (1993). Community structural change and fear of crime. *Social Problems, 40,* 374–397.

Taylor, R. B., Shumaker, S. A., & Gottfredson, S. D. (1985). Neighborhood-level links between physical features and local sentiments: Deterioration, fear of crime, and confidence. *Journal of Architectural and Planning Research, 2,* 261–275.

Tulchinsky, T. H., & Varavikova, E. A. (2000). *The new public health: An introduction for the 21st century.* New York: Academic Press.

United Church of Christ Commission for Racial Justice (1987). *Toxic wastes and race in the United States: A national report on the racial and socioeconomic characteristics of communities surrounding hazardous waste sites.* New York: United Church of Christ.

Wandersman, A., & Nation, M. (1998). Urban neighborhoods and mental health: Psychological contribution to understanding toxicity, resilience, and interventions. *American Psychologist, 53*, 647–656.

Webster-Stratton, C., & Hammond, M. (1997). Treating children with early-onset conduct problems: A comparison of child and parent training interventions. *Journal of Consulting and Clinical Psychology, 65*, 92–109.

Wilson, J. Q., & Kelling, G. L. (1982). Broken windows. *Atlantic Monthly, 249*, 29–38.

Wilson, W. J. (1987). *The truly disadvantaged.* Chicago: University of Chicago Press.

Zimmerman, M. A., & Perkins, D. D. (Eds.) (1995). Empowerment theory, research, and application [Special issue]. *American Journal of Community Psychology, 23*(5).

Zuravin, S. J. (1989). The ecology of child abuse and neglect: Review of the literature and presentation of data. *Violence and Victims, 4*, 101–121.

Afterword

Michael C. Roberts

The premises of prevention and promotion for optimal psychological and physical health have been well conceptualized and articulated, the actuality of implementation by community activities and professionals has increased dramatically, and the empirical bases for demonstrating the worth of prevention and promotion are becoming well established. The contributions of psychology and behavioral science to the prevention of various problems of children, adolescents, and adults are richly illustrated in the preceding chapters of this volume.

Where theory, practice, and research succeeded, the field has advanced and human lives have been improved. The value of conceptualizations in guiding research and action has been demonstrated in numerous venues of the community, school, family, churches, and other organizations. These serve as exemplars for future refinement and enactment. Where evaluative research has not proven the effectiveness of preventive interventions, the field also advances its understanding and seeks other routes to make prevention/promotion gains. Programming that started as good intentions and ideas, often poorly conceived or implemented under difficult circumstances, provides worthwhile case examples to instruct community action and research. With both success and limitation, the field has progressed immensely in the last several years; this book documents that progress and articulates research and implementation plans for the future.

When Lizette Peterson and I coedited *Prevention of Problems in Childhood*, published in 1984, we presented the position that "research and applications are intertwined since the prevention areas have typically employed an innovative and evaluative orientation when applying psychology-based programs to real-world problems" (p. 2). Our book documented the then current state of the field, noting "alternating states of frustration and optimism" while concluding that

345

the progress was encouraging and the prospects for future development in prevention were exciting for psychological research applications. The chapters in the present book by Drs. Jason and Glenwick, now close to 20 years later, demonstrate that many efforts have come to fruition and our earlier optimism and excitement were justified (notwithstanding the ongoing frustrations).

Drs. Jason and Glenwick note that the topic coverage in the book is illustrative rather than exhaustive. Nonetheless, as representative illustrations of this vibrant field, the conceptual richness, innovation, and emerging scientific base provide a context for action and growth, not just reflection on jobs done well. The range of prevention/promotion topics and problems, as well as the successes and limitations across the lifespan, are compelling.

Despite the seeming wealth of exemplars and research cited through the preceding pages, the question arises, "If prevention and promotion make so much sense, why is there not even more research and more action programming?" Americans seem to pay lip service to prevention/promotion concepts but all too often fail to embrace them (Roberts, 1994). As outlined by Roberts and Brown (2000), there might be noted several complex and interacting reasons for obstacles to prevention and promotion. Indeed, the successful programming documented in the previous chapters had to overcome many of these obstacles.

First, political and personal philosophies often defy intrusion by others, in that Americans hold the concept that they have a right not to do what others think they should do. Although this attitude hinders intervention and political support, it is not without its merits in some instances (usually defined as having others stay away from one's own vices and proclivities). Well-reasoned and better-justified "intrusions" must be articulated and marketed.

Second, Americans frequently engage in blaming the victims for whatever problems befall them and resent having to pay for programs to serve them. Often this involves a moralistic stance about the behavior of others and tends to muddle intervention efforts to improve the lots of those affected.

Third, Americans have acquired an orientation to short-term thinking. More often than not, prevention requires a longitudinal approach with consistent efforts exerted to achieve successful outcomes. American politicians look for short-term solutions, or patches, to problems that will get them through the next election based on appearance, not on actual solutions. Similarly, HMOs, which used to be "health maintenance organizations" with an orientation to health promotion because profits were accrued over the long term, are now an acronym almost without relation to health or maintenance. Short-term profits are typically taken in a managed care environment, and long-term prevention/promotion does not receive much interest or investment.

Fourth, as mentioned by numerous commentators in the prevention field, what is called prevention is often not preventive. Consequently, actions and expenditures may make it look as though the United States is engaging in preventive work, and the citizenry can feel good about that. (DARE and some restricted sex education programs are just a couple of examples, but a monograph could be written on such false prevention.)

Fifth, there seems to be an expectation that prevention of problems must meet a higher standard of proof and worth than does remediation of problems. American society and often our skeptical fellow professionals appear to expect perfection from prevention/promotion, making it more difficult to implement successful programming. This expectation of perfection from prevention also hinders the establishment of an empirical base of its merits.

Sixth, in the mental health professions, there remains a reliance on one-on-one therapy as the prized standard of worth. Changing a system, or a subunit of a larger system, therefore, is often not a valued goal; changing individuals one at a time is ingrained in the belief system (as well as the reward system). Correspondingly, mental health professionals have accepted the notion that, if particular activities are not reimbursed by an insurance policy, then those interventions must not be worthwhile to do. This is an insidious belief because it influences career choices, funding advocacy, clinical decision-making, and prevention activities.

Finally, unexamined "prevention" activities undermine the credibility of the prevention concept. Although it is sometimes necessary to conduct prevention interventions without an evidence base in the short run, for its future, American society needs to evaluate what is called prevention more assiduously and support those efforts that fulfill the mandate.

There are cultural, philosophical, financial, and professional obstacles to investigating and implementing prevention. To overcome these obstacles (and others), Roberts and Brown (2000) touched on five actions: (a) conceptualize prevention, (b) advocate prevention, (c) research prevention, (d) partner for prevention, and (e) practice prevention. The present set of chapters identifies and exemplifies these actions in a diverse set of problems and issues to help meet the needs of children, adolescents, adults, and their families through prevention and promotion activities.

REFERENCES

Roberts, M. C. (1994). Promotion and prevention in America: Still spitting on the sidewalk. *Journal of Pediatric Psychology, 19*, 267–281.

Roberts, M. C., & Brown, K. J. (2000). Overcoming obstacles to prevention in pediatric psychology. *Society of Pediatric Psychology Progress Notes, 24*, 11–14.

Roberts, M. C., & Peterson, L. (Eds.) (1984). *Prevention of problems in childhood: Psychological research and applications*. New York: Wiley.

Index

bnAchievement for Latinos through
Academic Success, 113
Acquired immunodeficiency syndrome.
See AIDS
Action-oriented prevention, perspective,
4–8
Adolescent Coping with Stress Course,
163
Adulthood, problems in
aging, 272–288
AIDS, 205–226
chronic health problems, 227–243
divorce, 245–271
HIV, 205–226
separation, 245–271
Advising programs, in high-school,
116–119
implementation issues, 117–119
Advocacy
by American Psychological
Association, 20
by Society for Community Research
and Action, 20
by Society for Prevention Research, 20
Aerobic exercise, effect of, 228
African Americans
depression, in youth, 157, 162–165
development of critical consciousness,
309
HIV/AIDS prevention, 217–220
Aging, mental health and, 272–289

AARP Widowed Persons Service, 282
Alzheimer's disease, 279–281
bereavement support groups, 281–282
description, 281–282
outcome studies, 282
rationale, 281–282
caregiver support groups, 282–283
description, 282–283, 284
outcome studies, 283, 284–285
rationale, 282–283, 284
case example, 286–287
dementia, 279–281
caring for elderly person with,
282–283
Friendly Visitors, 284–285
future trends, 287–289
grief, bereavement, 281–282
life review, reminiscence groups, 278
description, 278–279
outcome studies, 279
rationale, 278–279
literature review, 273–286
memory training, 279–281
description, 280
outcome studies, 280–281
rationale, 279
older medical patients, 285–286
description, 285
outcome studies, 285–286
rationale, 285
past experiences, evaluation of, 278

Aging, mental health and *(continued)*
  physical exercise, 276–277
    description, 276
    outcome studies, 276–277
    rationale, 276
  relaxation training, 274–275
    description, 274
    outcome studies, 274–275
    rationale, 274
  stress management, 275–276
    description, 275
    outcome studies, 275
    rationale, 275
  volunteering, 277–278
    description, 277–278
    outcome studies, 278
    rationale, 277–278
  volunteers at helpline, 286–287
  Widow-to-Widow Program, 282
AIDS prevention, 205–226
  case example, 217–220
  Community Demonstration Projects
    Research Group, 214
  database, Centers for Disease Control
    and Prevention, 19
  delivered to communities, 214–217
  delivered to individuals, 209–211
  delivered to small groups, 211–213
  effectiveness of, 209–211
  epidemiological history of, 206
  future trends, 220–222
  Information Motivation Behavioral
    Skills model, 206–209
  literature review, 206–217
  Multisite Prevention Trial, 212
  number of persons with, 206
  persons affected by, 206
  persons knowing they are infective,
    221–222
  small-group intervention
    African American men, 217–220
    information, 218–219
    risk reduction, 219–220
  social influence intervention, 215–217
  technology transfer, barriers to,
    220–223

  testing, effectiveness of, 209–211
  theory-based behavioral interventions,
    221
Alcohol abuse, 176–201
  academic failure, 189
  combination programs, efficacy of,
    186–187
  Communities that Care, prevention
    operating system, 187–192
  community protection profile, 190
  community risk profile, 189
  comprehensive interventions, 183–186
  environmental interventions, 182
  family attachment, 190
  family interventions, 181–182
  future trends, 192–193
  impulsiveness, 189
  literature review, 179–187
  media approach to curbing, 68
  Midwestern Prevention Project, 183
  mobility, 189
  moral order, belief in, 190
  neighborhood, 189
  phases of, 187
  prevention science, 178–179
  Project Northland, 185–186
  Project SixTeen, 1874–185
  prosocial involvement, 190
  prostitution, 177
  rebelliousness, 189
  religiosity, 190
  school-based programs, 179–180
  Seattle Social Development Project,
    183
  social skills, 190
  stages of drug use, 178
  transition, 189
Alternative messages, preventive
    intervention, competition
    between, 9
Alternative school settings, 111–112
  charter schools, 111
  Edison Project schools, 111
American Psychological Association
  advocacy by, 20
  criteria for interventions, 18

Anabolic-androgenic steroids, abuse of, 176–201
Antecedent behavioral change procedures, 9
Antisocial behavior, 126–152
    adolescent age, 128
    age of onset, 134
    antisocial youth, defined, 133
    case example, 139–141
    challenges, 133–139
    community-level factors, 129
    consequences, inconsistent use of, 128
    defined, 133–134
    developmental-ecological framework, 135
    ecological theory, 137
    family factors, 128
    family-focused approaches, 131
    future trends, 141–143
    gender and, 128, 136
    handguns, availability of, 129
    impoverished neighborhoods, 129
    indicated programs, 131
    interventions, 130–133, 138–139
    literature review, 130–139
    Metropolitan Area Child Study Research Group, 139–141
    models of, 135
    overly harsh discipline practices, 128
    peer factors, 128–129
    peer-group approaches, 131
    peer relations, 128
    population characteristics, 138–139
    prevention research, theoretical framework, 134–138
    problem-solving skills, 128
    protective factors, 130
    risk factors, 127–128
    SAFEChildren Program, 139–141
    selected programs, 131
    social class, impact of, 136
    societal factors, 129
    supervision, lack of, 128
    universal programs, 131
Anxiety, depression, in youth, 159
Assets, identification of, 337

Attrition, reducing, dropout prevention, 112

Battered Child Syndrome, publication of, 86
Behavioral control, risk of, 27
Behavioral parent training, 73–74
Bereaved older adults, support groups for, 281–282
Biological theories of depression, in youth, 158
Blueprints Project, Center for Study and Prevention of Violence, 18
Body image, negative, depression, in youth, 159
Building design, impact of, 327

Campbell Collaboration, 19
Cancer, prevention of, 227–243
Caregiver of elderly with dementia, support groups, 282–283
Center for Study and Prevention of Violence, Blueprints Project, 18
Center for Substance Abuse Prevention, 20
    Program Enhancement Protocols, 18
Certification, as prevention professional, 50–51
Change, coercion to bring about, avoidance of, 27
Charter schools, 111
Child abuse, 85–105
    Battered Child Syndrome, publication of, 86
    case example, 94–96, 94–98, 96–98
    defined, 85
    ecobehavioral model, 87
    future trends, 98–100
    literature review, 86–93
    older children, vs. younger children, learning from prevention programs, 92
    role-playing, 91
    self-report measures, 92
    social/ecological perspective, 86
    theories, 86–93
    young parents, 88

Child guidance movement, 40
Chronic health problems, 227–243
  aerobic exercise, effect of, 228
  case example, 236–268
  diet, cancer prevention, 228
  5–a-Day Power Plus Program, 232
  fruits in diet, cancer prevention, 228
  future trends, 238–240
  GIMME 5 program, 231
  Heart Healthy Cook-Off, 229
  literature review, 229–236
  lung disease, 227–243
  media-based programming, 232–236
  Pawtucket Heart Health Program, 229
  prevention of, 227–243
  San Diego Family Health Project, 230
  saturated fats, cancer and, 228
  Sports, Play and Active Recreation for
    Kids Program, 230
  vegetables in diet, cancer prevention,
    228
  Washington Heights-Inwood Healthy
    Heart Program, 230
  weight control program, 236
  youth-directed interventions, 229–232
Cigarette smoking. See Tobacco abuse
Class, impact of, antisocial behavior, 136
Class size, decrease in, 110
Coca-Cola Valued Youth Program, 113
Cochrane Collaboration, 18, 19
Coercion, to bring about change,
  avoidance of, 27
Collaboration
  in ecological model of prevention, 7
  between psychologist, other
    disciplines, 8
Collaborative to Advance Social and
  Emotional Learning, 20
Comer School Development Project, 115
Communication, divorce and, 251
Communications experts, collaboration
  with psychologist, 8
Communities that Care, prevention pro-
  gram, 187–192
Community, defined, 325

Community Action for Successful Youth
  Project, 71–74
  clinical intervention, 73–74
  direct mail, 71–73
  parent-child homework activities,
    71–73
  public health approach, 71–73
Community Demonstration Projects
  Research Group, AIDS/HIV, 214
Community development, 324–339
  assets, identification, utilization of, 337
  building design, 327
  case example, 332–335
  community, defined, 325
  community development corporations,
    330
  community problems, defined, 235
  comprehensiveness of intervention,
    336
  discriminatory housing practices, 328
  disempowering of community, 328
  Doris Duke Charitable Foundation, 332
  ecological framework, 333
  economic development, sustainable,
    337–338
  economic problems, 326
  empowerment, 336–337
  Family Partnership Plan, 335
  Free to Grow, 334–335
  future trends, 335–338
  incivilities, in distressed neighborhods,
    326–327
  literature review, 329–332
  political problems, 328–329
  population shifts, impact of, 329
  poverty, 326
  public health, 330–332
  Robert Wood Johnson Foundation, 332
  social incivilities, 327–328
  social problems, 327–328
Community development corporations,
  330
Community organizations
  parenting skills training, 70
  research on, 78

Community problems, defined, 235
Community psychology
  birth of, 5
  field of, development of, 4–5
Community Tool Box, University of
  Kansas, 20
Community-wide problems facing
  society, 3
Conceptual continuum, in prevention, 44
Consequences, inconsistent use of, anti-
  social behavior and, 128
Consultation Center, Yale University,
  54–56
Contextualism, 11
Controlled trials, randomized, use of, 23
Coping with Depression course, 160
Crime prevention, media approach, 68
Critical consciousness, in African
  American males, 309
Crowding, noise, impact of, 327
Curricula, return to basics in, 108
Customized educational plan, 108
Delinquency, 126–152
  adolescent age, 128
  age of onset, 134
  antisocial youth, defined, 133
  case example, 139–141
  challenges, 133–139
  community-level factors, 129
  consequences, inconsistent use of, 128
  defined, 133–134
  developmental-ecological framework,
    135
  ecological theory, 137
  family factors, 128
  family-focused approaches, 131
  future trends, 141–143
  gender and, 128, 136
  handguns, availability of, 129
  impoverished neighborhoods, 129
  indicated programs, 131
  interventions, 130–133, 138–139
  literature review, 130–139
  Metropolitan Area Child Study
    Research Group, 139–141

models of, 135
overly harsh discipline practices, 128
peer factors, 128–129
peer-group approaches, 131
peer relations, 128
population characteristics, 138–139
prevention research, theoretical framework, 134–138
problem-solving skills, 128
protective factors, 130
risk factors, 127–128
SAFEChildren Program, 139–141
selected programs, 131
social class, impact of, 136
societal factors, 129
supervision, lack of, 128
universal programs, 131

Dementia
  caregiver of elderly with, support
    groups, 282–283
  caring for elderly person with,
    282–283
Depression, in youth, 153–175
  academic grades, decline in, 159
  Adolescent Coping with Stress
    Course, 163
  African Americans, 157, 162–165
  anxiety and, 159
  biological theories of, 158
  body image, negative, 159
  case example, 162–165
  cognitive aspects of development,
    158
  cognitive-behavioral model, 160
  community entry, 163
  comorbid disorders, 153
  concomitant factors, 153
  Coping with Depression course, 160
  eating disorders, 159
  ethnic differences, 156–157
  etiology of, 157–159
  future trends, 165–166
  gender differences, 155–156
  goal identification, 163–164

Depression, in youth *(continued)*
  implementation of prevention
      program, 164–165
  literature review, 159–162
  major, risk of suicide with, 157
  media-based intervention, 161
  mental health resources, inadequacy
      of, 153
  prevalence, 154–155
  program design, 163–164
  psychological theories of, 158
  school-based intervention, 161
  self-esteem, 159
  suicide, 157
Design of buildings, impact of, 327
Developmentl model of prevention, 5–6
Diet, cancer prevention, 228
Discrimination, 303–304
Discriminatory housing practices, 328
Dissemination, empirically supported
      prevention practices, 20–24
Dissemination of program, challenge
      of, 11
Dissemination strategies, experimental
      research on, need for, 22–24
Diversity, respect for, 9
Divorce, 245–271
  communication, importance of, 251
  effectiveness of preventive interven-
      tions, 254–256
  first marriage, divorce rate, 247
  future trends, 261–264
  increase in rate of, 247
  literature review, 252–256
  prediction of, 250
  prevalence of, 3
  Prevention and Relationship
      Enhancement Program, 256–261
    components of, 258
    dissemination, 260–261
    materials, 259–260
    professional training, 259
    program content, 256–257
    program format, 257
  relapse rate, 250
  second marriage, divorce rate, 247

  sequelae, 248–250
  theoretical premises, 253–254
  therapy, marital, limitations of, 250
  United States, other countries, divorce
      rates compared, 248
Doris Duke Charitable Foundation, 332
Dropout prevention, high-school, 3,
      106–125
  Achievement for Latinos through
      Academic Success, 113
  advising programs, 116–119
    implementation issues, 117–119
  alternative settings, 111–112
    charter schools, 111
    Edison Project schools, 111
  attendance, improving, 112
  case example, 116–119
  Coca-Cola Valued Youth Program, 113
  Comer School Development Project,
      115
  future trends, 119–120
  grouping strategies, 108–109
    customized educational plan, 108
    heterogeneous ability tracking, 108
    interdisciplinary teaming, 108–109
  home-school partnerships, 114–116
  increase in dropout rate, 3
  instructional changes, 107–108
    curricula, return to basics in, 108
    school-to-work programs, 107
  literature review, 107–116
  structural reforms, 110–111
    class size, decrease in, 110
    smaller schools, 110
  teacher/student ratio, 112
  teaching, improvements in, 109–110
Drugs, illicit
  dealing, 177
  use of, 176–201

Eating disorders, depression and, 159
Ecological model of prevention, 5, 7
  collaborative relationship, 7
Economic development, sustainable,
      337–338
Ecstasy, use of drug, 176–201

Edison Project schools, 111
Education in prevention, 39–62
    certification, as prevention profes-
        sional, 50–51
    child guidance movement, 40
    conceptual continuum, in prevention, 44
    Consultation Center, Yale University,
        54–56
    educational settings, 49–50
    full-service schools, 49
    graduate training within universities,
        45–50
        community psychology, 45–46
        nursing, 48–49
        preventive medicine specialty, 47–48
        public health, 47
        social work, 49
        undergraduate medicine, 47–48
    history of, 40–42
    indicated preventive intervention, 42
    International Certification and
        Reciprocity Consortium for
        Alcohol and Other Drug Abuse, 50
    literature review, 45
    mental hygiene movement, 40
    post-degree professional training, 50
        addiction counselor training, 50
        dzergy, training in prevention
            skills, 50
        parent educators, training in
            prevention skills, 50
        teachers, training in prevention
            skills, 50
    President's Joint Commission on
        Mental Illness and Health, 40
    prevention professional, certification
        as, in mental health, 50
    prevention research, expanded defini-
        tion of, 44
    prevention science, emergence of,
        42–45
    preventive intervention research
        cycle, 43
    Project Head Start, 49
    risk, defined, 43
    science-based prevention, 51–54
    selective preventive intervention, 42
    settlement house movement, 40, 49
    teaching about prevention, usage of
        term, 39
    universal preventive intervention, 42
    Vermont Conference on Primary
        Prevention of Psychopathology, 41
Educational plan, customized, 108
Educators, collaboration with
    psychologist, 8
Effectiveness of interventions, research
    needed, 21
Elderly, mental health of
    Alzheimer's disease, 279–281
    bereaved older adults, support groups
        for, 281–282
    caregiver support groups, 282–283, 284
    dementia, 279–281, 281
    helpline, volunteers at, 286–287
    life review, reminiscence groups,
        278–279
    pharmacotherapy, Alzheimer's disease,
        281
    stress management, 275
    volunteering, 277–278
Empirically supported prevention
    practices, dissemination of, 20–24
Empowerment model of prevention, 5–6
Epidemiological Catchment Area
    Study, 24
Epidemiologists, collaboration with psy-
    chologist, 8
Ethnic differences, depression, in youth,
    156–157
Evaluation of programs, 25–27
Evidence-based prevention, 51–54
Exercise
    effect of, 228
    elderly, 276–277
        description, 276
        outcome studies, 276–277
        rationale, 276
Experimental evaluations, lack of, rea-
    son for, 23
Exploitation of population, avoidance of,
    27

Family Partnership Plan, 335
Family practice professionals, 71
Family well-being, ongoing monitoring, 78
Fats, cancer and, 228
Field of community psychology, development of, 4–5
First marriage, divorce rate, 247
5-a-Day Power Plus Program, 232
Free to Grow, 334–335
Friendly Visitors, 284–285
Fruits in diet, cancer prevention, 228
Full-service schools, 49

Gay community
    heterosexism, 305–306
    National Gay and Lesbian Task Force, 311
Gender
    antisocial behavior and, 128, 136
    depression, in youth, 155–156
GIMME 5 program, 231
Goals, organizing communities around, 74–75
Grades, decline in. *See also* Dropout prevention
    depression, in youth, 159
Graduate training within universities, 45–50
    community nurse, 48–49
    community psychology, 45–46
    preventive medicine specialty, 47–48
    public health, 47
    public health nursing, 48–49
    social work, 49
    undergraduate medicine, 47–48
Grief, 281–282
Grouping strategies, high-school, 108–109
    customized educational plan, 108
    heterogeneous ability tracking, 108
    interdisciplinary teaming, 108–109

Handguns, availability of, 129
Hate crimes, 307
Hate Crimes Statistics Act, 307
Health problems, 227–243

aerobic exercise, effect of, 228
case example, 236–268
diet, cancer and, 228
5-a-Day Power Plus Program, 232
fruits in diet, cancer prevention, 228
future trends, 238–240
GIMME 5 program, 231
heart disease, prevention of, 227–243
Heart Healthy Cook-Off, 229
literature review, 229–236
media-based programming, 232–236
media-based weight control program, targeting obesity, 236
Pawtucket Heart Health Program, 229
prevention of, 227–243
San Diego Family Health Project, 230
saturated fats, cancer and, 228
Sports, Play and Active Recreation for Kids Program, 230
vegetables in diet, cancer prevention, 228
Washington Heights-Inwood Healthy Heart Program, 230
youth-directed interventions, 229–232
Heart disease, prevention of, 227–243
Heart Healthy Cook-Off, 229
Helpline, volunteers at, elderly as, 286–287
Heroin, abuse of, 176–201
Heterogeneous ability tracking, 108
Heterosexism, 305–306
High-school dropout prevention, 106–125
    Achievement for Latinos through Academic Success, 113
    advising programs, 116–119
        implementation issues, 117–119
    alternative settings, 111–112
        charter schools, 111
        Edison Project schools, 111
    attrition, reducing, 112
    case example, 116–119
    Coca-Cola Valued Youth Program, 113
    Comer School Development Project, 115
    future trends, 119–120

grouping strategies, 108–109
customized educational plan, 108
heterogeneous ability tracking, 108
interdisciplinary teaming, 108–109
home-school partnerships, 114–116
instructional changes, 107–108
curricula, return to basics in, 108
school-to-work programs, 107
literature review, 107–116
structural reforms, 110–111
class size, decrease in, 110
smaller schools, 110
teacher/student ratio, 112
teaching, improvements in, 109–110
HIV prevention, 205–226
case example, 217–220
Community Demonstration Projects
Research Group, 214
delivered to communities, 214–217
delivered to individuals, 209–211
delivered to small groups, 211–213
effectiveness of, 209–211
epidemiological history of, 206
future trends, 220–222
Information Motivation Behavioral
Skills model, 206–209
literature review, 206–217
Multisite Prevention Trial, 212
number of persons with, 206
persons affected by, 206
persons knowing they are infective,
221–222
small-group intervention
African American men, 217–220
information, 218–219
risk reduction, 219–220
social influence intervention,
215–217
technology transfer, barriers to,
220–223
theory-based behavioral interventions,
221
Home-school partnerships, 114–116
Homework activities, parent-child,
71–73
Housing practices, discriminatory, 328

Howard Brown Health Center, Chicago,
sexually transmitted disease
testing, 313–316
Human immunodeficiency virus. See
HIV

Illicit drugs, use of, 176–201
Implementation specialists, need for,
21–22
Impoverished neighborhoods, antisocial
behavior, 129
Impulsiveness, substance abuse and, 189
Incivilities, in distressed neighborhods,
326–327
Indicated intervention, defined, 4
Information Motivation Behavioral
Skills model, AIDS/HIV prevention, 206–209
Instructional changes, high-school,
107–108
curricula, return to basics in, 108
school-to-work programs, 107
Interdisciplinary teaming
in high-school, 108–109
International Certification and Reciprocity Consortium for Alcohol
and Other Drug Abuse, 50
Internet
time spent surfing, 2–3
violence, sexuality on, 3
Intervention
indicated, defined, 4
selective, defined, 4
strategies, integration of, 10
types of, 4
universal, defined, 4
Involvement, of target population,
importance of, 8

Lesbian community
heterosexism, 305–306
National Gay and Lesbian Task
Force, 311
Life review, 278
outcome studies, 279
rationale, 278–279

Loneliness in older adults, support
    groups, 281–282
  outcome studies, 282
  rationale, 281–282
Lung disease, prevention of, 227–243

Major depression, risk of suicide with,
    157
Maltreatment, of children, 85–105
  Battered Child Syndrome, publication
    of, 86
  case example, 94–96, 94–98, 96–98
  ecobehavioral model, 87
  future trends, 98–100
  literature review, 86–93
  older children, *vs.* younger children,
    learning from prevention
    programs, 92
  physical abuse, 85
  role-playing, 91
  self-report measures, 92
  sexual abuse, 85
  social/ecological perspective, 86
  theories, 86–93
  young parents, 88
Marijuana, use of, 176–201
Marital distress, 245–271
  communication, importance of, 251
  effectiveness of preventive interven-
    tions, 254–256
  first marriage, divorce rate, 247
  future trends, 261–264
  increase in rate of, 247
  literature review, 252–256
  prediction of, 250
  Prevention and Relationship
    Enhancement Program, 256–261
    components of, 258
    dissemination, 260–261
    materials, 259–260
    professional training, 259
    program content, 256–257
    program format, 257
  relapse rate, 250
  second marriage, divorce rate, 247
  sequelae, 248–250

theoretical premises, 253–254
  therapy, marital, limitations of, 250
  United States, other countries, divorce
    rates compared, 248
Mass media, research on, 77
Medical patients, older, 285–286
Medical personnel, collaboration with
    psychologist, 8
Medical practitioners, educating in
    parenting skills, 71
Memory training, 279–281
  description, 280
  neurotransmitter acetylcholine, 281
  outcome studies, 280–281
  with pharmacotherapy, 281
  pramiracetam, 281
  rationale, 279
Mental disorders affecting population, 3
Mental health, in later life, 272–289
  AARP Widowed Persons Service, 282
  Alzheimer's disease, 279–281
  bereavement, 281–282
  caregiver support groups, 282–283
    description, 282–283, 284
    outcome studies, 283, 284–285
    rationale, 284
  dementia, 281
    Alzheimer's disease, 279–281
    caring for elderly person with,
      282–283
  Friendly Visitors, 284–285
  future trends, 287–289
  grief, 281–282
  helpline
    volunteering at, 286–287
    volunteers, 286–287
  life review, reminiscence groups, 278
    description, 278–279
    outcome studies, 279
  literature review, 273–286
  lonely older adults, support groups
    for, 281–282
    description, 281–282
    outcome studies, 282
  medical patients, older, 285–286
    description, 285

outcome studies, 285–286
   rationale, 285
memory training, 279–281
   description, 280
   outcome studies, 280–281
   with pharmacotherapy, 281
   rationale, 279
past experiences, evaluation of, 278
pharmacotherapy, Alzheimer's disease,
   281
physical exercise, 276–277
   description, 276
   outcome studies, 276–277
   rationale, 276
relaxation training, 274–275
   description, 274
   outcome studies, 274–275
   rationale, 274
stress management, 275–276
   description, 275
   outcome studies, 275
volunteering, 277–278
   description, 277–278
   outcome studies, 278
Widow-to-Widow Program, 282
Mental health professionals, teaching
   about prevention, 39–62
certification, as prevention professional,
   50–51
child guidance movement, 40
conceptual continuum, in prevention, 44
Consultation Center, Yale University,
   54–56
educational settings, 49–50
full-service schools, 49
graduate training within universities,
   45–50
   community psychology, 45–46
   public health, 47
   public health nursing, 48–49
   social work, 49
   undergraduate medicine, 47–48
history of, 40–42
indicated preventive intervention, 42
literature review, 45
mental hygiene movement, 40

post-degree professional training, 50
   addiction counselor training, 50
   clergy, training in prevention skills,
      50
President's Joint Commission on
   Mental Illness and Health, 40
prevention professional, certification
   as, in mental health, 50
prevention research, expanded definition of, 44
prevention science, emergence of,
   42–45
preventive intervention research
   cycle, 43
Project Head Start, 49
risk, defined, 43
science-based prevention, 51–54
selective preventive intervention, 42
settlement house movement, 40, 49
universal preventive intervention, 42
usage of term, 39
Vermont Conference on Primary
   Prevention of Psychopathology, 41
Mental health resources, inadequacy of,
   153
Mental hygiene movement, 40
Metropolitan Area Child Study Research
   Group, 139–141
Midwestern Prevention Project, 183
Models of prevention, 5
Moral order, belief in, substance abuse
   and, 190
Multilevel interventions, virtues of, 10
Multisite Prevention Trial, AIDS/HIV
   prevention, 212

National Advisory Mental Health
   Council, 3
National Center for Improving Tools of
   Educators, Univeristy of
   Oregon, 20
National Comorbidity Survey, 24
National Gay and Lesbian Task Force, 311
National Institute on Alcohol Abuse and
   Alcoholism, 19
National Institute on Drug Abuse, 18

Negative body image, depression, in youth, 159
Neighborhood disorder, defined, 326–327
Noise, impact of, 327
Nurse visitation programs, parenting, 71
Nurturing of children, as parenting skill, 63

Obesity
    prevention of, 227–243
    weight control program targeting, 236
Obstetric clinicians, training in parenting skills, 71
Older children, younger children, compared, learning from prevention programs, 92

Parental attitudes favorable to ASB, 189
Parental attitudes favorable to drugs, 189
Parenting
    alcohol abuse, 176–201
    antisocial behavior, 126–150
    child abuse, 85–105
    depression, 153–175
    education in, 39–62
    mental health professionals, 39–62
    parenting skills, 63–82
    school failure, 106–125
    sexual abuse, 85–105
    substance abuse, 176–201
    tobacco use, 176–201
    violence, 126–150
Parenting skills, 63
    access to intervention, lack of, 67
    alcohol consumption, media approach, 68
    behavioral parent training, 73–74
    case example, 71–74
    clinical approaches, 65–67
    Community Action for Successful Youth Project, 71–74
    clinical intervention, 73–74
    direct mail, 71–73
    parent-child homework activities, 71–73

public health approach, 71–73
community organizations, research on, 78
crime prevention, media approach, 68
dissemination, research, 75–77
family practice professionals, 71
family well-being, ongoing monitoring, 78
future trends, 74
goals, organizing communities around, 74–75
literature review, 65–71
mass media, research on, 77
monitoring, inadequate, 64
nurse visitation programs, 71
nurturing children, 63
obstetric clinicians, 71
pediatric clinicians, 71
physicians, 71
public health approaches, 67–69
    media, 68–69
    medical practitioners, 71
    schools, community organizations, 70
smoking cessation, media approach, 68
socializing children, 63
troubled families, participation of, 65
Past experiences, evaluation of, 278
Pawtucket Heart Health Program, 229
Pediatric clinicians, training in parenting skills, 71
Peer factors, antisocial behavior, 128–129
Peer-group approach, antisocial behavior, 131
Peer relations, antisocial behavior, 128
Personal control, of target group, fostering of, 8
Pharmacotherapy, memory training with, 281
Physical abuse
    of child, 85–105
    Battered Child Syndrome, publication of, 86
    case example, 94–98
    ecobehavioral model, 87
    future trends, 98–100

literature review, 86–93
older children, *vs.* younger children, learning from prevention programs, 92
physical abuse, defined, 85
physical abuse case example, 94–96
role-playing, 91
self-report measures, 92
sexual abuse, defined, 85
sexual abuse case example, 96–98
social/ecological perspective, 86
theories, 86–93
young parents, 88
defined, 85
Physicians, training in parenting skills, 71
Political problems, distressed neighborhoods and, 328–329
Population shifts, impact of, 329
Post-degree professional training, 50
addiction counselor training, 50
clergy, training in prevention skills, 50
parent educators, training in prevention skills, 50
teachers, training in prevention skills, 50
Poverty, impact of, 326
Practice Guidelines Coalition, 18
Pramiracetam, 281
Prejudice, 303–304
President's Joint Commission on Mental Illness and Health, 40
Prevention
current trends, 8–10
models of, 5
Prevention and Relationship Enhancement Program, 256–261
components of, 258
dissemination, 260–261
materials, 259–260
professional training, 259
program content, 256–257
program format, 257
Prevention field, challenges in, 10
Prevention professional, certification as, in mental health, 50

Prevention research, expanded definition of, 44
Prevention science
aging, 272–288
AIDS, 205–226
alcohol abuse, 176–201
antisocial behavior, 126–150
child abuse, 85–105
chronic health problems, 227–243
community development, 324–339
depression, 153–175
divorce, 245–271
ecological perspectives, 3–16
education in, 39–62
efficacy of, 3–16
emergence of, 42–45
heterosexist behavior, 301–318
HIV, 205–226
mental health professionals, 39–62
overview, 3–16
parenting skills, 63–82
racism, 301–318
school failure, 106–125
separation, 245–271
sexism, 301–318
sexual abuse, 85–105
substance abuse, 176–201
tobacco use, 176–201
violence, 126–150
Preventive intervention research cycle, 43
Problem-solving skills, antisocial behavior and, 128
Problems facing society, communitywide, 3
Program Enhancement Protocols, Center for Substance Abuse Prevention, 18
Programs, policies, framework for selection, 27–28
Project Head Start, 49
Project Northland, 185–186
Project SixTeen, 1874–185
Prosocial involvement, substance abuse prevention and, 190
Prostitution, 177
Psychological theories of depression, 158

Psychological well-being of society, decrease in, 3–4

Psychologists, other disciplines, collaboration between, 8

Psychology, community
birth of, 5
field of, development of, 4–5

Public health, 330–332

Public health approaches, parenting skills training, 70

Racism, 301–318
African American males, 309
community-level strategies, 310–313
critical consciousness, 30
discrimination, 303–304
early age initiation of prevention strategy at, 308
empowerment programs, 310–311
individual-level strategies, 308–310
literature review, 307–313
media, social marketing, 312
prejudice, 303–304
social support, 311–312

Randomized controlled trials, use of, 23

Rebelliousness, substance abuse and, 189

Redefinition, 6

Reeducation, 6

Relationship, collaborative, in ecological model of prevention, 7

Relaxation training, elderly, 274–275
description, 274
outcome studies, 274–275
rationale, 274

Religiosity, substance abuse prevention and, 190

Remediation, 6

Reminiscence groups, 278–279

Respect for diversity, 9

Risk, defined, 43

Robert Wood Johnson Foundation, 332

Role-playing, abuse and, 91

Safe and Drug Free Schools Program, U.S. Department of Education, 18

SAFEChildren Program, 139–141

San Diego Family Health Project, 230

Saturated fats, cancer and, 228

School-based intervention, for depression, 161

School dropout, failure prevention, 106–125
Achievement for Latinos through Academic Success, 113
advising programs, 116–119
implementation issues, 117–119
alternative settings, 111–112
charter schools, 111
Edison Project schools, 111
attrition, reducing, 112
case example, 116–119
Coca-Cola Valued Youth Program, 113
Comer School Development Project, 115
future trends, 119–120
grouping strategies, 108–109
customized educational plan, 108
heterogeneous ability tracking, 108
interdisciplinary teaming, 108–109
home-school partnerships, 114–116
increase in dropouts, 3
instructional changes, 107–108
curricula, return to basics in, 108
school-to-work programs, 107
literature review, 107–116
structural reforms, 110–111
class size, decrease in, 110
smaller schools, 110
teacher/student ratio, 112
teaching, improvements in, 109–110

:School-to-work programs, 107

Science-based prevention, 51–54

Seattle Social Development Project, 183

Second marriage, divorce rate, 247

Selective intervention, defined, 4

Selective preventive intervention, 42

Self-report measures, abuse, 92

Separation of marital partners, 245–271
communication, importance of, 251
divorce, increase in rate of, 247
effectiveness of preventive interventions, 254–256

first marriage, divorce rate, 247
future trends, 261–264
literature review, 252–256
prediction of, 250
Prevention and Relationship
    Enhancement Program, 256–261
  components of, 258
  dissemination, 260–261
  materials, 259–260
  professional training, 259
  program content, 256–257
  program format, 257
relapse rate, 250
second marriage, divorce rate, 247
sequelae, 248–250
theoretical premises, 253–254
therapy, marital, limitations of, 250
United States, other countries, divorce
    rates compared, 248
Settings, complexity of, 11
Settlement house movement, 40, 49
Sexism, 301–318
  community-level strategies, 310–313
  early age, initiation of prevention
      strategy, 308
  empowerment programs, 310–311
  gender, 304–305
  individual-level strategies, 308–310
  literature review, 307–313
  media, 312
  social support, 311–312
  stereotypes, 303–304
Sexual abuse, 85–105
  Battered Child Syndrome, publication
      of, 86
  case example, 94–98
  defined, 85
  ecobehavioral model, 87
  future trends, 98–100
  literature review, 86–93
  older children, *vs.* younger children,
      learning from prevention pro-
      grams, 92
  role-playing, 91
  self-report measures, 92
  social/ecological perspective, 86

theories, 86–93
young parents, 88
Sexuality, on television, Internet, 3
Sexually transmitted disease. *See also*
    AIDS; HIV
  testing, howard Brown Health Center,
      Chicago, 313–316
Smoking, 176–201
  academic failure, 189
  combination programs, efficacy of,
      186–187
  Communities that Care, prevention
      operating system, 187–192
  community protection profile, 190
  community risk profile, 189
  comprehensive interventions, 183–186
  environmental interventions, 182
  family attachment, 190
  family interventions, 181–182
  future trends, 192–193
  illegal sales of tobacco, 28
      disseminating program in Oregon,
          29–31
      future trends, 31–32
      generic features of effort, 31
      initial dissemination efforts, 30
      subsequent efforts, 30–31
  impulsiveness, 189
  literature review, 179–187
  media approach, to cessation, 68
  Midwestern Prevention Project, 183
  mobility, 189
  moral order, belief in, 190
  neighborhood, 189
  phases of, 187
  prevention science, 178–179
  Project Northland, 185–186
  Project SixTeen, 1874–185
  prosocial involvement, 190
  rebelliousness, 189
  religiosity, 190
  school-based programs, 179–180
  Seattle Social Development Project, 183
  social skills, 190
Social class, impact of, antisocial behav-
    ior, 136

Social competence model of prevention, 5–6
Social Development Research Group, University of Washington, 20
Social incivilities, 327–328
Social skills, substance abuse and, 190
Socialization of children, as parenting skill, 63
Societal issues
  heterosexist behavior, 301–318
  racism, 301–318
  sexism, 301–318
Society, community-wide problems facing, 3
Society for Community Research and Action, advocacy by, 20
Society for Prevention Research, 19
  advocacy by, 20
  assistance to communities, 20
Sports, Play and Active Recreation for Kids Program, 230
Stages of drug use, 178
Standards, setting of, 19–20
Steroids, abuse of, 176–201
Stolen goods, selling, 177
Street economy, 177
Stress management, elderly, 275–276
  outcome studies, 275
  rationale, 275
Stroke, prevention of, 227–243
Structural reforms, high-school, 110–111
  class size, decrease in, 110
  smaller schools, 110
Substance abuse prevention, 176–201
  academic failure, 189
  combination programs, efficacy of, 186–187
  Communities that Care, prevention operating system, 187–192
  community protection profile, 190
  community risk profile, 189
  comprehensive interventions, 183–186
  environmental interventions, 182
  family attachment, 190
  family interventions, 181–182
  future trends, 192–193

impulsiveness, 189
literature review, 179–187
Midwestern Prevention Project, 183
mobility, 189
moral order, belief in, 190
neighborhood, 189
phases of, 187
prevention science, 178–179
Project Northland, 185–186
Project SixTeen, 1874–185
prosocial involvement, 190
prostitution, 177
rebelliousness, 189
religiosity, 190
school-based programs, 179–180
Seattle Social Development Project, 183
social skills, 190
stages of drug use, 178
transition, 189
Suicide, 157
  with major depression, 157
Supervision, lack of, antisocial behavior and, 128
Surfing Internet, time spent in, 2–3
Sustainable economic development, 337–338
Synar Amendment, 28

Target population, importance of involving, 8
Teacher/student ratio, 112
Teaching. See also School
  improvements in, 109–110
Teaching about prevention
  certification, as prevention professional, 50–51
  child guidance movement, 40
  conceptual continuum, in prevention, 44
  Consultation Center, Yale University, 54–56
  educational settings, 49–50
  full-service schools, 49
  graduate training within universities, 45–50
    community psychology, 45–46

preventive medicine specialty, 47–48
public health, 47
public health nursing, 48–49
social work, 49
undergraduate medicine, 47–48
history of, 40–42
indicated preventive intervention, 42
International Certification and
    Reciprocity Consortium for
    Alcohol and Other Drug Abuse, 50
literature review, 45
to mental health professionals, 39–62
mental hygiene movement, 40
post-degree professional training, 50
addiction counselor training, 50
clergy, training in prevention skills,
    50
parent educators, training in
    prevention skills, 50
teachers, training in prevention
    skills, 50
President's Joint Commission on
    Mental Illness and Health, 40
prevention professional, certification
    as, in mental health, 50
prevention research, expanded
    definition of, 44
prevention science, emergence of,
    42–45
preventive intervention research cycle,
    43
Project Head Start, 49
risk, defined, 43
science-based prevention, 51–54
selective preventive intervention, 42
settlement house movement, 40, 49
universal preventive intervention, 42
usage of term, 39
Vermont Conference on Primary
    Prevention of Psychopathology, 41
Television
time spent in viewing, 3, 12
violence, sexuality on, 3
Testing for HIV/AIDS, effectiveness of,
    209–211
Theoretical prevention perspective, 4–8

Theory-based behavioral interventions, 221
Therapy, marital, limitations of, 250
Tobacco, reducing illegal sales of, 28
disseminating program in Oregon,
    29–31
future trends, 31–32
generic features of effort, 31
initial dissemination efforts, 30
subsequent efforts, 30–31
Tobacco abuse, 176–201
academic failure, 189
combination programs, efficacy of,
    186–187
Communities that Care, prevention
    operating system, 187–192
community protection profile, 190
community risk profile, 189
comprehensive interventions, 183–186
environmental interventions, 182
family attachment, 190
family interventions, 181–182
future trends, 192–193
impulsiveness, 189
literature review, 179–187
Midwestern Prevention Project, 183
mobility, 189
moral order, belief in, 190
neighborhood, 189
phases of, 187
prevention science, 178–179
Project Northland, 185–186
Project SixTeen, 1874–185
prosocial involvement, 190
prostitution, 177
rebelliousness, 189
religiosity, 190
school-based programs, 179–180
Seattle Social Development Project, 183
social skills, 190
stages of drug use, 178
transition, 189
Trials, randomized controlled, use of, 23

Understanding, importance of, 8
United States, other countries, divorce
    rates compared, 248

Univerisity of Oregon, National Center for Improving Tools of Educators, 20
Universal intervention, defined, 4
Universal preventive intervention, 42
University of Kansas, Community Tool Box, 20
University of Washington, Social Development Research Group, 20

Vegetables in diet, cancer prevention, 228
Vermont Conference on Primary Prevention of Psychopathology, 41
Violence, on television, Internet, sexuality on, 3
Violence prevention
 adolescent age, 128
 age of onset, 134
 antisocial youth, defined, 133
 case example, 139–141
 challenges, 133–139
 community-level factors, 129
 consequences, inconsistent use of, 128
 defined, 133–134
 developmental-ecological framework, 135
 ecological theory, 137
 family factors, 128
 family-focused approaches, 131
 future trends, 141–143
 gender and, 128, 136
 handguns, availability of, 129
 impoverished neighborhoods, 129
 indicated programs, 131
 interventions, 130–133, 138–139
 literature review, 130–139
 Metropolitan Area Child Study Research Group, 139–141
 models of antisocial behavior, 135
 overly harsh discipline practices, 128
 peer factors, 128–129
 peer-group approaches, 131
 peer relations, 128
 population characteristics, 138–139
 prevention research, theoretical framework, 134–138
 problem-solving skills, 128
 protective factors, 130
 risk factors, 127–128
 SAFEChildren Program, 139–141
 selected programs, 131
 social class, impact of, 136
 societal factors, 129
 supervision, lack of, 128
 universal programs, 131
Violent Crime Index, increase in crime in U.S., 126
Volunteering, by elderly, 277–278
 at helpline, 286–287

Washington Heights-Inwood Healthy Heart Program, 230
Weight control program, targeting obesity, 236
Well-being
 monitoring of, 24–25
 of society, psychological, decrease in, 3–4
Widow-to-Widow Program, 282
Widowed Persons Service, AARP, 282
Willingness to understand, importance of, 8

Yale University, Consultation Center, 54–56
Young parent, physical abuse of child, 88
Younger children, older children, compared, learning from prevention programs, 92
Youth
 alcohol abuse, 176–201
 antisocial behavior, 126–150
 child abuse, 85–105
 depression, 153–175
 education in, 39–62
 mental health professionals, 39–62
 parenting skills, 63–82
 school failure, 106–125
 sexual abuse, 85–105
 substance abuse, 176–201
 tobacco use, 176–201
 violence, 126–150
Youth Risk Behavior Survey, 24